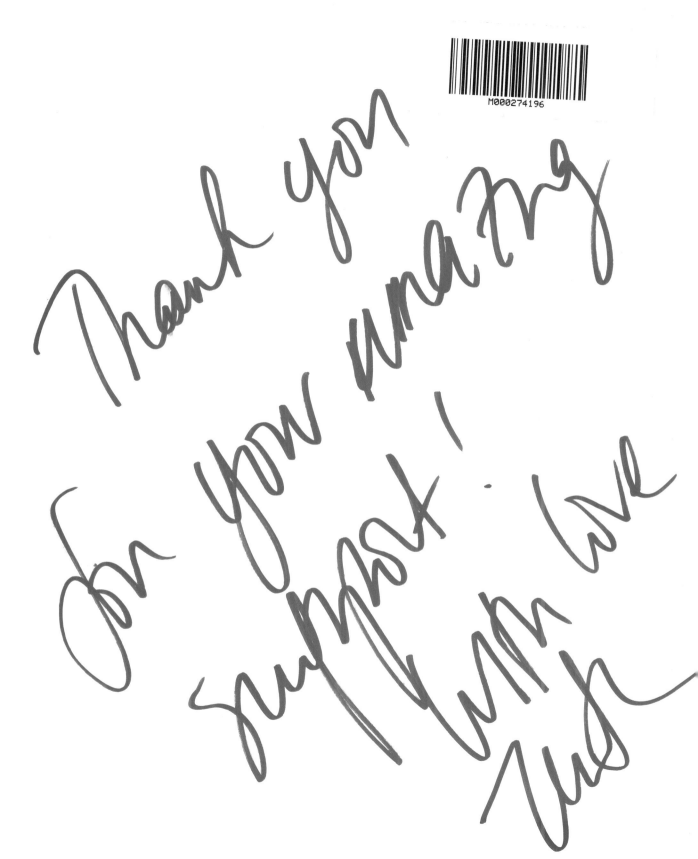

Thank you

for you amazing

support !

with love

Lisa

PRAISE

"Sexyfit is different, it's a lifestyle, it's about being proud of yourself and transforming your body into something you would look in the mirror and feel truly proud of. I'm 55, and at my age I didn't think I could ever see myself as "sexy." But I've taken it on because I do feel sexy now."

— Susanne Rose, 55

"I lost 40 pounds and got my confidence back! This is so much more than just a diet because I've tried every diet under the sun before. I've overcome big obstacles, like the fear of failure or investing money in myself. It turns out that with Sexyfit I could never fail because there are Zlata and the [Sexyfit] Community always there to support me, motivate me, and keep me accountable."

— Amanda Kempker, 32

"I thought I was signing up for a weight-loss program, but I've grown so much mentally and spiritually that the weight loss is just a bonus! I'm seeing my body respond in amazing, long-lasting ways that bring joy to my mind, body, and soul. I've had such great results that I told my parents about the Sexyfit approach, and they have lost over 50 pounds collectively at the age of 75!"

— Mistie Haybob, 42

For information about permission to reproduce selections from the book, please write to Sexyfit Ventures at info@sexyfit.com www.sexyfit.com

The Sexyfit Method
Your Step-by-Step Guide to Complete Food Freedom, Loving Your Body, and Reclaiming Your Life
Hardcopy ISBN 978-0-9985372-3-8
Ebook ISBN 978-0-9985372-7-6
Self Help/ HEALTH & FITNESS

Cover and Book Design by Jenni Wierzba
Editor Amy Reid
Food Images/Exercise Images by Kirk Hensler and Hale Productions
Food Styling by Alexis Asquith
Prop Styling by Irina Georgieva

Printed in the United States of America

To my dear mother, thank you for sacrificing many things in your life to make sure I live my best.

I love you.

GRATITUDE

"All accomplishments in life, both great and small,
can be traced to the influence and efforts of many."
— Katherine Woodward Thomas

I believe in miracles. And I know for a fact that they happen every day. Sometimes they come in the form of a message from a fortune cookie, or a strange coincidence, or perhaps as someone brought into your life to teach you a universal lesson. This book is the collective effort of many experiences shaped by a collection of extraordinary miracles and remarkable human beings.

I want to extend a special thank-you to many who have walked this journey with me. First and foremost, Samantha and Wyatt, thank you for your enthusiasm, open hearts, and willingness to share your knowledge without ever asking for anything in return. To Rea Bavilla and Cari Leyva, for being phenomenal pageant directors and helping shape me into the woman I am today. A huge, special thank-you to my best "horrible" boss Lori Brandt, for your endless faith, infectious positivity, and for being my guardian angel — and for somehow always showing up in the right place at the right time. Thank you for your kindness, generosity, and your gentle nudges in the right direction. To my darling best friend Valeria, I'm forever grateful for our friendship and for your constant love, support, and being my partner in crime in any endeavor, and for showing me what health and fitness are truly about. Thank you Natalie Jill and Brooks Holland, for your inspiration to share my story and for your faith in me. A special thank-you to Lori and Chris Harder, for your wisdom, commitment, and leading by example and for standing in your authentic power to do the greater good in every situation. Thank-you to my loving and kind friend Megan Gjovig, for your encouragement, loving support, and spiritual guidance. To my spiritual teachers, Eve Ellie, Andrew DeGregorio, and Gabby Bernstein, I'm grateful for your courage and willingness to share your universal gifts with me and the world. Thank you for always being in the right place at the right time. Thank-you to Bobby Agron, for your kindness and your special talent of being a fantastic listener, and for your hidden talent of asking the best questions to help guide me toward all of the right answers. Thank-you to Kirk Hensler, for investing your creative super-ninja powers to create the visual experience of the Sexyfit brand, and thank-you to Alexis Asquith, for your food styling expertise to make simple food look like magazine-worthy carb cover models. Your love for your craft is infectious. To my editor, Amy Reid, thank you for your inspiration, encouragement, and magnitude of talents and for your ability to catch all of my mistakes to help me best craft my message. I appreciate you above and beyond what words can express. To my designer, Jenni Wierzba, thank you for your endless patience, creative inspiration, hard work, and dedication to the Sexyfit message, and for bringing this book to life.

A big thank-you to a certain someone who had quite literally put my faith in this message and this book to the test. Thank you for your challenge to lead the way into the endless expansion of my goals and talents that serve thousands. Thank you for the much-needed fuel to fire and for helping me to transform into the woman I am today.

Thank-you to a perfect stranger whom I met at a coffee shop, who became an endless inspiration, support, and source of kindness, care, love, and compassion, and my "vision keeper" — Irina Georgieva. Thank you for being the best manifestation and goal-setting partner in crime, and thank you for being a solid compass and a fellow wild soul, and for always having my back.

An overwhelmingly sincere thank-you to my mother. I thank you for the eight evil years of music school you had dragged me through. It taught me to finish what I start. Very much like this book that I started two years ago, when every page felt like it took a year to write, but now it's here because because of that life lesson I learned. Thank you for dragging me out of a foreign country to give me a bed, a warm shower, food on the table, and even a walk-in California Closet® but most of all for giving me the chance to create endless opportunities. Thank you for not driving me to school in the morning but instead insisting that I take the evil school bus. It taught me to deal with people, face adversity, and always have my big girl panties on. Thank you for not buying my first car for me. Now I know the value of a dollar and that I must find a way to get the things I want. Thank you for not paying for my college education because that's exactly what I needed to be able to assume financial responsibility for my future. Thank you for the best advice when I called you saying that I wanted to shut down my podcast because it was "too much work." Your advice was that it takes a pro to produce episode #1005 with the same enthusiasm as episode #1, regardless of how you "feel" that day. I turned pro, and the Sexyfit podcast has transformed hundreds of thousands of women to date. And one big, final thank-you for telling Mr. Trump to "stand where you are and not move until I take a picture" during the post-pageant party. It was a lesson I needed to learn: that nobody is better than anyone, regardless of the price of their suit.

Dad, thank you for all of your love, support, and sober way of looking at every situation. Thank you for your endless business and life advice that's more useful than any self-help book I could ever read. Thank you for reading my mind, and knowing exactly what to say and how to say it. Thank you for your endless fatherly love.

Thank-you to my first client Visjna, who gave me a chance, and every client thereafter who gave me a chance to be their guide on their journey. Thank-you to everyone who has trusted me with their fears, hearts, and stories, and who has inspired me with their growth and transformations. It's my joy to watch you walk your path with courage, enthusiasm, and grow into the best version of yourself with every step. My biggest cheerleader and incredible Sexyfit Community manager Amanda Kempker, thank you for being the motivation and the validation to write more than a book of shrimp recipes, and something that was big and transformational to many. Thank-you to every podcast listener who keeps me committed to my work, my mission, and our big message. A big thank-you to our large virtual community that feels like a sisterhood and the tribe of women I longed for all of my life.

Finally, the biggest thank-you is to you, my reader. I wrote this book for you, and I believe it's no coincidence that you have it in your hands. I thank you for your willingness to learn and grow, to explore and heal, to stay open-minded and willing to dive deeper into your journey of transformation with me. I hope this book brings relief, clarity, certainty, and endless inspiration for you to live Sexyfit.

INSPIRATION

"Stay afraid, but do it anyway. What's important is the action. You don't have to wait to be confident. Just do it and eventually the confidence will follow."

– Carrie Fisher

AMANDA KEMPKER
40 pounds fat loss and learned to invest in herself.

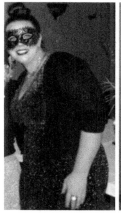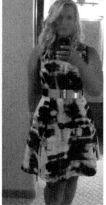

"I joined because it was finally time to put ME, first. I always put everyone else ahead of me; family, friends, co-workers. I'm always doing for others. I needed to start doing for me. So I decided it was my moment to be a little selfish and focus on just that. ME. It's like making deposits into the bank of Amanda!

What I loved most when I started was access to the community is amazing and every is like on big family, heck I even became a community manager after my transformation! I also love that the fitness and nutrition plans are realistic. I haven't encountered one workout I couldn't do. Or a meal plan that left me feeling hungry or even worse — broke! Everything is reasonable. Plan the work and work the plan!

I am really proud of myself for my current weight loss and running my first marathon EVER!!! But there are so many other things to be proud of, too. Like learning more about nutrition and fitness. Learning how amazing my body is. Learning more about myself: my whys and my motivations. Learning how to hold myself and others accountable. Learning that if I put my mind to it, I can achieve my desired results."

KRISTIN BUTLER, ICU NURSE
Beat work stress and got pregnant!

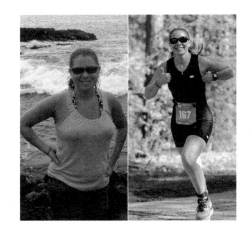

"The biggest reason why I joined was that I wanted to allow myself the best physical and emotional health possible. I wanted to have a healthy body because my husband and I want to start a family and part of getting ready for that step is being healthy. I've changed the way I manage stress of my job as a nurse. Usually, when I would get home and get really anxious after work and instead of sitting on the couch and eating, I'd go for a run and listened to Sexyfit Podcast. If I found myself eating emotionally, I'd get still after work and really slow down with my thoughts and feelings. My major win is having confidence in myself, doing a Spartan race and completing a triathlon. The things you can accomplish when you have confidence are amazing! My advice to anyone starting doesn't feed themselves with negative thoughts, just take one day, one hour, one minute at a time and ask for help."

LILLY VAN DRIESSCHE
Beat Anxiety and Ran her First Half Marathon!

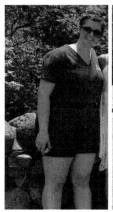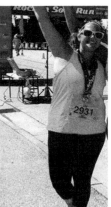

"Before starting Sexyfit, I was very good at giving up and not finishing what I start. Then I saw a great friend achieving amazing success with Sexyfit and I wanted to try it. Sexyfit was both what I expected and what I did not expect. My biggest win was also a surprise for me. I had a physical transformation of course, but the mental transformation was what surprised me and what I've been most proud of. I'm a completely different person now and I refer to myself as the New Lily. Now I laugh about the things that "Old Lily" did.

I was dealing with a lot of anxiety and depression and I was on medication. Over the year, I gave up all my medication. I'm happier and more carefree than I've ever been in my life. I love myself enough to go to the gym, hit my macros, stick to my workout program and be involved in the community. I've realized I'm doing all that for myself, that loving yourself is not selfish and that's a total mind shift. I've come a long way and I'm proud of that."

DR. IZABELA CHROBAK
From heart attack at 31 to Spartan Finisher

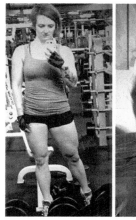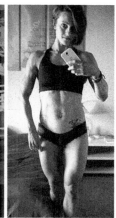

"I have a very My background is quite specific. I come from Poland and I was a cardiopulmonary scientist, doing my scientific job for 14-18 hours a day. I didn't eat properly, I would have milkshakes, candy and energy drinks. I burned myself psychologically, emotionally and physically, and ended up having a heart attack at 31. I got really serious about my health and hired a trainer. I later got into bodybuilding. While I was achieving great success it turned out not to be healthy at all. I was on the same meal plan for 18 weeks. Eventually, I couldn't sleep, had no energy, I could barely walk and didn't know what these symptoms were, but something was definitely off. Being a scientist, I researched and I found out I had adrenal fatigue and was ruining my metabolism once again with strict dieting. I found Sexyfit when I really needed a sustainable method to get my health back together. My life changed a lot in the last 1.5 years. I'm not competing but I love bodybuilding. I don't need to compete to look healthy, sexy and fit. My biggest lesson was how hard it was to overcome a huge mindset obstacle related to body image. I wish I didn't waste 10 or 15 years pleasing others instead of asking myself what made ME happy. I would rush my younger self to make the changes faster and be more committed to my idea of beauty. It took us 6-8 months to rev up my metabolism, get lean again and I feel so great now!!! Thank you!!!"

MACKINZIE SHRIVER, MASSAGE THERAPIST
Got her athletic drive and motivation back

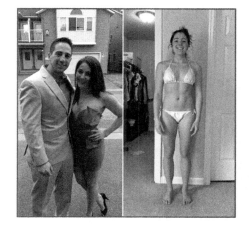

"Growing up I did gymnastics and was in great shape both functionally and aesthetically, but since quitting I hadn't kept up my athleticism. One of the things I like most about Sexyfit is that it isn't about selling a product for some quick, secret weight loss trick. Sexyfit teaches you what you should do and why for your individual body, for both diet and exercise, so that when you're done with the program you're able to be self-sufficient and lead a healthy, sustainable lifestyle. Consistency is key. You will never regret investing time, energy, effort, or money for your health. You may be surprised at how making a lifestyle change in regard to your health will also result in positive changes in other areas of your life"

JOANNA WILLIAMS
Husband and wife losing 120 pounds after nothing seemed to work.

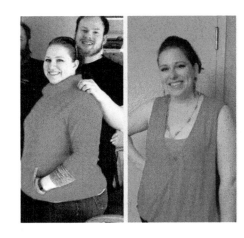

"I used to be in the military and got out 6 years ago. I have 2 sons and I've been working full-time and going to school full time for 4 years now. The reason I joined Sexyfit was because I was at my heaviest weight and I tried so many things and the weight never stayed off. NEVER!

My biggest win was that I went from size 20 to size 12 and then I'm now under 160 pounds, which I haven't seen in over 6 years. That's huge for me. I was also able to change my lifestyle and nutrition and now my family does it with me. My man lost over 60 pounds too! That's 120 pounds between the both of us! If I were to give myself a piece of advice, I would say to stop all the fad dieting and that there is a better way out. I was so defeated because I was so big. Starting was hard at first, but I wanted it and it's honestly what you make of it. I had committed. That was a big thing for me. I had to stick with it even when I felt like giving up. The results are worth every bit of sweat and effort you invest."

MARGIT JENSEN-COOK, Marketing Manager
Best example for her family and her baby Jensen.

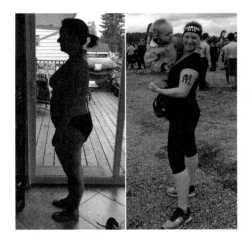

"I love Sexyfit because all makes sense, the journey, the process, the focus on your lifestyle, the desire for change. Work smarter, not harder, right? Why spending 1.5 hours in the gym when you can be in and out in 30 minutes, and accomplish exactly what you need to get your body moving and face the challenges? I didn't want my son to get the idea that we sat on the couch all day. My body desperately needed to move and I needed a coach. I knew I needed this! Not without bumps on the journey but I am happy I committed myself to this journey. My best advice for someone just starting out, Don't beat yourself up. If today is the day you decide, then today you're making the change. If it's tomorrow, then tomorrow you will make the change. But if you know in your heart that the change needs to happen, then you have to put your energy into that and design a plan. Ride those emotions, jump on board and go after that"

DR. VIVIAN BURK
Beat yo-yo dieting and ran her first relay race!

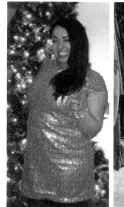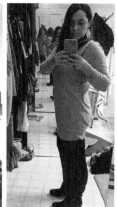

"I was tired of hating every picture I was in, not feeling comfortable in any of my clothes (and thus having each night out almost ruined). I was also feeling really lethargic and I felt like I was not heart healthy. I was terrified of having a heart attack, and every time I tried to run even a little I was completely out of breath. This was my WHY for starting! What I like most about Sexyfit is the community. The Sexyfit family is amazing motivation and support. It's so helpful to not only see people succeeding around me, but to hear about their shortcomings too. I think when you're out of shape and you see "fit" people you think they're just perfect little gym goers that never eat unhealthy. I truly have no idea what I was doing with weights when I started. It can be so intimidating when you're just starting out. To get me started and to keep me going, I like having a set plan to follow and that I can do my workouts at home and not have to be in a gym. Recently, I ran my first race ever, and even though I'm a self-professed non-runner, I went all 6.5 miles without stopping! I also have found myself feeling the need to run or work out when I've had a rough day — a trait I thought you had to be born with, I NEVER thought that would be me! The physical results are just a side effect of all the great habits I created and what I was able to achieve"

SUSANNE ROSE
"Don't use your age as your excuse, make it your reason."

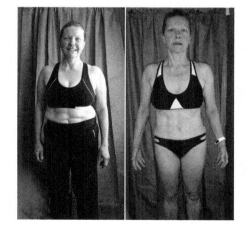

"I started exercising when I was a teenager and I've exercised all my life. For me, exercising was a way to control my weight because I love to eat. I did that until I've realized that exercising makes me feel great, that I sleep better and it affects my overall well-being more than it works for weight control. I exercised by myself for many years but I realized I needed a professional coach and finally, I invested in myself. I found Sexyfit program though the Sexyfit podcast. I gave it a go and realized it's a whole new lifestyle for me! Now, it's all about being proud of myself and feeling great in my body. At my age I didn't think I was going to go this way, I never thought I would be "Sexyfit." But I do take it on now because I feel sexy and healthy."

MY STORY

INTRODUCTION

STEP I: TRAIN YOUR MIND

STEP II: FOOD FREEDOM

TABLE OF CONTENTS

PREFACE

WELCOME TO THE SEXYFIT FAMILY, SISTER! I'm thrilled and beyond grateful that you've trusted me and the Sexyfit Method on your journey to transformation. You're about to embark on the most beautiful path, the best gift you could have given yourself.

I created Sexyfit as a result of being frustrated with the norms of the dieting industry and unrealistic standards of the fitness world. You see, we live in a world of diets and deprivation. We've labeled and demonized food over time. This is clean, this is dirty, this is "good," this is "bad." The industry says that we can get washboard abs in three days, a bikini body in seven. Beauty trends change so fast that we can hardly keep up. Five years ago, it was in style to be thin, and now we're obsessed with the idea of a big behind. And we're looking at magazines and social media for validation of what we "should" look like.

See, I'm not interested in selling you another "diet" to give you short-term results on MY terms and projecting MY set of "breakthrough" rules onto you. I'm also not interested in polluting your mind with more comparison messages, with the intention of shrinking your "fat zones" in hopes of sexier arms, leaner legs, and shredded abdominals just to give you a boost of short-term motivation that will then send you into a downward spiral of self-loathing, while dying on the StairMaster.® And I'm sure also not interested in selling you detox teas, magic wraps, waist trainers, or fat freezing.

We both know that all of that doesn't work. When women like you come to Sexyfit, they're usually fed up and done with fad diets, voodoo super foods, seven-day cleanses, and the latest fitness trends. I lived in that world of the fast food version of beauty for far too long, and none of it worked. You, too, probably picked up this book because you're done with all of that.

The journey you're about to take is a result of a decade of my experience as a fitness professional and coach, coupled with research from more than 300 top nutritionists, trainers, and doctors throughout the world. And it has already transformed thousands of women just like you. Together, you and I are going to walk through the steps of this Sexyfit Method book to discover and create what works best for YOU so you can experience complete food freedom, create the body you love, and, ultimately, reclaim your life.

In my years of lifestyle coaching, I haven't met two women who are alike, have the same life story, the same schedule, and eat the same type of foods. As your coach, I recognize that I can't put you in the same diet box with other women and expect equal results. Your story, your lifestyle, your body is going to require something a bit different, and we get to create it together walking the steps of the Sexyfit Method. Me and my team of coaches carefully tested, sampled, and tweaked the methodology to guide you on your own journey, and give you the results you'll love and you deserve.

I made a lot of mistakes on my fitness journey to sexy and fit. I lived under the false pretense of wanting to appear perfect, so I held back some of these stories for years because I wanted it to look as though I had it all together as a coach. I have to admit that it makes me feel very vulnerable, exposed, and downright embarrassed to share my story with you in the first part of the book before we even dive into any strategy. But I strongly believe that our life unfolds directly in proportion to our courage. And I'm beyond grateful that I get to share my story with you by writing this book to inspire and motivate you to shine your true colors and find perfection in your imperfections.

We're led to believe our journey to health and fitness is a linear path. That's the furthest thing from the truth. It's more like a hero's journey of a thousand miles, where you get to slay dragons and take a narrow, winding road to magic land, which is okay so long as you have faith and continue to show up for yourself. Then you, too, will make progress and get incredible results. Because in the wake of making these mistakes, I also uncovered many practices that work incredibly well and have worked for hundreds of you.

If you're feeling timid and hesitant, and feeling "sexy" doesn't quite sit so well with you right now, I want to share this beautiful quote with you by Leonard Cohen: "There is a crack, a crack in everything, and that's how the light gets in."

As women, we try to keep a perfect facade and always act as if we have our stuff together. I did for so many years! We were told from a young age that crying is bad and showing our emotions is terrible, too, and that we must be 100% in control of everything around us. The pressure in our head is enormous. We think we need to have it all. We watched our mothers take care of everyone and everything; and we learned to do the same, while putting our needs on the back burner. We've forgotten to experience who we are and how to find the "I," to stand strong on both of our feet in the ever-changing world around us. We've forgotten about ourselves, and what makes us unique and sexy in our own way. Emotional eating, self-sabotage, burnout, anxiety, endless dieting, over-exercising, or over "Netflix and wine-ing," drinking, non-stop movie marathons, clearance shopping – all of these are side-effects of not having a strong "I" and are our way to "check out" from the world we feel no control over.

So, what's the solution?

LOVE. IT'S ALWAYS LOVE.

The answer is falling in love with ourselves, with our body, with our story, with our imperfections and the way we do things. And I'm in deep, caring, meaningful, forgiving, unconditional love with the wounded, cracked, tiger-striped, broken-hearted, lonely, single, imperfect selves.

I've worked with a lot of women. And I mean A LOT!

I've never met a woman who isn't strong or beautiful or sexy.

We are so much more than what we see.

More than we ever imagined or believed was true.

I look at every woman in our community, and every time I'm in awe of how they handle life.

Faith.

Gratitude.

Kindness.

Compassion.

Positivity.

Determination.

Perseverance.

Forgiveness.

Acceptance.

ENDLESS MOTION.

It's infectious.

It's beautiful.

It's beyond sexy.

See, we have it all wrong.

Sexy isn't a size of your pants or a title or a trophy. It isn't achieved by external validation from a man or peers. Sexy isn't the perfection or the convenient truth behind an inconvenient story. Sexy isn't a number on a scale or a dress size. Sexy isn't the media-projected ass obsession that earns Instagram likes.

Every single one of us is sexy in our own way, and every woman is a masterpiece because of her cracks and the battle wounds she's endured in her lifetime. So you, too, get to claim the term "sexy" with pride and own it.

Sexy is having a strong sense of "I," cultivating radical self love, and feeling at home in our body. I hope my stories serve as a motivation for you to know that you're capable of many great things, that your story is what dictates your reality; that you can live at home in your body and create the life you deserve from there, knowing that health and fitness are the foundation for your success.

I created Sexyfit to help you cultivate self love for the body that you have, and, as a result, live your best life. Here are the steps to your Sexyfit lifestyle:

STEP I: TRAIN YOUR MIND—Clear away the obstacles that are holding you back from creating the body you've always wanted. Create a strong "I" and sense of self.

STEP II: FOOD FREEDOM—Overcome emotional eating, break free from the dieting roller-coaster, and experience complete food freedom. Get recipes and a meal plan to support your transformation.

STEP III: SIMPLE FITNESS—Understand how to get lasting results and feel at home in your body. Get super-effective workout routines that you can do at home or at the gym to get your sexy back.

STEP IV: ACCOUNTABILITY—Unleash your potential, and stay motivated with simple accountability tips and tricks for lasting fat loss.

STEP V: POWER OF COMMUNITY—Cultivate a sense of community to support your journey. Join thousands of women who support you, create a community, and maximize your results.

Each section is equally important. There are also helpful links, resources, and tips, so when you're not reading you can listen to the tidbits of my podcast and the audio I put together for this book. You can take me with you anywhere. I dare you to NOT get addicted to the podcast. It's sooo good! I also suggest that you get prepared and grab a journal, a pen, headphones, some tissues, a cell phone, and a healthy dose of motivation. You also have the Sexyfit virtual Community as a trusted resource of hundreds of like-minded women to walk the journey with you, so you get the support and motivation you need. I recognize that having a tribe of women whom you can trust and lean on will reap tremendous benefits for you. To find a group in your city or to start a book club, you can find your fellow sisters at sexyfit.com/community. I truly believe in the enormous value of being #StrongTogether and encourage you to get the support you need from your Sexyfit sisters.

At the end of this book, I included a 21-Day Transformation Plan you can use to guide you as you begin. Just because it's 21 days doesn't mean you can only do it for 21 days, though. In fact, for best results, do the nutrition and fitness section a few times.

And since we're going to dig and dig deep for the real you, if at any point you find yourself feeling really uncomfortable, choose to move past it. Great things are ahead for you. If you feel like you need more support and are ready to take the plunge, you can always talk to one of our coaches. This isn't a pitch, this is the truth. Some of us need a deeper level of understanding and accountability to make the shift.

I'm beyond grateful for the opportunity to be a part of this journey with you. No matter how disappointed you've been in the past, how many diets you've tried, how many times you've failed, I know that you can choose a new path that will enable you to feel at home in your body. Take the journey and don't be discouraged. You deserve this, and I believe in you.

With love,

MY STORY AND THE BIRTH OF SEXYFIT
CHAPTER 1

WELCOME TO AMERICA

HOW DO YOU SAY YOUR NAME? You can probably imagine that with a name like Zlata I'm not from here. I'll help you out because you probably have no idea how to say it. It's pronounced Za-la-da. Usually the next few questions I get are: Where's it from, and what does it mean?

It's an old Russian name, and it means "Gold." My name was supposed to be "Olga" until my mom met a lovely lady named Zlata at the hospital and changed her mind to name me Zlata.

I was raised in Moscow, Russia, and moved to the U.S. when I was 16, only knowing two English words: "Hello" and "Big Mac." I didn't speak English when I moved, and neither could I write nor express my needs without an extensive amount of gesturing and pointing. In fact, just explaining how to say my name became such a struggle that I swore to myself I would do ANYTHING to not have a Russian accent.

My mother was a traveling journalist and ended up in Alaska after getting a movie documentary assignment. I moved there to join her but only after a long journey of immigration, endless paperwork, motherly tears, and lots of waiting.

Growing up in Moscow was an interesting time. Mainly because it's an obnoxiously large city of more than 15 million people, and I wasn't necessarily born with a silver spoon in my mouth. At the time, I didn't really have anything to compare my life to other than my friends' lives, but looking back at it now, we were, ahem … poor.

I knew we weren't exactly rolling in money, but the fact that I didn't have an actual bed growing up didn't strike me as odd at the time. My dad, step-mom, sister, brother, aunt and uncle, their daughter, grandma, and I all lived together. Since it was so crowded and we had to manage to house all of us in such a tight space, I slept on one of those cots with a flower pattern on it because I alternated a bed with my step-sister. I would wake up every morning and I'd have to put away the cot and fold it so we had room to move around. That's probably why making my bed is one of my most favorite daily rituals nowadays. We had two fridges; took turns sharing one bathroom; and our washing machine ran on a legit schedule, with a clipboard to "reserve" laundry time. Talk about tight spaces and interesting family dynamics!

My parents did their best, but unfortunately in countries like Russia your "best" is limited by the situation. Politically or historically, Russian "best" isn't what we're even remotely used to here in the States. My dad was a serial entrepreneur, whose businesses rose and fell due to economic times or the political regime. My mom was a journalist, who constantly worked long hours and odd schedules, and had to keep up with the ever-changing new staff of younger, ambitious anchor woman wannabes. They divorced when I was young, mom moved, and I ended up living with my dad and crazy big fam.

I remember not having food at home when times were really tough, and we had to get super creative with what we could do with rice. Or we could make macaroni and cheese, or something out of potatoes. Either one of the three was in abundance. It really wasn't about what we wanted to eat, it was mostly about what we got to eat, and if we didn't want to eat that, then we just didn't eat. I remember coming home from school one day, opening the fridge, and just seeing a package of lonesome seaweed salad. I don't remember ever being a particular fan of seaweed salad at the time, but when it was really my only option, it went well with the rice I made. I think this is how I learned to make meals literally out of nothing. You see an empty fridge, and I see 15 dinner options.

Because of our financial situation, American chocolate was a treat for a very special occasion. I have a special relationship with Snickers® candy bars because that's what my daddy used to get me when we had money or when something really major happened. My childhood memories of happy times include just me going to McDonald's with Dad and treating it like it was an experience more precious than eating at any Michelin five-star restaurant. "Happy Meal" had a different meaning for me because it really meant happiness. Dad would always get a Big Mac, and I was a fan of chicken nuggets.

Another thing I remember vividly is that I wasn't an active kid. My extra-curricular activities included two to three hours of playing piano, plus singing in a choir. All after-school programs that involved sports were really out of the question for me because skipping P.E. was my hidden talent. To be honest, I don't remember a non-terrifying fitness experience from my youth: falling down on the gymnastics rings … never being able to hit a volleyball … frequently being hit in the face by a soccer ball during a class game. Not to mention, in the winter we were required to do cross-country ski laps around the school, and if we skipped class the teacher would wait until spring and make us carry the skis around the school to assure we got all of the laps in … while holding 20 pounds of ski gear. In fact, my P.E. teachers were like terrifying creatures to me, constantly yelling and making me take laps and complaining that I was so weak, while giving me pitiful B- grades just to make sure I kept my grades up. I remember feeling so absolutely worthless in those classes; like I just wasn't made for it. I guess, though, it was because my family wasn't really active either. My mom dabbled in tennis and to this day believes that sports are bad for you. Dad could win an Olympic medal in sweet-talking, but that's about it.

Since my mom and dad were separated for quite some time, and mom spent a lot of time traveling, which eventually led her to settle down in Alaska, I knew it was inevitable for me to move with her … eventually. Because she moved right around 9/11, you can only imagine how long immigration took. By the time I got the green light to move, five (six … seven) years had passed, and I was already a full-grown adult by Russian standards, with a boyfriend and a life of my own.

I'll never forget the subway ride to the airport. There was a giant pit in my stomach, and I was tightly hanging onto the stuffed baby cow toy my step-sister gave me the night before as a sign of our friendship. Why a baby cow? I have no idea, but it was so cute and the only thing that kept me comforted for many months after I got to Alaska.

The only thing I knew about America was what I saw in movies like "Mean Girls," "Charlie's Angels," and "Gone in 60 Seconds." I knew Americans were obsessed with green lawns, lived in neighborhood homes that all looked the same, drove big cars, and that girls in school were mean.

I remember being in complete shock. I was excited to see my mom, but I was sad to lose everything that I ever knew was my life. To be honest, until the last second I didn't believe that I wasn't ever going back to my life in Moscow. It was probably my way of calming myself down in the time of extreme uncertainty.

The first few weeks were okay. I felt like I was on a big, fun vacation I never had.

And I remember my first day of school like it was yesterday.

I was excited! SCHOOL!!! FRIENDS!!!! Shenanigans!!!!

So, first day of school …

The first obstacle to overcome was the school bus. First, I had to find it. When you don't know anyone under age 40 and Google doesn't exist, finding a school bus was an issue. At 6:45 a.m., I walked out on the road where it was sort of supposed to be, but the bus was already passing me.

I ran after it.

The bus stopped, the driver let me on. He yelled something, which I assumed meant "Don't be late." I finished a lot of sentences for people in my head because I truly didn't understand a thing they said.

It was a rainy morning, the bus was dark and cold, I squeezed myself next to a kid with a mouthful of braces. He smiled, I cringed. Those look like they hurt, I thought — I'd never seen braces before. By the end of that bus ride, he called me "weird" for wearing pink high tops. I thought he was weird and didn't understand Russian fashion.

First hour started in the auditorium of 2,000 high-schoolers. Some guy, who I later learned was the principal, was proudly blabbing into the microphone, and the only word I truly understood was "WELCOME." Woohoo, I thought.

When the bell rang, it was time for class. Imagine what it would look like when 2,000 new students exit four doors of an auditorium. It was an ant house. Everybody was walking down the bleachers, and I knew no one. Not. A. Single. Soul.

I was the last one to leave, and I'd never felt so alone and lost in my life … until lunch.

The classes I was taking were AP chemistry, AP biology, dance (because other P.E. classes sounded more awful), history, and by the time 5th period rolled around I didn't even know what class it was. During my school orientation, I refused to take English as a Second Language classes because a girl told me only uncool kids took it, and since I didn't want to be uncool I told my advisor "I got it." Another phrase I added to my vocabulary, after "Hello" and "Big Mac."

By the time lunch rolled around it was clear that "I didn't got it." I understood it was lunch hour because I saw kids sitting down at tables; some were pouring out of the school doors to drive to get lunch. Which, for me, was just wild — driving to get lunch — wow! I grabbed my food, which was something my mom made for me, and tried to sit down with two people at the big lunch tables. Both of those seats ended up being "taken." As a result, the only place I could get cozy was … the bathroom. It was quiet for the first time in four hours, and nobody called me weird for my shoe choice. Pink Puma high tops were my favorite choice at the time.

I ate lunch in the bathroom for a few days. Okay, a few weeks. I later upgraded my lunch spot to the highest flat of stairs away from the noise, and that's where I listened to Benni Benassi's new album so nobody would talk to me.

I went from an outgoing, fun, self-sufficient adult to a child whose mom had to sign papers for me to watch a movie in school. It was devastating.

If I didn't understand someone, people would just YELL louder in my face, as if there's a correlation between the volume of speech and my level of understanding. I suffered from horrible headaches because of hours of studying and translating every line in the AP Chem book so I wouldn't feel quite so lost the next day. I prayed that no one would speak to me because gesturing and trying to explain myself would land me in the "weird" category again. If someone asked what my name was, it would take what seemed like hours of explanation of how to say it, what it meant, and where I was from. And all of that would bring memories of my former life, and how much I loved and missed it.

I was weird and different.
My name was strange and difficult to say.
Outfits I wore weren't what the popular girls were wearing.
Boys didn't look at me anymore.
Girls raised their eyebrows.

I was lonely and sad. And it was a deep sense of emptiness because eventually I would just go home and shut down in my room. I couldn't even watch TV because it was ALL IN ENGLISH!

Many nights I cried myself to sleep. At the time, I didn't realize it, but I was suffering from depression.

One day when I was in school, I passed a vending machine. Guess what was in it? SNICKERS!

OMG!

My favorite candy! So I took some money out of my pocket and got it. It seemed like I had a magic wand in my hands. The perfect solution to my typical crappy day. At lunch I did my usual thing: got my Russian food from my locker (which I was still struggling to open at that time), planted myself on the stairs, plugged in my CD player, kicked back, and took a bite.

It seemed like the world stopped for a minute.

I closed my eyes and remembered the times my dad would bring one of those magic candy bars home. It wasn't something we could afford to eat everyday, and it wouldn't happen often. But now it was like I went home for a moment, and got to hang out with dad and the fam. I imagined his big fatherly hug wrapping around me like a soft blanket. It brought back the good times.

I started getting a Snickers on a daily basis. And everyday the world seemed to stop for a moment. It felt nice. It felt like life had some soft of balance and meaning again.

Shortly after I began that daily ritual I made some friends. Because I didn't want to seem weird, I spent lunchtime with them eating whatever they were eating, which for an average high-schooler is pizza, mac 'n' cheese, something from Taco Bell, or at best a Subway sandwich. And still, everyday when I would come home, I would find those pieces of chocolate and have them with tea. My grandma used to do that once in awhile, and it was nice to have that same feeling and reminder of my grandma.

Life was better. Junk food was making it better because I could take myself back as if in a time machine to when I felt loved and included.

One day, I was in my mandatory gym, a.k.a. DANCE class, and a teacher came up to me while I was tying my shoelaces while sitting on the ground.

She said, "You need to change out of this outfit. Your gut is hanging out, and it's not appropriate."

I looked up and asked, "What's gut?"

I could see the vein on her forehead popping out. She slowly and loudly said, "GUUUUTTT" while pinching her stomach, so everyone could hear her.

I was mortified.

Gut is FAT, fat stomach. Got it.

Kids laughed. She walked away throwing her hands in the air with a sense of disgust because I didn't understand her.

She left me ashamed, sitting there on the ground wondering how I could hide my "disgusting" stomach. I remember wanting to disappear in that moment. She showered me in shame and judgment, and left me feeling worthless.

I thought, "Greeeeeaaattt, now I am going to be weird and fat, too. I might as well just go die in the locker room right now."

What am I supposed to do?
Am I supposed to find a shirt?
Where am I supposed to find a shirt?

"Hey, I have a shirt you can borrow."

I turned around, and it was a girl named Samantha. Tall, blonde, beautiful. She was a cheerleader and track runner. Samantha was also ridiculously good at dance, unlike me who still struggled with the first set of steps we learned months before. She was the "it" girl. And I was now the fat girl. Until then, she didn't know I existed.

"Here." Samantha handed me a white tee. "Bring it back next time."

We went back to class. I was sweating through the "it" girl's tee and simultaneously plotting a world takeover in my brain.

So what was I thinking? I knew that wasn't just a shirt; it could be something more. Maybe even my chance to hang out with the "it" girls and not eat my lunch in the bathroom.

I clung to the sweaty shirt like a lifeline.

The shirt experience almost made yet another terrifying gym experience a little better. I came home that day and asked my mom if we had a scale. But I didn't tell her the story because she would have gotten really upset.

I remember jumping on the scale expecting maybe five to 10 pounds of weight gain, since my pants did fit a little tighter.

I was 26 POUNDS HEAVIER! I had to do the calculations from kilos to pounds in my head, and I was absolutely mortified once again. By that time I had been in the States for about eight months, so that was averaging three to four pounds per month that I was steadily packing on. It came on so gradually, I didn't even notice how it all had happened. It just crept up!

Admittedly, I secretly knew I was gaining weight but didn't know how much I had let myself go. That revelation meant that I had to stop my escape into the time machine to access the happy times. I was scared to let go, knowing that I could no longer visit my happy place on a regular basis.

The next day—after eating my bodyweight in mini candy the night before, while drowning in self-pity—I had to do my duty of returning the life-saving t-shirt to Samantha. I could have waited a few days and returned it in dance class, but, NO, I had another plan in mind that I had carefully worked out in my head. And it was GENIUS!

I thought that I'd go up to her during a long break to return the t-shirt. That meant that I'd have to go up to all the big tables where football players and other blonde cheerleaders hung out. HOLY COW! It was terrifying, but there was HOPE for my plan.

I remember that while on the bus on my way to school I wrote out the exact sentences of what I wanted to say. Even brainstorming every word she could say back. Because I didn't want to sound weird, dumb, or stupid. It was very important that THIS went smoothly! I only had one chance.

After third hour, I had precisely four minutes before class to do the deed.

My palms were sweaty, my knees were shaking, I rehearsed my lines for the last three hours in every class. I headed downstairs while doing deep-breathing exercises.

I walked up to the table and with every step I took, my heart beat faster. I squeezed my way between the big boys, Drew and Blair, and faced the cheer crowd.

I tapped Samantha on the shoulder, and said in my trick Russian accent, "Hi, you gave me shirt yesterday. I want to give back now."

So far so good.

"Yes, thanks!" She reached out.

I got the next words out the best I could ... "I have a question. Teacher said I have gut, and you helped me with this." I pointed at the shirt. "Can you help me with gut, too? Maybe?"

She broke into a smile.

"Can you do today after school? I'll show you some things. Meet me on the track after school."

Me: "But I have bus ..."

I started to get sad; my heart sunk because I had to catch the damn bus with brace face!

"I'll drive you home. Talk soon. Baaaaaaaaayeeeeee."

She turned back around to tell her story. I squeezed out of the crowd of people who treated me as if I were invisible.

OH MY GOD what just happened?? It was a feeling I'd never felt before. It was a blend of anxiety, happiness, and a heart-attack state of mind.

I was so excited I nearly skipped to class. For the next three hours, anticipation was building, and by the time the final class bell rang I'd already played out every single scenario in my head. I wrote out the scripts for what to say, and, most importantly, I still had her shirt! YES, YES, YES, half of my plan had worked! You know why I kept the shirt? She would have to talk to me again!

That was the most exciting thing that had happened to me in America over the past eight months! It meant that I could actually have a cool friend who would hang out with me! It also meant that I didn't have to face bus weirdos, my unpleasant driver, and, well, brace face for at least a day.

When we met, she put me through the most excruciating 10 minutes of crunches in my life. It felt like hours and hours had passed. It was the hardest thing I'd ever done. I was embarrassed, uncomfortable, lost, confused, afraid, and all of the feelings you could think of all at the same time. I couldn't really keep up with her, but I could keep a straight face, and that was already a win.

When we were done, she started to explain things. I couldn't really understand, but then she said the words that changed my life forever: "I am doing this bodybuilding show next month, you should train with me. It will be fun."

ME? WHAT? My heart started racing again, then fell near my feet. I stood there and couldn't say a word. Even the few that I knew.

"You think I can do?"

The bodybuilding show that Samantha was talking about was what every senior and junior girl talked about for months prior. I heard that it was very hard and only a few people could actually train for it. It was for athletes and cheerleaders, and lots of football boys were doing it.

My mind was racing. I CAN'T DO THIS?

"I will help you train for it. We can do cardio every day, and I will drive you home. You have six weeks, you can do this," she said.

I agreed on the spot without knowing what I agreed to. I'd never seen a bodybuilding show, and I didn't know what to expect, but I knew I had to jump on the opportunity for two reasons: Right then, Samantha was the only friend who didn't think I was the weird Russian girl, and I knew it was time. It was time for a major change.

Up until that minute, the only good emotions I experienced were when I ate a Snickers in the dirty school stairway. What I was feeling at that moment was different, exciting, strange. It was a positive emotion I didn't have to chew.

For the past eight months I'd been walking around like a zombie and eating away my feelings. My weight was the reflection of all of the emotions I was hiding from. I never told anyone how alone I was. When my dad or step-sister would talk, I'd tell them that everything was fine and that I was taking all sorts of really fun classes and about my part-time job at the beauty supply place. I'd never once mentioned to my mom that I cried every night before going to bed because I missed everyone so much. Up until that moment, I was the weird girl, and I was going to continue being the weird girl who eats lunch alone on the stairs or in the bathroom unless I said "Yes" to Samantha.

I DON'T WANT TO LIVE THIS WAY ANYMORE! More than a thought, it was a soul-wrenching outcry to finally break into something that gave meaning to my existence.

Yes, I was afraid I was going to be humiliated while standing in a bikini in front of my high school peers. But honestly, I was already at the bottom. Nothing worse could have happened to me. I had nothing to lose because I was already weird, and I already didn't have friends, and it just didn't matter. Yes, I was 30 pounds overweight at that point. Yes, I had "gut," and I was already shamed in public by even my teachers. No, I had no idea what I was doing, but being at rock bottom sucked worse than the possibility of actually doing something significant.

She drove me home after our first crunch-off session.

"We'll run a mile tomorrow. Bring your shoes to school for after school. I'll drive you home after."

OH, ok! BYEEEEE.

I slammed the door of her tiny sports car, with the license plate "IMTRBLE," and I was liberated.

I got home and told my mom about what had happened and how excited I was about the show. I had no idea what it meant, but I knew I had to train really hard and eat certain foods.

Over the next few weeks, I dug into training and nutrition and understanding the world of bodybuilding. The only thing I knew about nutrition at the time was that Snickers and emotions give you a "gut," and the only thing I knew about fitness was that I knew nothing about fitness. I didn't even run my first timed mile until I was with Samantha. I only had six weeks to get ready, and that meant embracing every aspect of what it would take to step on stage. I thought that crunch-off and first mile were hard. RIGHT! Samantha introduced me to the weight room and resistance training. Imagine a tiiiinny, tiny high school gym with sweaty, pimply football players and two chicks trying to lift weights. Sam lifting and me trying to not die. I was so happy she was with me, and I could count on her help because I was sooooo embarrassed to go in by myself. One day she was 10 minutes late for our set time to train, and since there were no cell phones back then I really had no idea where she was. It was just me, the weights … and about 10 sweaty boys in the weight room. I had to work up MAD courage just to get off my butt to do squats. I couldn't really go anywhere. Sam was my ride, and I wasn't about to just sit there and wait for her. So that first time I lifted by myself I remember feeling like a total BEAST! Look at me! I am doing the DANG thing. I'm lifting! I know what I'm doing! I'm the boss! Watch me squat! It was like a powerful force outside of myself lifted the weights for me. I won't ever forget that feeling. I truly "got it," and that was the day I fell in love with training. It stopped sucking after I realized I kind of knew what I was doing.

In the following few weeks, Samantha took me to the first bodybuilding meet-ups in our school. She also introduced me to the high school coach, Wyatt, who was the organizer, seasoned bodybuilder, and also running Mr. Anchorage that year. I grew more fond of attending the meetings and group workouts, maybe because there was a sense of finally belonging to something and having a goal, or perhaps because Wyatt — a perfect Magic Mike lookalike — was the best-looking man I'd ever had the chance to speak to in my lifetime. Samantha and Wyatt gave me books; gave me a diet to follow; and spent hours with me posing, training, and making sure that my uncoordinated, non-athletic self could actually lift a weight off the ground and eventually step on stage.

I liked that new lifestyle.

See, in its own way, the bodybuilding community was weird, too. No sane teenager would voluntarily stand in front of their high school peers in their underpants, covered in orange paint, flexing their muscles in hopes to earn a trophy. I was now a part of a whole different group of "weirdos" who ate the same strange food, and spent before and after school in the weight room. Leading up to the show, I had noticed that our group was thinning out more and more. But everyone was right: What we were doing wasn't for everyone. It was hard, and every moment in the weight room was a challenge since I didn't know what all of the machines did. So everyday I repeated what Wyatt and Samantha taught me. I was living, breathing, and dreaming about the day of the show. I ate what I was supposed to, I showed up to every meet-up, I listened to Wyatt like he was a bodybuilding god. It was the most intense period of my life to relearn my old habits. And instead of reaching for sugar and candy to make myself feel better, I had to stay mentally strong and exercise every bit of willpower to stick to my new regimen. I didn't realize because I had been rapidly gaining weight and all of the candy had kept me full, that I had stopped eating much real food or meals in general and just picked up bites all day. That was the habit that had to change quickly because Wyatt and Sam told me my body needed fuel, and to grow muscles I needed to eat! As a good student, I obeyed the rules and even ate according to alarms in order to remember to not skip meals. Having a plan gave me focus, having a date gave me the dedication I needed to push through the times I didn't "feel like" training, having Wyatt and Sam on my side gave me confidence. Their belief in my success gave me motivation and inspiration because I didn't want to fail them since they had invested too much in me.

Competing in the show gave me an insane amount of confidence and hope in the fact that the whole American journey and my zombie life had some sort of meaning.

My clothes started getting looser. One day as I was pinning my work pants in the breakroom at my job at the beauty supply shop, my witch of a boss walked in. Her name was Lori, and I'd worked for her for nine months by that time. I thought she was going to be pissed that I was just hanging out in the breakroom trying to fix my pants. I didn't want to buy new work pants yet because I knew I would lose more weight.

I think she hated me the entire time I had worked there; but even if she didn't, she certainly acted like it. Most of the time she would look at me and just call my Russian co-worker friend over to explain what I was messing up rather than attempting to explain it. Nine months after I started my job I was still cleaning shelves, and there was nothing glorious about my job. I wanted to sell. I knew I could because I actually knew what the products did. I read labels everyday I cleaned them, and I translated every word. None of the other girls did.

She asked me what I was doing in there. I told her I was going to do a bodybuilding show, so I had lost weight and needed to pin my pants before I "show butt to people on floor."

She kind of laughed. It was the first time she ever laughed at one of my jokes. It turned out that Lori was a huge fan of bodybuilding and had recently lost the Max Muscle store next door in her divorce … from a bodybuilder. She offered to sponsor some products for me to try, and all of sudden we were laughing like two best friends in the breakroom. Later, my witch of a boss ended up being one of my most incredible mentors, who constantly invested her time, money, resources, and connections so that I could make my competing dreams come true. She traveled with me, she paid for me to travel. She was there for every show and every moment. I eventually ran the beauty supply and became her right-hand woman. We spent five years side by side. You never know who you'll find to be your biggest supporter and your biggest cheerleader.

By the time the show day came, I had lost about 25 pounds in a matter of six weeks. I did it for me, to prove to myself that I could actually do something. Since before I had signed up for the show, gym class had been a terrifying experience every time, and I was sick and tired of saying "It's not my thing" or "I can't do that." Finally, for the first time ever, gym was MY thing. I divorced my old story that I sucked at sports. I sucked at sports because others told me I did. Not anymore.

I was so proud to be around those who believed in me. It was because of my coaches; and my supporters, like Sam and Wyatt and Lori; and all of those orange weirdos backstage who worked their butts off to show up on the day of the show. Whether I won or lost, or was humiliated in front of the school, I didn't care. I worked so hard to get where I was that it didn't matter what happened. I embraced the journey and the learning curve, and I was truly doing it for me, my new self, my most confident and best self. The previous six weeks of my life in America had been more exciting than the nine months I'd spent in my zombie state. I found my smile again. I had friends I could wave to in the hallway. And that's all that mattered.

The night before the show I had one of the salon stylists change my hair. It had been blonde with red highlights because in the midst of my identity crisis over the last nine months my hair color was the only thing I could actually control. I wanted to change who I was because I was no longer that girl; I wanted to be someone different. I had lost weight. I felt good about myself. So I colored my hair from blonde to brunette and it's been the same ever since.

I was the new me.

It wasn't just my hair color that changed, but with the weight that came off, I gained a new sense of confidence, and being the fitness girl became my new story.

Then it came down to showtime!

I remember the smell of the backroom — the combination of musk smells of sweaty high school boys who haven't showered in days due to their couple layers of spray tan, cheap Victoria's Secret perfume from all the cheerleaders, and massive amounts of spray tan. It's quite delightful, as you can probably imagine. If I were to bottle it, it would forever be on sale for 99 cents at Walmart.

Everyone was running around; they were nervous. I was nervous, but in my head I'd visualized the moment so many times, I'd walked those steps with Sam hundreds of times that I was really beyond ready! It would be the first time I would show my new body to the whole school, "that teacher," and my coaches.

Samantha said she liked my hair and that it went well with my tan and suit. She was really proud of me. I knew it in her eyes.

I stood backstage in my clear heels and black bikini that I had borrowed from a friend, shimmying back and forth trying to keep my nerves down. It was SHOWTIME! When they called my name, I took the first step. The lights were bright, it was hot, and it smelled really bad. I couldn't see anyone, not even my mom. I proudly took turns in line with all of the girls that I was competing against. I didn't care about my placement. I just remember smiling with all of my 32 teeth because I was SO proud in my new body and my newfound identity and a sense of control in my out-of-control situation.

When I received my last-place trophy, I remember crying on stage.

My first happy tears while in America.

That last-place trophy didn't mean failure in my eyes.

Failure would have been not trying at all and accepting my story of a chubby kid with a gut, who got called names by her bully teacher. Failure would have been giving up and buying into the fear-based story that I couldn't do it, and that I wasn't athletic, and that that sort of thing must be for others who are better and more capable than I was. Failure would have been quitting, like many kids did when they got sore, missed a cardio session because of homework, or used their after-school job as an excuse to not do something challenging. Failure would have been not showing up on the day of the show because I was terrified of how I might have been perceived by my peers.

I chose to do something about it, and that was a win in my book. Yes, I looked great. But the moment of the show defined many things for me.

It made me realize I was in control of my mind, and body, and what I was truly capable of when I focused. It showed me the true power of community and importance of being led by those who believe in me and possess the expertise. With every pound I had lost I was able to separate more and more from my victim story of depression and sugar addiction. More than anything, I attributed my success to my faith, as well as my willingness to fail as many times as necessary for me to succeed and then to be led in the direction I consciously chose. I cultivated that faith in my next show a year later, where I had won the overall title in the high school show. I went on to win the Junior State Bodybuilding show that year and took 2nd in my class in all of the state. This was my gateway into my eight-year-long career in fitness competitions.

To date, I've won or placed in the top five in more than 26 state, national, and international fitness shows. The only thing that got me through every show prep, hours of training, and months and weeks of strict dieting — no matter how difficult or how smoothly it went — the one and only solution to everything in spite of my fully loaded schedule, has always been my faith, and my unbeatable belief in myself and my ability to make it happen.

BRACE FACE AND WINNING
MISS ALASKA TEEN USA
CHAPTER 2

My first year in college wasn't nearly as awful as my first year in high school. Nobody made fun of me, and I wasn't weird. I could actually express myself, and I got to choose my classes. Everyone was new to college, green, and excited, unlike high school with its very tight-knit communities. After the first semester, I quickly realized that I couldn't afford school. I'd been making decent money to support myself and my car expenses, but since I hadn't grown up in the States my parents didn't really have a college fund, so I had to fork out my own money to cover the tuition bill.

One day while at work I got a text message from my friend Samantha (a different one but total coincidence on the name) asking if my mentor Lori could sponsor her for the upcoming Miss Alaska USA pageant, and since I was already a store manager at the time she figured I could help her out with the fees.

I was really excited for her and started firing off an endless stream of questions. It turned out that the winner would get a full-ride scholarship to the university I'd been attending.

BINGO!
SCORE!
DING, DING, DING!

I was immediately sold on the idea. There was no hesitation in my mind. I gained a significant amount of confidence through competing, and the possibility of having a full-ride scholarship instead of paying out-of-pocket for school was far beyond enticing. I figured that I would do my practice run as Miss Alaska Teen USA and the next year would run for the MISS title. At the time I'd just gotten a brand-new set of shiny braces (who was brace face now?) and still had a very thick accent. I don't remember being particularly nervous about the competition. I borrowed a dress from a friend, completed my application while sitting in the most boring math class ever, and didn't really spend all that much time preparing for the interview portion. I figured that I'd just show up, and since it was a trial run anyway I would just have fun with it.

The show went smoothly. Shiny lights made it all a quick blur. The smell of the fake cloud dust made it seem like it was all unreal. I knew my mom was there, and so were Lori and my best friend from high school Valeria, so that made everything a little less scary … even the dance routine we had to do in the beginning (and we all know how great I was at dance).

When I made the top five I was in shock. I remember pacing behind the thick black curtains thinking, "CRAP, CRAP, CRAP, I have to answer an onstage question! What will it be? Why didn't I practice? UGHHHHH! NOOOOOO.

When it was my turn, I walked onto the stage and with a smile as wiiiiiide as my cheeks permitted at the time, showed the world my shiny new braces.

I drew a question out of a fish bowl. It read: "What does it mean to be a patriot?"

Oh. Crap.

The only question I hadn't really thought about until that moment.

I had to think quickly, and only the truth could pour out of my mouth.

Un-coached, raw, real truth.

With a thick accent, I proudly announced ...

"You have to love YOU country" (not a typo, ladies, not a typo) and work very hard to be the best version of yourself."

After sounding extra Russian under the pressure of a tough question and the stress of bright lights, it came time for the winner announcement. I was sure the girl in the yellow dress won.

"And the winner is ...

The world seemed like it had actually stopped for a moment. I felt my heart sink to my feet. The bright lights got brighter, my vision got blurry. So. Many. Lights. I held my breath for what felt like hours.

"... the winner is ...

Zlata Sushchik!"

WHAT??

I WON!! I WIN, I WIN, I WIN, I WIN!!

WHAT??

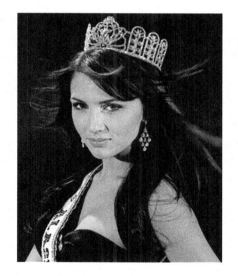

I was in shock. A state of paralysis. And the bright lights got even brighter. I was euphoric, and for just a second I left my body and traveled to the happiest place I'd ever been.

Winning.

It left me speechless.

Different thoughts raced through my head but mostly that I'd never have to pay for school again.

YES!!

While in rehearsal, I was so unsure of winning that I had missed what to do during the whole crowning ritual, which made me look cute/clumsy on stage when it actually happened. Typical Zlata; go figure.

I heard my name and had a celebratory dance to follow. It's really funny; you can Google it.

I walked to the middle of the stage so that the former queen could stick four bobby pins into my head to hold the five-pound shiny, bright Swarovski crystal crown to my head.

I shed the mandatory crowning-moment tear.

It was beautiful. Like a movie. My mom was proud. Lori was exhilarated. Valeria was excited, too!

I knew that what had just happened was significant. I was unsure of how or why, but I knew that life wouldn't ever be the same.

The next morning there was a mandatory meeting with the director to walk us through what lay ahead. The only thing I vividly remember was signing a contract that said I wouldn't wear black eyeliner or yoga pants in public.

Both of which sounded equally devastating.

I still wanted to know why because I'd just recently perfected my flawless cat eyeliner skills. So I asked. The answer was simple: "It's just not what Miss Alaska does."

Okay ... good to know.

Something irritated me so deeply that day. But it wasn't about the eyeliner or the yoga pants. No. It was about not having the freedom to choose what I did or didn't want to do. And I guess I knew that something that silly wasn't the only thing that I wouldn't get to choose throughout the next year.

I felt confused.

That year was filled with events, people, fund-raisers, more events, more people, political balls, and benefit galas. And at every event I had to show up and put in the work, whether it was selling tickets or raffles, or smiling enough to get people to sign fund-raising checks, or holding babies and dancing swing with the elderly, or visiting wounded soldiers in the hospital. There's a common misconception that the titleholder goes to galas, and sits at the head table looking pretty and eating filet mignon, or just perhaps smiling and waving.

It's the furthest thing from the truth.

As you can imagine, as a titleholder you see many people. And with every event, fund-raiser, gala, parade, and person you meet comes the baggage of opinions.

For some odd reason, when you become Miss Alaska, or hold a title of any kind, everyone around you — friends, family, directors, and even random strangers — have some sort of criticism and opinion about what you should and shouldn't do, wear, or say because you're supposed to be something they envision in their eyes.

About you.
About pageants.
About the crown.
About your hair.
About your outfits.
About the dress you chose for nationals.
What your political views are.
Even what you did or didn't say.

And every one of those opinions is likened to chopping down a tree.

Opinion ... WHACK!
Opinion ... WHACK, WHACK!!

You should ... WHACK!
Maybe this will ... WHACK, WHACK!!
Maybe that ... WHACK, WHACK, WHACK!!!

WHACK!
WHACK!
WHACK!

It got exhausting.

Battling with stereotypes, stupid jokes about seeing Russia from the backyard since that was the year Sarah Palin ran for office, endless "should haves," and the molding of the next queen.

The only thing that became authentic to me was my inauthentic pageant smile while trying to hide my braces.

Hugs.
Hello's.
Practices.
People.
Opinions.

"Hi, my name is Zlata Sushchik, and I am Miss Alaska Teen USA." That was all I was for a year. I was defined by my title and what I "should do" as a result of having a sash across my chest.

I realize that I sound ungrateful, but that's not the point. I'm very grateful. Beyond grateful because it was a fascinating experience and I got to do truly fascinating things, and the opportunities that emerge are none like you've experienced before. You get to touch people in a different way because there's something truly special about walking around with a crown on your head. That year we racked up more than 400 hours of community service, participated in 74 events, and raised thousands of dollars to benefit organizations like a women's shelter, the American Heart Association, the American Cancer Society, the Muscular Dystrophy Association, and, honestly, so many more that at some point I lost count. It was all a blur of endless events, massive amounts of hair spray, and a bleeding head from wearing the crown for hours on end. I honestly think I still have a dip where the crown sat. We toured Alaska, teaching goal-setting workshops, with the title "There is no one road to success," to kids in middle school and high school.

It was a lot of work. On top of the job and a full school schedule, my plate was full. I had no room to complain, though, because I took on that mission, and even though I didn't fully realize what the title would entail beyond a school scholarship, I had a duty to uphold, and mama didn't raise no quitter. So I pageanted. Pageanted hard. I don't remember a single day where I was "tired" or "bored," and I somehow managed to stay strong.

That's the good side of things. But just like they say, if it sounds too good to be true it probably is.

So back to the opinions ... and nationals. Like the kind you see on TV.

THE DARK SIDE OF PAGEANTRY: behind the glitz and glamour, photoshoot lights, and flowy dresses, big hair, sparkly crowns, and parade caravans. The dark side of pageantry involves the behind the scenes of getting ready for a national competition.

It also means that you might as well plead temporary insanity during the time you're prepping. And if you think Bridezilla is bad, it's like Bridezilla meets dance moms, and there are 50 brides in one room. They should make a show leading UP to nationals. That would blow NBC's ratings out of the water. "Desperate Pageant Contestant of the MISS USA." Man, that would be a great show.

But why is that the case?

Because life's meaning becomes about making it into the top 15 or taking home the crown. Even if it means the impossible, since Alaska hasn't ever won in the history of the Miss USA or Teen USA.

Nationals prep is the time when the contestant works closely with the pageant team to get "molded" (that's exactly what it's called) into the best version of "yourself." That basically means being transformed into the perfect version of what the judges want to see representing Miss Teen USA — what a titleholder must look like, speak like, act like, and what they do and don't do.

As it turned out, the black eyeliner and yoga pants were the least of my worries. "I knew it. I flipping knew it." That intuitive, confused state that I felt at the first meeting was living out its reality.

That was truly the first time I was introduced to the pressure of meeting a certain beauty standard. It was also one of the first times I was faced with so much pressure from family, friends, coworkers, and perfect strangers to be everything that I'm not — and they're not either but seem to have a very set opinion about it.

In bodybuilding and all of the shows to that date, I'd been focused mostly on the feeling of the "stage high" that I would get from receiving a trophy and accomplishing a goal. It made me feel powerful and in control and like I could take over the world. Even for weeks afterward when I was still covered in orange spray tan. So the standard of beauty — as heavily and as vividly as it was in pageantry — hadn't been projected onto me until that time.

We can both imagine what a beauty queen looks like right?

Think about it …

Close your eyes and envision a beauty queen. What do you see?

She has big, long hair; white teeth; is thin with long legs and most likely a 6-pack. She laughs and smiles and usually waves and mentions world peace. She doesn't have any flaws. And when you look at her it's almost like a walking Barbie doll except she's a real person.

But what if she has braces, semi-short hair, a Russian accent, and believes in world peace but just clearly doesn't fit in? And she's far from looking like a Barbie doll.

That was me to a T. Again, I didn't fit in.

So, I had to get molded. In pageants, anybody who's a square peg can be made to fit into a round hole with enough hair extensions and spray tan.

I had to meet a perfect standard of beauty, as well as everyone's self-projected expectations and daily dose of public opinion.

Since I was also competing with 50 other gorgeous women, most of whom had grown up in the lifelong culture of pageants, comparing myself to Miss Texas (or whomever) became a part of my daily to-do's. In bodybuilding, there wasn't ever an obsession for weeks and months in advance about looking at whom I was competing against. I was competing against myself, and what I was able to do, and it really didn't matter who showed up on competition day.

In the first meeting, we were also told that we weren't allowed to be friends on social media with any current or past titleholders. But like every dedicated and resourceful teenager, by the time you get to nationals you know the exact details of everyone's life, like their favorite color and pet's name.

The combination of both is pretty toxic because it leaves you feeling like you're not enough, and then the endless self-criticism starts to kick in due to the criticism and pressure of everyone about your every move. Speaking of pressure, not only does everyone have an opinion about you and your actions, but directors, sponsors, family, and friends all have a certain expectation of you representing your state, and if you mess up it'll be a reflection of the entire state.

So ... let the pressure begin and the molding along with it.

Leading up to nationals we had weekly coaching to make sure that I had the perfect talk, the perfect smile, the perfect turn, the perfect speech, the perfect talking points, and the perfect hair. In coaching I'd go through an array of questions from "Who do you want to be when you grow up?" or "How are you positively impacting your community," to less trivial matters, like "What do you do for fun?" or "What will you take to space with you?" I really mastered the art of dodging questions that didn't matter at the time; as well as the simplicity of answering a question with a prepared talking point, whether it was "Who do you want be when you grow up?" or "What's your favorite ice cream?"

Let me demonstrate ...

What are your political views on the recent election, where Governor Sarah Palin was chosen as VP?

Sarah Palin was a great leader of our state. We're excited that she was chosen as VP and hope that she'll lead our nation to success. You know what else will help our country become a success? If I'm Miss Teen USA, I'll make sure that teens have the opportunity to reach their goals by learning that there's not one road to success. When I was Miss Teen Alaska, we toured the state with a series of workshops under the slogan "There is no one road to success."

Lets' try something else ...

What's your favorite ice cream?

It's vanilla. There are hundreds and thousands of teens who love vanilla ice cream, too, and if I'm Miss Teen USA I'll make sure that every teen gets to have vanilla ice cream. You know what else I'll do? I'll make sure that teens have the opportunity to reach their goals by learning that there is not one road to success. When I was Miss Teen Alaska ...

You get the point right?

I was a good student. Very coachable.

But deep down in my heart I knew there was no way for me to win the national title. As I had mentioned before, in the history of the pageants Alaska hadn't won a national title and very rarely placed in the top 15. I had felt so out of place in the whole pageant world that I had pled temporary insanity and started doing things like spending $2,700 on a pageant dress when my monthly salary was half of that. Just to make sure not to look out of place in the national line-up. I flew to Tennessee to meet with top pageant coaches, and spent half of my hard-earned sponsorship money on the best of the best just so I could make sure my walk was perfect. Even insane things like whitening my teeth so white that I couldn't eat for a week. What kind of pageant queen would I be without a perfect, pearly white smile? Speaking of eating, this brings me to the special subject of eating while you're a pageant girl. And since my walk, interview skills, and many other things needed massive amounts of coaching, what I could do was control my weight and the fitness part of the competition.

That was truly the only thing that made me feel like I was in my element because the other things felt completely unfamiliar to me. I focused on the diet and the fitness part like I'd never before.

At the time, food was divided into two categories: on a sheet of paper from the trainer and off a sheet of paper, a.k.a. food limits, a.k.a. evil food. I was so focused that I ate by alarms, and I had the same thing every day for 12 weeks leading up to the show. I'm talking about the same thing, not just the same food; the same meal every single day and at the same time, no less. The food was plain-chicken, rice, broccoli, eggs, cottage cheese, apple, chicken, rice, broccoli, eggs, cottage cheese, apple, chicken, rice, broccoli, eggs, cottage cheese, apple, chicken, rice, broccoli, eggs, cottage cheese, apple. You get the point. There were no quinoa or fish, and vegetables that weren't green didn't exist; fruit, pure evil! I never slipped, not once. I was in control of it. I was given free range in fitness on what I could do, and I took that very seriously.

I eventually dieted down to 108 pounds. All of the photos of me that you see now are where I was at about 130-135 pounds at 15 percent body fat. Being 108 pounds is being thin; very, very thin. I was skin and bones, but proud as hell because I got the "body" part down. I kept getting compliments that this was the best Miss Alaska has ever looked in the fitness category. At some point, my mom and others voiced their concern that I was skin and bones, for which we both knew the answer at the time — the ball was already rolling, and there was no stopping it. I kept dieting because I had to and because a perfect body doesn't just happen and because it was soothing to be in control of something.

Did I "feel" good? Like did my body physically feel good?

I don't remember because food wasn't fuel for me at the time, and fitness wasn't a way to make myself feel better. I didn't have time for "feelings." Exercise and food was one thing and one thing only: exercise of control and certainty, while keeping my fingers on the pulse of constant events, dress rehearsals, walking practices, and feeling inadequate in the world I was so uncomfortable with.

It was finally time for nationals.

I remember arriving at the Atlantis Paradise in the Caribbean islands. Nervous. So nervous. I was about to face everybody for the first time. I was about to reveal what Alaska had to BRING this year. Since they were all so perfect, I made sure I showed up looking perfect, too, and I had better get across that I'm worthy of this crown and this title.

I had planned outfits for everyday.

I needed to project the perfect beauty queen I was, and everything I'd rehearsed in pageant coaching was finally coming in handy. I had the answers to everything. My walk was cute and energetic. My teeth finally perfect without braces. We were assigned a hair stylist and makeup artist, and were treated like queens. I got endless questions about Sarah Palin, but I had rehearsed the answer to that, as well.

I started opening up a bit after falling in one of the rehearsals, as I tripped over my feet trying to twirl.

"JESUS CHRIST, ALASKA, know your steps. I can't put you in the back because you're ALASKA. Otherwise, I would. Come on!"

What's with all of the dance teachers hating on me?

Come on!

Yes, you heard that right, he called me Alaska because that's what happens at nationals: You lose your name, and you just become your state sash. Another side effect of the reality of pageant life. In the moment it becomes okay, and everyone is doing it, so it takes the pressure off of trying to remember everyone's name.

In pageants the morning of the show, there's an interview portion, where judges get to meet you in person and ask questions. I was convinced I had it down. I'd rehearsed those talking point just like I'd rehearsed my lines on the school bus before trying to talk to Samantha the cheerleader. I knew what I was saying.

The first judging panel went really well. They laughed, they loved me. I was charming, cute with a little Russian accent.

Second panel, not so much. I was grilled on political questions and my job. Some dumb question about my favorite flower. It was going okay, but it wasn't a hit. But nor was it a disaster, until some judge in his late 40s who looked like he was absolutely hating life while waiting for his coffee refill. I had appeared to be an inconvenience in his morning routine. He bit on a croissant, lifted up his head, threw down the rest of the delicious pastry (my mouth was watering; that damn bread and butter stick looked delicious), wiped his face with a sleeve, and almost yelled.

"So, YOU, Zlata" — he pointed his finger at me, waving his wrist in disgust, looking through the top of his glasses. "Your life sounds sooooo great. WHY do you want to be Miss Teen USA anyway."

I don't know if it was the powdered sugar on the damn croissant that took up most of my attention because I was absolutely starved by that point or the pressure of the moment, but I stood silent, as that was the talking point I hadn't rehearsed all that much. Why would they ask the most TRIVIAL question?! NOOOOO, NEVER.

He drew his fingers through his hair in utter frustration and threw both his hands into the air. His face said, "See, I told you guys ... NEXXT! BYYYEE ALASKA."

Well, that was stupid but I walked out relieved in a way. The worst part was behind me. I was 100% sure I didn't need to talk anymore for the final on-stage question and, needless to say, I was NOT the next Miss Teen USA.

When it came time for the show, I remember feeling so beautiful standing in front of the mirror right before going on stage. That was the first time I had the full "get up" on and felt like a total princess. If Instagram had existed at that time, I would've posted 15,000 selfies, for sure.

Fake hair extensions.
Fake volume.
Fake curls.
Fake lashes.

Fake makeup.
Fake nails.
Fake tan.
Fake white teeth.

It only took a team of four to dress me, do my makeup, volumize my hair, and rub butt glue on my bikini to avoid any mishaps.

Mostly fake. But beautiful.

"AAAAALLLLLAAASKKKAAA" the announcer announced in his deep voice.

I walked out and there were those bright lights again. I could see my mom, and she was crying. It was the first time I'd ever seen my Russian mother cry. She was proud, and I was proud too.

I felt like I belonged on that stage, and I wasn't weird brace face girl.

It felt right. I was one of them, and I was skinny and that felt awesome. I worked hard to be there, and it was a moment to remember for life.

Until I stumbled and ripped my dress on stage ... and dropped my sarong during the swimsuit competition ... AND decided to pick it up ASS to the audience in all of my glory.

It was a disaster to say the least. Everything I could have messed up, I did. At least I didn't fall, and even though I wasn't going to win, at least I didn't fall. And mom got good pictures.

I didn't win.
I didn't place in the top 15.
I was a wreck, and my heart wasn't in it.

You know why? I never wanted to win. It wasn't my vision for myself. It's not what I actually wanted to do that year of my life, but did so because I felt obligated to want to do well and even win because when I take on a job, I take it very seriously. And being a titleholder is exactly that: a job. I felt obligated in front of my wonderful director, my mom, my sponsors, my friends, my state. I felt the enormous pressure of opinions, commitment, everything I'd needed to do — and at 19-years-old. I still didn't have a strong enough sense of self, though, to stand in my "I" and figure out what I wanted to do.

After not placing, I cried. Mainly because when 36 girls who didn't place are crying, you better damn well cry, too. So I shed a mandatory tear again and went backstage to find the damn croissant I'd been wanting all day since the asshat judge decided to have a standoff with me.

Upon returning home, I'd experienced something I'd never felt before.

Total emptiness.

In my chest, in my heart, in my head. It was all empty. And the once-cheery, fun, driven, non-stop, no-excuses Zlata became a certified couch potato. It was like I was competing in the food-/mouth-shoving Olympics. It really didn't matter what the food was, but at the time vanilla ice cream went really well with extra-butter popcorn while watching Netflix marathons. I was planted on the couch for about a week. I didn't leave the house. I didn't go to the gym. I only talked to Valeria. Within the first three weeks, I'd gained most of the weight back that I'd worked so hard to lose. There was no longer a goal, a date, a "thing" to work toward. I would never need to whip out another talking point from my pocket.

I didn't know what I was feeling back then. I thought it was the post-pageant blues that all of the girls had talked about. How they would reminisce about pageants being the best time of their life. I wasn't reminiscing. I was lost because my sense of self was nowhere to be found, and I could finally let go of the control and the pressure and the obligations and chill out for a second. I spent nine months dancing to someone else's thoughts and in a false identity that didn't align with whom I was. I felt like I failed myself and folded under the pressure of what others wanted me to do. The overly perfect world of beauty queens and perfect walk, perfect talk, perfect everything got the best of me. But after a year of molding, that was all I knew. I learned to play a role, and I got really good at it, and all of sudden I didn't need to act anymore. And that was harder than I would have imagined.

On top of that, my body was so exhausted. It was completely burned out from endless dieting. Now granted, I looked phenomenal, and that's exactly what I got praise for. But I knew I couldn't keep up with that schedule. I remember being really proud but really sad at the same time seeing myself slip away from my thin Victoria's Secret model look. Don't get me wrong: The fact that I can talk, walk, write, ask questions, and conduct myself nowadays comes from the pageant world. Many positive things came from it. But I didn't quite know how to deal with myself and my "I" at the time.

With hopes of keeping busy after the pageant, I fully immersed myself in school work. Taking advantage of my full-ride scholarship, I decided to breeze through college, taking as many classes as I possibly could.

MY NOT BOYFRIEND AND A NEW RELATIONSHIP ... WITH PIZZA
CHAPTER 3

This is when the story gets really interesting. There's no great story without a great love story, right?

Our romance was brief, like every text message he ever sent. He was tall, with dark blue eyes, long hair, and tattoos, and he had that whole "swag" thing going for him. He was like one of those guys you see at a bar and think, "Damn, he's bad news, sister," but you go for it anyway. Nothing about that guy said boyfriend material. I knew he was all sorts of bad for me, but the idea of dating a bad boy sounded so fun and so rebellious after being a perfect "goody girl" for so long, who couldn't even wear black eyeliner without permission.

Coincidentally, at that time a whole new division was emerging in the bodybuilding community. Lori, my coaches, and my friends encouraged me to step in. After the pageant world, I had so many skills that I could put to good use. I thought about it and decided to step in. Truthfully, I was once again in a predicament about the uncertainty of "who do I want to be when I grow up?" With just starting to live on my own, and sorta dating the bad boy, having a goal like a show sounded SO comforting amidst the constant change and madness of it all. When I talked about my plans with the la'boy, whom I was so desperately trying to turn into la'boyfriend, he loved it and was totally stoked for me. I saw the pride in his eyes, and it made me want to compete even more!

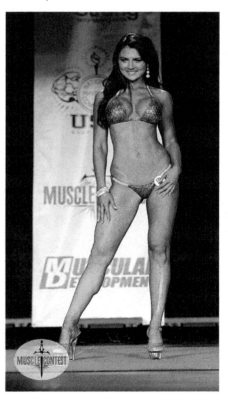

In the next six weeks, I went full-on Zlata mode over that fitness competition. I was IN my element again. My community was there, my weight was going down; closer to 110 again, where I felt like a total rockstar. That number somehow became the new standard where I felt great. If I was over, it totally controlled my mood. I would feel upset all day, drink less water, eat a bit less. The next day, it would be 110, and I was happy. I had to be at that weight. It was my "mojo" weight that I started to associate with everything going well in life because it was!

When it was time for me to step on stage, I felt good. I owned it. It was soooo my jam. All the prep seemed like child's play in comparison to the national pageant. On the show date, I was stoked. Mostly for la'boy to see me "do my thang" and hopefully move me a step closer to girlfriend status. Big hair, fake spray tan, clip-on nails, blingy suit. IT was just like the pageant, except I didn't have to talk to anyone looking all high and mighty, chewing a croissant in front me.

Pre-judging, the first part of the show in the morning, went screamingly well. When it was time for the night show, I peeked behind the black curtain and saw HIM! I whispered to Valeria, "HE IS HERE!" I was so excited. When they announced the top five, I was IN IT! Cool, let's take that 1st place trophy home!

When it was time for the final judgment and for the five girls to do their mandatory terms, I stood in the lineup with Vaseline on my teeth, astonished at what was happening. Not because I was about to win the show, but because my not-boyfriend took a phone call and disappeared from the room right before I walked out on stage. I was so PISSED off that I messed up all my steps, took the 3rd place trophy, stomped off the stage, and broke down in tears to Valeria.

I was livid. How could he?! Who called that was THAT important?!

Right there's where you'd think a girl would get a clue and tell that "boy BAH," in the words of Queen Beyonce, and so I did afterward.

But instead of letting the boy GO and moving on with my life like a normal human should, I did the complete opposite. I embarked on a crazy quest for what I called a "revenge body" at the time. I know it seems totally Khloé Kardashian right now, but I was on that ride long before it became a thing.

Totally irrational thoughts went through my head: make him MISS me; make him LOVE me; and, I'll be SO hot, he'll totally want me; since I'm 110 again and fucking unstoppable, let's do this. Competing had given me a false sense of control over someone else, when in reality he probably didn't even care.

Totally logical if you ask me, right?

Since I was already in complete Zlata mode, upset about that boy, unsure about my future after graduation, I went on to compete in every show I could sign up for. I won state, collegiates, placed 3rd at nationals, placed in the top five internationally, came back to state, and took another overall. That season, I ate more tilapia any human should eat in a lifetime. I was all cardio, carbs, tilapia, training. My life was competing. Sure I worked, sure I passed my classes with honors, and somehow that boy was in and out of the picture every time I won a show.

Looking back, I realize that fitness had became a way for me to control the things that I couldn't really control in life, and 110 was a visible validation that I indeed was in control.

Don't know what to do with life – compete!
Not having much fun and don't know what to do – compete!
Not sure about your next career choice – compete!
Not getting love from a man – compete! DUH!

Uncertainty = competition = control = 110 pounds = feel good, certain, loved.

It was all great and under control, until the off-season came around. Between every show I had incentive to stay on my rigid plan. But with no show in sight for the next six months, I could finally let go a little – still be healthy, of course, but at least it didn't have to be green beans, tilapia, broccoli 24/7/365. I could spice it up a bit, and actually have a slice of bread here and there. I deserved it; after all, I worked so hard all that time! It was my ultimate reward for the seven trophies I collected that year! But what I hadn't considered was that when you eat like normal people, you no longer get to be 110 because normal people don't walk around at 9-11% body fat all year-round. My body was doing something I'd never experienced before. Not even after the pageant. I ballooned up to 150 pounds in a matter of three weeks. That was 40 pounds in three weeks. FORTY!!!

It literally felt like the end of the world.

It was a disaster. I didn't want to go anywhere, I didn't want to show up at the gym because everyone would know how fat I had gotten. I was so self-conscious, and I noticed myself hiding from any male creature that I encountered. I don't have any photos from that year. I thought I was SO FAT! Fat became the adjective to describe all of my emotions at once. Mostly to express shame, guilt, and feeling like I had completely lost control, and that I was consciously and subconsciously so afraid that someone would call me out on my gut again. I thought that I had been doing everything right, and eating some bread here and there shouldn't have been such a big deal. With 110 pounds fading from the scale and nowhere in sight, so was my confidence and mojo. I did everything in my power to wrestle my body back to normal. I didn't get what my body was doing. Wasn't fitness good for you? Wasn't eating clean a good thing, too? What do you like now, body?

I so desperately wanted to get a hold of the situation that I decided I would go back to my pre-stage diet again and screw the whole rest thing. It wasn't working for me! So what did I do? I trained more, I ate less. I cut carbs even more. I didn't eat fat. I didn't eat cheese. I did DVDs in the living room.

At first, the weight budged a little, but despite my best efforts it just wasn't coming off as quickly as I had hoped. By the time I was about to get ready for a show, I was already exhausted, still 20 pounds over my goal weight, and already in a serious mental struggle after three months of fatness. All I wanted was my body back. I wanted my confidence. I worked so hard, and it just wasn't helping. I felt like my body betrayed me. Why couldn't I just have a Pinterest model body? I would spend hours on Pinterest looking for motivation and trying to figure out how much "leaner" I could cook. At the time, social media was just emerging, and I would spend hours scrolling, trying to get the secrets of the pros. I wanted to become pro more and more because of the bodies they had. It all seemed so happy and glamorous on the other side of where I was.

I hired a new coach to help me solve that puzzle. He was THE best, the number one. I put that payment on my credit card and thought, "How in the world am I going to pay this off?" It didn't matter how much it cost. He trained pros, and he would make me pro, too. And he thought I had a chance at it. So began the roller-coaster of the same dieting cycle, more cardio, less carbs. More hours spent on Pinterest, more negative self-talk, more comparison games with fitness models, more expectations, more "team no day off" inspirational messages, and more dreaming of the glitz and glamour of that pro card.

It was all going better. Until one day when I was sitting at my new dream corporate job that I had gotten after college. It was lunch hour, and the thought of tilapia and green beans for one more meal seemed revolting. I grabbed my keys and escaped the office on a secret mission to commit the ultimate crime that would cost me hours at the gym. I was fed up. Well, I was under fed up, really, with not seeing results fast enough, meal after meal of the same food, the meal plan, check-ins, cardio, and my body failing me. I had no 6-pack abs like the other girls,

I had no muscles like the other girls, and I was working so hard. I just thought, "FUCK THIS, I'm just going to eat whatever the FUCK I WANT."

I embarked on a mission to find pizza and ice cream that I'd dreamt about for a month. Because WHY NOT? And while I was at it, I'd get some candy, too.

I pulled up to the nearest strip mall that had a pizza place and a grocery store all in one. I ninja'ed my way into the pizzeria so that nobody could see me, and ordered a pepperoni pizza and cheese sticks. I felt slightly embarrassed but mostly rebellious. If my body could be rebellious and not comply with my diet, I would be rebellious, too. I even thought of an excuse in case someone saw me. I would say it was for a work party! Brilliant! I walked out of there with the forbidden cheat meal and headed into the grocery store next door. After a careful, yet swift, assessment of the candy aisle, I got a Snickers, Starburst, jelly beans, and something else I don't remember, but it was about 40 dollars worth of candy. It was the only time I could do that, so I had better get it all now! It was like I was possessed by the junk food gods.

And then I sat in my car and ate it all. Yes, the whole pizza, the whole thing of cheese sticks, a few Starburst, and whatever else I had gotten at the time. I was once again in outer space, like in high school on those stairs, alone, sad, and about to be fat-shamed. I couldn't tell my coach. I couldn't tell anyone.

So I didn't. In fact, I've never told anyone ... until I just wrote the words here. I can't believe I'm actually sharing this with you because it wasn't the original story at all. I was deeply embarrassed about that for almost six years, but if you're about to get real honest with me and yourself, I better get real honest with you.

You can only imagine what happened next ... I got insanely sick. So sick that the next logical thing was to just open my car door and let it all out.

"I can't go back to work like this," I had thought. I took a look in the rearview mirror. Blood shot eyes, smeared makeup, and the evidence of my crime left on the passenger seat in the form of an empty greasy pizza box and colorful wrappers.

I called in sick, went home, prayed to the porcelain god for awhile longer. And after I was done, just to make sure there was no evidence of the evildoing on my progress photos, I performed an exorcism of the fat that could potentially end up on my ass: I went to the gym and lapped imaginary miles on a treadmill for a few hours.

But that didn't happen once, not even twice ... actually, quite a few more times than I care to count.

By the time I had stepped on stage again, I was so wrapped up in my meal plan, workout schedule, color of my suit, and goal bod, that I hadn't realized that I had developed a full-blown eating disorder. Since I hadn't told anyone, it wasn't real. I wrestled my body to stage weight. I placed, I won. I would keep it all under control. I was so invested in my goal, in my world, and in my identity — not to mention wrapped up in the magic number 110 to give me the much-needed sense of self-worth — that I missed all of the signs.

I was sick. Like really sick.

I looked great. I was 11% body fat. My suit was shiny. My fake smile was semi-real. The world was under control as long as I was doing that. The pressure to get the pro card grew stronger. My coach really thought I had the chance. I started to get fitness jobs and got offered a sponsorship from a big supplement company. The ball was rolling in the dream direction, but I was rolling downhill fast without wanting to admit the inner struggle I had.

DR. SOMETHING AND MORE ON FAITH
CHAPTER 4

The roller-coaster of competing, self-oathing, and eating disorder continued until I visited a doctor's office for an annual check-up for my insurance. The lady in a white lab coat, Dr. Something, asked me how I felt. I said, "Fine."

Oh boy. Anytime a woman says, "Fine," brace yourself because she's not FINE.

She said, "Fine? Okay. You have dangerously low levels of T4 and T3 in your body, and are low in iron, magnesium, vitamin D, and vitamin B. Date of last period?"

I didn't have an answer for her because I hadn't had one in awhile. Having a period in bodybuilding meant that you weren't working hard enough. It was frowned upon.

"You know, I'm just fine. Can I go now?"

At that moment, she sat down next to me with the sweetest motherly look. You know, when a doctor sits down next to you in a movie-like fashion, as if something is seriously wrong.

"Zlata, what's going on? You have a hormonal panel of a post-menopausal woman who's 50 years old. I'm seriously about to send you in for cancer screening."

Thank god that at that moment I was smart enough to tell her basically the whole story of what had been happening, and once I said it out loud it sounded SO TERRIBLE. Almost as terrible as it sounds typing it for this book. Like I'm some sick, crazy woman with an eating disorder, who's obsessed with every bite I eat, and has no life because I spend it on the treadmill with an iPad.

Oh wait, that WAS me.

"I am going to write you a prescription, come back for an adrenal test. I bet there is more going on. I suggest you rest, go see someone for the eating stuff, take it easy, and come see me again in a few months?"

I smiled and nodded, but at the same time I was thinking, "HA! ME? You think I don't have this under control. You think I'm crazy or sick? I don't need a prescription. Like I said, I am FINE!"

In full-blown denial, I exited her office and threw the damn Rx in the trash. (NOTE: *I'm here for you to learn from my mistakes, so please do as I say, not as I did and don't throw your prescriptions in the trash.*)

But the truth was I wasn't fine. I spent the next few days staring at the wall at home, with tea, pretending to be very sick and calling in sick to work. I think my roommate at the time knew what was going on but didn't really want to get in the middle of it.

My false sense of control about life had crumbled before my eyes. All of the masks of roles I had played came down. There was no more hiding from myself and what had happened. Something that once gave me joy and certainty, and had made me feel so confident was lost, and I wasn't sure where or how I could find it again, or even try.

I surrendered my shiny bikini after a serious powwow with myself. I wasn't going to compete for awhile until I got better or at least until I got the eating thing under control. I knew that what I had been experiencing was common among fitness models and competitors — many don't have their menstrual cycle for months, end up on thyroid medication, or use unauthorized prescriptions just to get down in weight for the show. It was real and it was everywhere.

And since I'm an unstoppable force when I want to solve or fix something, I decided that I was going to dig in and learn more about that fitness thing. Because if I was having those issues I obviously needed to know more about fitness. So I studied, researched, read, interviewed, and Googled my way into learning more. I needed to figure out how I could have the body I wanted, while still being married to the 110 number and actually eat. Basically, I wanted the impossible and figured that other fitness people must know the answer.

What I discovered was quite interesting and disturbing all at the same time ...

The very team members, coaches, competitors, and fellow models I trained right next to — the ones with eating issues and constant negative self-talk — were the very people teaching the fitness thing to normal people like you and me. Eat clean, train mean, team no days off, six meals a day, clean eating, cardio ... wait! I'm trying to leave that world, and that's what you're teaching people? I knew that most models in those magazines and on the pages of any fitness book at the time, or on Instagram, only looked like THAT on the day of the show. Other times, they were just like me: disordered eating and living wrapped up in their stage-weight identity.

I didn't want to go back there. Not with my mind or with my body. I couldn't get back on that train.

The more I looked into fitness, the more I realized my problem wasn't fitness. I knew how to train, but that wasn't enough. So i started researching everywhere else but fitness: nutrition, digestive health, hormonal health, sleep, the brain, behavioral psychology, cognitive psychology. I started to connect the dots more and more.

Around that same time, my dear friend Valeria approached me and asked if I would help her train for a show. At first I was completely against it. I knew what crazy mind game she was about to walk into. I resisted for awhile, and she actually had gotten really upset with me. You see, she had supported me all of those years, and now it was time for me to be that friend to support her. I'd done that 26 times by then, and she had always been there. It would have been incredibly selfish of me to just say "NO"! AND also selfish of me to not let her have her own experience. But Val didn't really know the extent of my struggles, since I'd just abruptly left the stage, disabled my social media accounts, and pretended I was busy with my new job and master's degree.

But I did know a ton, and I really did want to help her, after all. We started going to the gym together. The first time we worked out, her arms had been giving out doing the shoulder press exercise with 5-pound dumbbells. Her cringe face was priceless, but she was on a roll! We did grocery shopping together, we prepped meals together, we ate out of Tupperware® together. I remember having to explain that chicken nuggets were not an appropriate protein substitution for grilled chicken. Then before it came time to hit the stage, we posed together, we walked together, we huuuuur-flipped together. Since I was recovering at the time, I knew the exact rabbit holes I wouldn't want to send her down. I hadn't wanted to teach her the very things that broke me.

She had this childlike joy, excitement, and nervous laugh, and one day she had said, "I know I'm not placing Zlata, but I just want to do this, to prove to myself I can do something THIS big. I've always envied you in a way for doing this, and thanks for giving me the courage to try. I'm doing this for me because I was scared shitless to do it for so many years." I loved her sober outlook on the whole situation. She wasn't chasing her pro card, she wasn't trying to win, there was no pressure, she was happy with every pound she lost and didn't obsess over those pounds she didn't lose.

And, like with every transformation, it wasn't just me helping her, because it takes a village to transform! But that once-timid Valeria had started flourishing into a whole new woman. With pounds melting off, she grew more and more confident everyday. Not just her body, but her attitude, bubbly personality, how she handled life. It brought out parts in her that I'd never seen and probably would've never seen if she hadn't embarked on that journey.

In order to compete in the upcoming state show, Val had lost more than 70 pounds. When stage day rolled around, I was the one in the audience being the supportive friend with a glittery sign, donuts, and flowers.

When she walked onto that stage, it was like Valeria 2.0 emerged out of nowhere.

She floated onto the stage in all of her glory and confidence. Every step, every move. Step left, step right, hair flip, cute smile, a wink to the judges.

SHE NAILED IT!

She had placed in the top five; won best transformation; and schooled my bitter, overworked self who had given up on fitness altogether. See, for her it wasn't about the 6-pack abs or getting a trophy or placing at nationals or buying a $2,700 dress to please everyone around her. She didn't care that she was a size 6 or that she had some cellulite that showed once she stepped on stage. For her, it was about feeling sexy in her own skin, her own way, for her health, for her confidence, to fight her fear and stretch her comfort zone and push herself to a new level ... even when your arms give out doing the easiest exercises. It was about how she felt in her own skin and proving to herself that she CAN do it.

She did it her way, for herself.

Through her transformation, she had restored my faith in the journey and mirrored what I had so desperately needed to learn at that time. To this day, I don't think that she knows that I owe her, and it's not the other way around.

Valeria was my inspiration. Once I'd seen how she had been transformed, my heart and soul had been set on fire. I'd been filled with an overwhelming urge to help women achieve that kind of transformation, and avoid the traps and rabbit holes I'd gone down and hadn't needed to go down in hopes of getting a sexy bod. I saw how much the knowledge and skillset of everything I'd learned helped her to transform. And I then knew that I could help more women do the same.

When it came time to pick a name for my business, "Leanfit," "Skinnyfit," "110fit" were obviously the wrong ways to describe what kind of outcome I wanted women to achieve. I wanted to help them feel better in their body and in their skin without the pressures of meeting ever-changing beauty standards, social media pressure, and the opinions of others.

In the midst of brainstorming, all I could think about was Valeria's face on stage and her attitude about life off stage. She took that attitude with her everywhere. To her job, to school, eventually meeting a man she loved and moving out of state in pursuit of more. And fit, obviously, because she had become one fit mama! "Sexy" and "fit" were the best ways to describe her transformation.

So the idea of "Sexyfit" was born.

I wanted to avoid the traditional weight-loss messaging about losing 10 pounds in five days or any agenda that makes women feel like they need more "ER" in their life: thinnER, leanER, strongER, implying that they'll be MORE when they buy this "thing." And implying that they aren't enough as themselves right now. Neither did I want to promote shakes, powders, red pills, tea detoxes, "clean eating," or anything in that manner. I was also desperately trying to get away from the usual M.O. of the superficial fitness world and "wear" Sexyfit with pride.

Case in point: Life threw a test of faith at me in the first two months of running "Sexyfit" as a business. One day while working on my lap top at a coffee shop, I bit down on a baby carrot I had packed for myself as a snack. I heard a loud crunch, and it turned out that my left front tooth had got bit off with that carrot. YES! I had lost my front tooth!!!!! And because it was a crown already, there was no quick fix for it. I ended up doing all of my speaking gigs, coaching calls, and online training sessions with a fake flipper, which gave me a crazy lisp for almost eight months! There was a time I had to hold my loose flipper with my tongue while speaking on stage to hundreds of women about living a confident lifestyle. I look back at that and when times get tough I remember it could always be worse. At least I still have all of my teeth!

To this day, I remain dead set on the agenda of removing the superficial part of fitness as much as possible, despite many marketers, branding agencies, and people telling us that we really need to shift the focus.

I want Sexyfit to be different, as well as a unique experience for everyone because not one of us is the same. We're built differently; we have different genetics; different skin color, body shape, body type; everything about us is different, and that shit is the best. But most importantly, we have a different story of where we came from and what we struggled with and why we struggled with it.

It's all different here because I don't want you to be more like me. I want you to be more like you. The 2.0 version of you — certain in self, healthy in your body, mindful, strong, confident, sexy, and fit.

Since starting Sexyfit, we've transformed hundreds of women to complete food freedom, loving their body, and reclaiming their life to be healthier, happier, and more confident. I took everything I learned over a decade of fitness experience and combined it with endless research about hormones, as well as my personal experience overcoming hypothyroidism, adrenal fatigue, an eating disorder, and body dysmorphia. I started hosting a radio show with the best of the best in the fitness industry and interviewed more than 300 experts on the same topics. I am to the core obsessed with our message, our method, and what it does for women. I know what it did for me, I know what it did for my best friend, I know what it has done for other women. I know what it can and will do for you. No matter where you've come from, no matter where you are now, if you want to experience what it's like to be at home with your body, this is the way. No judgment, no comparison, no in-the-box thinking.

Your lifestyle, your way.

Sister, we're ready to dive in now!

INTRODUCTION

Something as natural and as simple as eating and moving our body has become a seriously confusing chore. We have become too outward focused on the next best diet and DVD, we're in constant search of new "rules" and new gurus, and Google our way into "how to's, and the ins and outs of a healthy lifestyle. So if you're feeling overwhelmed and confused, and have spent an enormous amount of energy trying to figure out what's best, you're not alone. The more we get inundated with information, the more we seek stricter rules for how our body is supposed to work. This book wouldn't be one of those cases.

As I previously mentioned, your transformation isn't a linear path, and not a "one size fits all" or one truth for all. Discovering what's right for you, as opposed to what's right for me, or what's right period, is what we're about to do with this book and this method. You'll find no harsh rules, no over-complicated plans, or secret formulas to magically transform you overnight.

What you WILL find here are the basics of what you'll need to know about health and fitness that I believe have been over-diluted for "general" consumption and packaged as the fast-food version of what health/beauty is. You'll also get the steps to help you transform your life, your relationship with self, and your relationship with your body and your food.

Before diving in, there are three basic premises I would like to share with you that will serve as a great foundation for your success with the Sexyfit method. These three principles are necessary, and, when in doubt, you can apply any of them to seek out a solution. At its core, a premise is something you don't necessarily need proof for. Whether you agree with them or not, they exist for a reason. For the purpose of walking through this journey together, I ask that you give them a test drive. You can always shy away from them after you're finished with the book, but for the sake of working together, I believe these are important. If you allow these to sink it, I have no doubt that eventually you can apply them to create an enormous amount of success in your life.

PREMISE #1

In the beautiful words of George Bernard Shaw, "Life is not about discovering yourself, life is about creating yourself."

We live life by design, and we choose our way into the outcomes. You and only you create your life, your experiences, and your transformation.

The truth is, we create our experiences through beliefs, actions, and thoughts, and everything that we're surrounded by was chosen by us at some moment in time. This might come as a surprise to you, it might even make you angry at me for a moment, but it's true. In one way or another, we chose our circumstances, our lives, and our situations. Ultimately, only you are responsible for your actions, and have to take responsibility for your experiences and the outcome. Many of us live our lives thinking that massive success, a hot body, an amazing job, and a happy, fulfilled life is for someone else "out there."

We go through life with a victim mindset, as if everything happens to us. Some of us have chosen this mindset as the default, or have accepted it after years of someone telling us that, without taking full responsibility for whom we are and what we're capable of. You might feel like you didn't have the right resources, the right support system, you didn't have time, or you had an illness or an injury that defined your current situation. All of those reasons sound understandable and rational to continue living in the victimhood mindset. You can choose to continue to do so if you wish, but it will ultimately cost your transformation and your best life.

PREMISE #2
There are two most powerful emotions: love and fear.

All positive emotions, like compassion, contentment, passion, excitement, acceptance, peace, and joy, all flow from a place of love. When we're in love, we open up to the world of joyful opportunities and creative possibilities.

All negative emotions like anger, hate, anxiety, guilt, expectations, self-loathing are rooted in fear. When we're in fear, we pull back from life. And every choice we make is either an expression of love or an expression of fear. Where there's fear, there's an absence of love. We can't be both in fear and in love at the same time; they're opposites.

Unfortunately, because we're so unaware of our patterns and our subconscious brain loops, we choose fear every day. Especially when it comes to how we look. Virtually any successful viral fitness campaign on the Internet has been spun out of fear. All fitness magazine headlines make sure that you feel like you have FOMO. Unless you're strongER, leanER, or any other "ER," you're not good enough and must push for more. No good thing can come from fear, and no life-changing breakthrough can take root in a place of fear or negative pattern. That's why revenge bodies don't last, why proving someone wrong by getting in shape doesn't stick, and why fear-based fitness marketing of products just leaves us more dissatisfied.

We must relearn to default to love in every situation if we want our results to last and for us to be fulfilled, proud, and excited about the changes we're making. I don't necessarily mean some froufrou self-love, like painting your nails on a Sunday afternoon, which, too, is an important act of self-care. I'm talking about strong, deep-rooted love in your "I" and in your "SELF." Where there's love, there's no failure.

PREMISE #3
There's a fundamental and universal truth that masculine and feminine energy exists in our relation to everything. I'm not talking about bodies, men and women, husband and wife, parent and child, or lovers. I refer to your nature, and the expression of personal masculine and feminine energy. Without understanding masculine and feminine energy, we can become very much out of balance. This is exactly what's happening within ourselves in our relationship to self and, for that matter, in our relation to others. Whether you call it left brain/right brain, yin and yang, this energy connection exists, and we must pay much attention to it when it comes to feeling at home with our body.

Take a look:

MASCULINE — DO, GIVE, THINK.

Masculine energy is primarily based on logic, reason, energy of action, firmness, ease of achieving material goods, common sense. Masculine says, "I think." It's focused, disciplined, active, with a purpose, has a vision. Healthy masculine energy needs a bit of feminine energy to give it softness, depth, joy, and wisdom. In nutrition and fitness, masculine energy loves the idea of rigid meal plans, workout schedules, and certainty in what and when a meal comes next. In an imbalanced state, the masculine aspect could manifest as over-intellectualizing food — dissecting it to calories, grams, and an endless deciphering of ingredients; eating too fast; indigestion; overeating; and at risk of being stuck in "analysis paralysis." Or as an over-controlling life with rigid workout schedules.

FEMININE — FEEL, RECEIVE, NURTURE.

Feminine energy is primarily based on intuition, nurturing, healing, calmness, emotional awareness, expression of emotions. Feminine says, "I feel." It's open, patient, caring, wise, flexible, compassionate. Healthy feminine energy needs a bit of masculine energy to give it focus and structure. The feminine aspect of nutrition and fitness shines through, honoring the beauty and nourishing qualities of food; and tapping into the sensual properties relating to eating, such as taste, touch, smell, and sight; gathering food; and food preparation. The female inclination is to follow intuition. Feminine loves the idea of intuitive eating, being guided by intuition, and making decisions from the place of "I feel." Having too much feminine can cause to become unfocused, depressed, unmotivated, and over-nurturing, and could unfold as over-emotionalizing food — connecting it to fear, anger, worry, sadness; eating copious amounts of fat (or fearing eating fat); and using food to show love to self and others.

The problem is, many of us have disowned our feminine parts of self in perception as if it's the "weak" side of us. Since as long as I can remember, I've thought that being an alpha female was my superpower. I thought being in masculine energy was what made me successful in life. There was no time for the feelings nonsense. But it was only separating me from myself, and disallowing the connection with my true essence and the relationship with my body.

I'm going to say this with every ounce of love and respect for the recent major strides of the feminist movement. It has brought enormous benefits to our society, and we as women enjoy many benefits of equality as a result. In some cases, though, I believe that we've taken the idea of being a strong, independent, alpha woman to the extreme in the sense of treating femininity as a weakness and shunning away from our emotions. With the recent development of our feminine rights, we've started to take on more and more masculine roles: getting jobs, pursuing higher education, become breadwinners in the household. We now function in the masculine energy of "doing" and "thinking" and "achieving," and, as a result, we settle to be a lovelier version of a man. If we're constantly giving to everyone around us, we're thinking our way out of problems and into new problems. This why we grow angry, resistant, and dissatisfied, and at some point crash, burn, and lose all control ... because we aren't meant to control everything all of the time. We've taken ourselves out of our natural "receiving" seat and somehow got on a roller-coaster of constantly giving and giving and giving. And feeling worse and worse and worse.

Right now we're seeing this shift mostly in how we treat our body, with trying to restrict certain food groups, seeking rigid meal plans, and eating on the go. We're starting to feel this in relationships, too. You've heard women say,

"Where are the real men at?" The dissonance is everywhere, and the more we disown our feminine, the more it's going to seem impossible to make any progress in our physical transformation.

As much as I'm a feminist and I love equality, we can't function equally because we're different, and that's what makes us unique in our own way. A healthy feminine is always going to default to 60% feminine emotions and feeling, and to 40% masculine. The sooner you apply this concept, the easier it'll be for you to dance between the balance of both and create a relationship within yourself in regard to every part of self. My life has completely changed as a result of it — with work, relationships, friends, and, most importantly, with SELF. If in general you're looking for balance in life, this is the only balance you need to know.

I know that all strong, independent ladies like you and me take incredible pride and joy in being really good at separating thoughts and emotions, or not having any at all and being a "doer." But as women, it's in our nature to be highly sensitive, emotional beings. Emotions are what make us different from a toaster or a vacuum cleaner. The danger of denying the universal gift of "feeling" by shunning away from feelings yields an unprecedented danger of becoming overweight and unhappy, or losing a sense of purpose for whom we are and what we do. We as women are designed to rely on our feelings as a guide, a compass, a universal map to steer us in the right direction. Being strong and powerful doesn't mean not having feelings; strong and powerful and a high sense of self comes from mastering our emotions and how we manage our state of mind on a regular basis.

All emotions must be felt and granted otherwise they go straight to our waistline; it doesn't matter if you're doing it with Snickers, perceived healthy peanut butter binges, or sweet potato fries that you're well aware are not good for you in excess.

The bottom line is that to have a healthy relationship with self, we need a healthy relationship within self in respect to both masculine and feminine energies. Learning to receive instead of constantly give is a new way to feel and act. It feels selfish at times. But remember the announcer on the plane who's always telling us to put on our oxygen mask first? This is exactly what they're talking about. We can be a better mother, wife, daughter, nurse, lawyer, dentist, marketer, business owner when we allow our relationship with ourself to default to our feminine superpower.

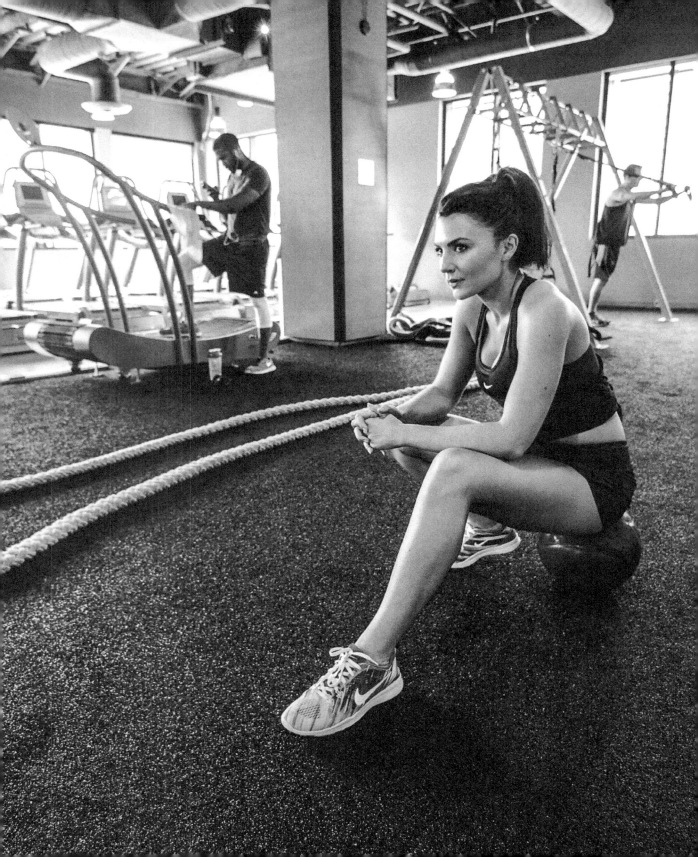

STEP I
TRAIN YOUR MIND

Clear away the obstacles that
are holding you back from
creating the body you've
always wanted.

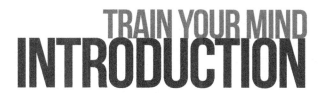

TRAIN YOUR MIND
INTRODUCTION

"The future depends on what we do in the present."
– Mahatma Gandhi

Your transformation and the joy of your journey is deeply rooted in the quality of your mindset. Having the right tools and the right foundation will help you not only achieve the results you're looking for but also keep them for life. Physical transformation without a mindset transformation is like building a house on a marsh. Sure, you can build a home, but there are only so many sandbags that will help you sustain it. Sandbags in this case are external motivators we're used to, like Instagram, Pinterest, magazines, or the usual source of fitspiration.

This section of the book will help you build a firm foundation for lasting change.

IN THIS SECTION OF THE BOOK:

- We'll explore the beliefs, stories, and thoughts that are holding us back from creating the body we've always wanted.
- We'll create a new mindset which will shape our desired outcome through compassion, acceptance, kindness, faith, gratitude, and self-love.
- We'll overcome our adverse relationship with specific body parts and practice radical self-acceptance and self-care.
- We'll set conscious goals, and create a vision of the body and the lifestyle we love.
- We'll begin by taking specific, consistent actions to show up for ourselves and our goals in support of our vision.

THE STORY OF YOUR STORY
CHAPTER 5

In the wise words of Mahatma Gandhi, "Your beliefs shape your thoughts. Your thoughts become your words. Your words become your actions. Your actions become your habits."

What we believe or rather what we allow ourselves to believe will either propel us to new heights or keep us stuck where we are now. Achieving sustainable fat loss, just like any transformation, requires a new mindset and a new set of beliefs to create a new story. Meal plans, fitness plans, and trainers are a dime a dozen. With all of these tools and resources — available anywhere, at any time — it has never been easier to get these resources in the fast-paced virtual world we live in. But it doesn't start with a plan. If it were that easy, we would all we walking around with 6-pack abs.

It starts with our beliefs, thoughts, and our stories.

Here's a list of the most common thoughts that are holding us back from achieving what we want. At any given time, we've all used them to clip our own transformation wings.

I don't have time.
I don't know what what I'm doing.
I don't know how.
I'm not a runner.
This isn't for me.
Someone else is more capable and has more time, and it's for them.
I have kids.
I'm too busy with my job.
This is too hard, and I don't think it's for me.
I've failed so many times before, why would I try again?
I've tried everything, and nothing works.
Nobody supports me or gets me.
I'm older, and now my metabolism is for crap.
It's time for medication and weight loss surgery, or something to fix me.
When I do this _____, then I'll start again _____.

The more we subscribe to this playlist, the more it starts to make sense. And the thing is, on the surface, all of these stories actually seem to have merit. "You tell a lie big enough, loud enough and long enough, the people will believe it." You know whom those words belong to? Adolf Hitler.

See, all of these statements are merely a story that's standing in the way of us getting the transformation we desire. We're wrapped up in some sort of story about something we haven't yet achieved — why we haven't moved, gotten a job, made a million dollars, or aren't dating Brad Pitt. And no matter how rational, logical, and "wise" it sounds to us, it's just a story.

This is where it all starts.

"I've tried everything."

Yes? You say you've tried everything? What have you tried? Name the things you did try. Most of us have tried two to three of the same things over and over again, failed, and expected different results. If you lost a bunch of weight and gained it all back, or didn't even get that far, perhaps you just found a way that didn't work for you. And if you really, really wanted to make it happen, you'd have really done it.

"I don't have time."

I'm sure you have a busy job. I'm sure Johnny needs to be dropped off at school and picked up from soccer practice. But if you really wanted it, you'd find the time. Some statistics say that the average adult watches between 24-36 hours of TV per week. Some stats also say that we spend an average of 40 minutes per day on social media. So if you can find the time to be on Facebook, you really could do less Netflix-ing and more lifting. And if you really wanted to, you could order a salad at the drive-through rather than that double-double that just somehow ends up in your hands.

"I don't know what I'm doing."

Hypothetically, if there were a gun to your head, could you really find a way to become a runner? I think so. You'd just run. Slow as hell, but you'd run.

And I love this one: "It's just not a priority right now."

If taking care of your "home" isn't a priority, then what is? Your friend's birthday party? A new episode of "Orange is the New Black"? The real question is why your health isn't a priority at all.

Okay, you get it. I could go through the list of "The dog ate my homework"-type of excuses all day.

"Okay, well I'm just lazy then, and I can't do it!" is the next thing I typically hear. Well, news flash, sister, I don't think any of us is lazy. Not you, nor your friends who have been trying to lose weight for years. No lazy person in the world would pick up this book — you go to work; you do things all day; if anything, you're overbooked! You aren't lazy in other areas of life.

If you have been working out or attempting to find a diet that works for you for quite some time now, you have a different set of stories that's wrapped up in fears and anxieties due to information overload and not trusting your body to know what's best.

Food makes me gain weight.
I don't eat _____ because it makes me "fat."
I heard gluten is bad for you, so I stopped eating it.
I can't give up food, I LOVE food too much.
Unless I work out for 45 minutes it's useless.
I'm afraid to get hungry because I don't want to binge eat.
I can't stop doing cardio, I'll gain weight!
I'm afraid to lift weights, I don't want to get bulky.

I get it.
I get it.
I get it.

But all of these statements come from the same playlist that we subscribe to that's not serving us in the best way.

See, every one of these stories actually has a story behind it. It's like reading between the lines. You tell me one thing, and I actually hear something else. Behind every one of these excuses — and that's what these stories are — there's an actual story that's ruling your subconscious mind.

The real question is WHY do you think you don't have time … WHY do you think you don't have money … WHY do you think your health isn't a priority?

We usually mask the real story with some sort of "easy-to-tell story" that's just an excuse or stories we tightly identify with based on "experience." However, the real story is typically tightly sealed, labeled "not for anyone's eyes," and tucked away in a back of our mind, where we're hoping nobody notices and we don't either.

So what's the real story of your story?

THAT'S where the block is. That's what really has been preventing you from getting where you want to be. You're not lazy. You don't need a kick in the ass. And neither do you need the latest weight-loss supplement that your neighbor is trying to sell you.

Many of us aren't even aware that this story exists, and that our subconscious story has a powerful hand in about 95% of the decisions we make on a regular basis. Weight loss is no exception.

This means that somewhere along the way we made a subconscious decision to avoid some sort of thing that has caused us great pain, wrapped that pain in fear, packaged it up as universal wisdom, and now it's running our thought process.

Don't believe me yet?
Let me give you an example:

I was once a guest on a radio show, and a woman called in to ask a question about why she couldn't seem to get results. She had one of those really thick Southern accents.

Caller: "Hi ya'll, I hope you can help me. I think I am doing everything right. I am going to the gym, ya know. I eat real good ya know, and I bought all these diet books. I listen to the show every week, and I tried all kinds of stuff. Lost some weight but then something happens. I just gain it back because I get so busy. I just can't stick to it long-term. It all creeps up on me. It's like I have no self-control or something. What is the next thing you think I should try?"

Since the show was co-hosted by a dear friend, I let her take over the conversation for a bit. We found out more and more about the caller. Her name was Chelsea, and she had been overweight her whole life; not by much, like 30 pounds or so, and had been trying to lose the same 30 pounds for over 15 years. She had been on every diet under the moon ... and the sun ... and the whole solar system. The lovely co-host gave her some tips on what new green juice to drink and what new seeds to try in her salad.

The whole time I was sitting on live air, fuming more and more. In my mind, I was like:

"IT'S NOT ABOUT THE DAMN GREEN JUICE OR THE DAMN SEEDS!"

(Imagine me screaming this in my head.)

There was more to the story than we were being led to believe.

I grew more impatient and decided to take the matter into my own hands. See, I'd heard hundreds of those stories. I'd heard hundreds of ya'lls stories about diets and DVDs and juices and what seeds to take.

I took over the mic and kindly said:

"Chelsea, I have a feeling that you're a hard-working, smart, and strong woman. I also know that a woman like you will do whatever it takes and try whatever it takes, including the green juice and the seeds. But what's really the story here? What are you really afraid of?

The pause was long. I pointed a finger at my co-host to not say another word until Chelsea wrapped her mind around the question. They really hate dead air on radio, but questions like these require time to be answered truthfully.

Some of us would laugh and say, "It's really nothing!"

Some of us would freeze in disbelief of what we were about to say.

Some of us would be so shocked that we'd want to run out of the room.

With a tremble in her voice, Chelsea put herself together, took a deep breath into the microphone, and said:

"When I lost 30 pounds my family started noticing, and everyone was giving me compliments. I thought I would love it, but all the attention made me feel uncomfortable. My family started acting differently around me and thought that I was all full of myself, so I didn't want to stand out anymore. It sounds so stupid, I know, but what if they won't accept me at this new weight?"

"So what are you afraid of?" I asked.

She said, "That they won't love me if I continue to lose weight."

Now we were getting somewhere. We went from the timid statement of "I lack self-control sorta" to the real issue. The true story and the true fear lay much deeper than any amount of green juice or chia seeds could fix. It was about her being loved and accepted by loved ones. Her diet and her health journey were directly in competition with the most important need in life: to be loved, especially by those whom we love.

Another client, Lisa, confessed in our first few sessions that she was sick and tired of all the weight she had gained through yo-yo dieting, and that she was finally ready for something strict and would do whatever it took. Everything else in her life was right. She had the house, the job, the man, the everything she had ever wanted, but her weight was always something she had struggled with. She wasn't lazy. She worked hard for everything she had.

I like to ask questions. Maybe that's why I host a podcast; to really figure out where the block or belief is that has been stopping women for all of that time.

After walking her through a series of questions, she realized that it wasn't that she needed a strict plan to follow but that she was scared of her weight loss. Yes, actually afraid of weight loss because every time she would lose weight something bad would happen to her. When she lost weight the first time, her fiancé left her. When she lost weight again, she got accused by her friends of using drugs and supplements to help her. As a result, her weight kept her safe and without negative attention.

Other women I've coached used dieting as a way to control their environment out of a deep dissatisfaction with life or lack of anything else going on. Perhaps they were on a journey of leaving a job they felt they couldn't get out of or a relationship they felt trapped in. Or maybe an injury had caused weight gain, and they were so fixated on fixing it that they forgot that friends and family even existed. That was very much the story of my story, of weighing 110 pounds as validation of being in complete control of my life.

Another client was so wrapped up in all of the rules she learned after two decades of dieting that she became gluten-free, lactose-free, gave up red meat even though she loved steak, stopped dining out with friends, and was living in a world paralyzed by self-imposed rules to the point that she couldn't even go out on a date and enjoy her time. Her fear was letting go of control over her food because her mother put her on her first diet at age 13, saying that unless she was thin, no man would have a romantic interest in her. As a result, at age 33 she perceived herself as overweight, and sabotaged every relationship in her life due to her rigid approach to food and the many rules for herself.

So what's common in these stories?
F
E
A
R

Quite simply, it's our subconscious fear.

Fear of not being loved and accepted.
Fear of failing because we've tried so many things before.
Fear of success.
Fear of loving ourselves and putting ourselves first.
Fear of uncertainty
Fear of the unknown.
Fear of gaining it back.

But the biggest fear of all is the feeling of failure that surrounds weight loss if we fail. "Tried a thousand things and failed. Might as well not start now because I know I'll fail anyway." And every time you think you've failed because you ate something or missed a day at the gym, it's just easier to say, "Oops, I fell off the wagon again. Guess I'm a failure." But that's just lazy thinking right there. It's just a reason to get yourself off the hook. It doesn't mean you've failed.

You have an opportunity to analyze what happened, why it happened, and how you can get out of that pattern. If you don't do this, it'll feel like you keep starting over and over and over again because your desire to transform wouldn't go anywhere. You only fail when you stop trying. PERIOD. Just because you ate something that you perceive is bad, or missed a day or a week at the gym, picking yourself up and making it work FOR you not against you is what's going to keep you IN the game.

Our subconscious fears show up because somewhere along the way, whether in our childhood or recently, we had an experience that we treated as wisdom about how we should act. But it's really not wisdom. It's a fear in disguise that rules the way we think and approach fat loss and everything else in life, for that matter.

My need to control everything definitely comes from a having a childhood where I didn't have enough certainty of even the basic needs, like food and shelter. I crave certainty. I yearn for it, like a heroine addict, so competing and controlling my weight was the outlet to get the certainty I longed for. Did I stop because I said, "Well, I made all these mistakes, nothing works, let's quit now! ... I failed"? So. Many. Times. Over and over and over again. There's only one difference between you and me right now. I treat failure as my asset, and you better start, too. The obstacle IS the way, and as long as you keep showing up, you'll eventually nail it for yourself.

One day we have to look that fear in the eye and decide which we want more: to be paralyzed by the convenient fear or rise above it to achieve a great transformation?

We don't get to have both.

⚙ CHAPTER PRACTICE

IDENTIFY—Together we're going to increase your awareness around the core beliefs you subscribe to and operate from. To identify your story, first outline the belief system around self, food, and exercise that you currently subscribe to. Take out your journal and answer the following questions:

- What do you believe about yourself when it comes to fat loss?

- Where did this belief come from?

- What's your belief system around "dieting" and healthy nutrition?

- What's your belief system around fitness and working out? What's your belief system about the gym?

- My last plan didn't work out because_____.

- But it really didn't work out because _____.

- What evidence can you find that may suggest that your negative beliefs about yourself might not be true?

RELEASE—On a separate sheet of paper, I ask you to write down the beliefs you know of that are holding you back from achieving the results you want and creating the body you love. You can also analyze previous statements and look for patterns of behavior.

Write on a piece of paper:
I release the (thought/belief/pattern) _____.

AFFIRM—I ask you to write affirmative, positive statements to yourself about the negative beliefs you just released in Step 2. Affirmations are designed to transform old negative beliefs into new positive thoughts. Make sure to write all of your affirmations as positive.

Example: I'm not terrible at sports. Correct affirmation: I am gifted at sports.

I am_____.

I am_____.

I am _____.

I am _____.

I am _____.

⚙ PODCAST ALERT

Reference the www.sexyfit.com/resources page to listen to the "What Are You Afraid of? Conquering Your Fears Through Faith" podcast.

THOUGHT PATTERN AWARENESS
CHAPTER 6

"The mind is everything. What you think you become."

-- Buddha

I used to wake up every morning, step on the scale, look in the mirror, take out a pocket knife, and start my day by giving myself multiple stab wounds.

Okay, I didn't really actually stab myself every day, but it sure felt like I did.

Every morning began with a similar narrative of the self-destructive, judgmental, negative self-talk, and thought patterns dissecting every part of my body. It would continue on as the day went by, and as I caught a glimpse in the mirror all I could focus on was how big my stomach was or how gross my legs looked that day in a skirt. When we would get together with friends, we, too, would talk about each others' flaws and envy the body parts we didn't have. Every day, endless scrolling meant polluting a mind with garbage motivational messages of "no pain, no gain," Instagram models, and making sure to pin the bodies that could truly make me feel you're less like enough and more like an unrealistic fitness model.

Ever looked in the mirror in the morning and said:

"Good Lord, you should lose 10 pounds"

Or maybe looked in the mirror after a long week of work and thought:

"Damn, you look like crap."

We women do this all day, every day. And this is somehow the new norm; to be stuck in these negative thought patterns. It's like we live with a frenemy who's constantly comparing us, judging us, sets unrealistic expectations, doubts us while expecting us to be perfect, and as a result feel like we're never good enough. The sad thing is, we have NO idea that we're even doing this to ourselves.

When we wake up every morning, our world is neutral—we choose to give it meaning. Every day, and really every minute, we get an opportunity to start the day fresh with a new mindset that will set us up for success, endless self-love, consistent progress, and feeling like we're enough. It's up to us which choice we make. Or, we get to continue down the path of self-loathing. In a way, we choose which beast we get to feed.

I want to shine a light on the five most common ways that we feed the wrong beast and walk you through the solution for each one.

Let's take comparison as an example. Ever gone on Instagram, checked out one of your friends, and thought, "Damn, must be nice to be you!"? Her life is perfect, her dog is perfect, her husband is the spitting image of young David Beckham, owns a million dollar mansion, and is just a goddess. It's SO incredibly easy to feel completely inadequate in a matter of seconds on social media.

We parade the best part of our life and who we are and what we do.

No Instagram account is going to show you that your goddess friend works 14-16 hours a day in her pajamas with no makeup on and hair in a bun to afford that mansion. Or that her and her husband are going through fertility issues because she's too lean, and that 6-pack you see is her lifelong struggle with her own body image. You don't know the full story. Compassion is the thief of joy, and everyone, EVERYONE has a struggle. Just because it looks shiny and perfect doesn't mean it is. The only difference between you and her and everyone else on social media is that they just know how to take better pictures. Chill.

Now let's leave the comparison game in the dust and make a beeline to the next item on the list: judgment. It's something we do all day, every day. Judge our hair, outfits, and actually everything else around us, too, because why not. We judge our thighs for being too big, our belly for being too round, our arms for being too jiggly. Our self-judgment is denying the very part of ourself that needs the most love.

And the standards and expectation hangovers—that has GOT to be the favorite way to constantly be disappointed with ourselves. Oftentimes we'll look at others, or flip through too many magazines, and point out every woman with 6-pack abs and commit to the journey of having 6-pack abs, too! But, like ... tomorrow. After all, it says 6-pack abs in seven minutes! So you crunch away for seven minutes a day in hopes that it'll happen for you, too. But I have to tell you this: I've spent a fair share of my time with fitness models who've graced magazine covers. Even the girl on the cover doesn't look like the girl on the cover come three days after the shoot, and they spend hours, and I mean HOURS, a day working on a physique like that.

Remember the famous quote by Cindy Crawford: "Even I don't wake up looking like Cindy Crawford." Exactly.

Many models you see on covers take months to get ready for that very cover. Many tear sheet models spend weeks on the StairMaster and eat tilapia around the clock to be chosen for a photoshoot. This is their job; they're MODELS. It's toxic to compare where you are now with the body of a 25-year-old single model living in L.A., while you have two kids, a full-time job, and a husband you love.

Directly related to the last point—but on the flip side—is seeking perfectionism. We feel an enormous amount of pressure to be perfect. We walk on eggshells trying to plan our way into a perfect future, and when it doesn't work, it's a classic case of expectation hangover. It creates an all-or-nothing thinking with nutrition and fitness. Unless we can eat "perfectly clean," we don't bother with healthy eating all. Unless we can go to the gym every day, we don't bother showing our face at the gym at all for months. We wait for the "perfect moment" and the right time to start our "new diet" when "things slow down," but the truth is that being a little less perfect will make us a lot more consistent. We wear our perfectionism as a badge of honor—I'm a bit of a perfectionist as if it's a good thing. At times, yes, it's a great thing, but not when it comes to looking for perfection in regard to food and exercise. Perfectionism shows up everywhere, at times for a good reason. If we're performing heart surgery, building a skyscraper, or trying to paint a straight line; when risks and the stakes are high, that's a good time for us to pull out the perfectionist tendency. Making a regular weeknight dinner, folding laundry, heading out to grab a cup of coffee with messy hair—not necessary and exciting if we always try to be perfect. Low stakes, medium to low reward. Sure, there's a time and place for it, but mostly perfectionism is a form of lazy thinking because we don't actually get to make any mistakes, and it purposefully keeps us small so we don't have to try new things.

Oh, and there's more … there's the guilt of spending money or time on ourselves; the mommy guilt; the guilt of not being in a hundred places at once; oh, and the doubt over if we're doing this right; and saying that we "should," "probably," "most likely," and "hopefully" will "try" to do something.

How did we get here?

How did this become the new norm?

How did this frenemy creep into our life?

It's exhausting to live in our own head and none of this is real. If we lived in this mindset for way too long, we don't think another reality exists. The thing is, where our focus goes, our energy flows, and we've conditioned ourselves to live this way because we don't know anything else. We don't really know WHY we do it, but we don't really know another way of existing. This is all we see, and the state of self-hate becomes our reality. What we don't know is that our brain is incredibly smart, and in an effort to keep our attention it isolates certain experiences and amplifies that experience to have the grasp on life.

But we don't see the full picture. Want proof?

Look around the room right now. Look for everything that's orange — QUICK! Close your eyes. Name a few things that were orange?

QUICK, QUICK, QUICK.

Don't just keep reading, look around.

What do you see?

Look to the left, look to the right.

Now, name everything that you saw that was blue?

What was it for you?

I see a chair, a pen, a book, a light on my mic.

Name what you saw that was blue.

Now, while you were looking for blue, how many things did you see that were orange? Or yellow? Or purple?

Not very many, I bet. Your brain was given a task to look for blue, and that's all it was seeing.

We choose comparison, judgment, expectation, perfectionism, and guilt and doubt because that's all we know. It's a way for us to default to fear because that's how we've been conditioned to live. In other words, all we see is blue. In a society that profits from self-doubt, fear, and unrealistic expectations, loving yourself is a rebellious act.

How do you reprogram your brain to see more colors like orange, yellow, and purple? What's the answer to see more? Again, the answer is love. Love is really always the answer. The more you choose love as your new default to untangle yourself from the fear-based thinking story, the more you'll be drinking the self-love cool-aid.

Your daily practice now is to default and cultivate love-based thinking when you're referring to yourself and others. Here are love-based antidotes to fear-based thinking. You get to choose compassion, acceptance, kindness, trust, and gratitude as your go-to thoughts.

COMPARISON — COMPASSION

When you catch yourself in comparison, exercise as much kindness and compassion for yourself as possible. Say a compassionate statement to yourself from a place of a kind heart. You never know the full story; you can only focus on your story and your great effort.

JUDGMENT — ACCEPTANCE

Judgment is a way for us to disown a part of ourselves that we haven't yet accepted. Judging others is seeing a disowned part of ourselves in that person. Whether you're judging yourself or others, make it a point to say something nice that you like about yourself or others. It'll help you to eventually work into accepting self as you are and others as they choose to be. If you're hyperfocused on one particular part of your body that you dislike, hold that body part on a daily basis and affirm accepting statements in your mind as you touch it. I have to make another comment on judgment …Many times as you start progressing and seeing results, others will attempt to comment on your weight or "how quickly you're melting before their eyes." They'll choose to judge and make comments about your appearance and request that you stop, say how they're "scared for you," or say, "it must be nice to be healthy/young/your age/ in your 40s/to have time" — implying that you think you're special in some way. Projected judgment of others makes us doubt ourselves and our journey. It will diminish our efforts and make us feel like we're doing something wrong. Please know, these statements have nothing to do with you. They have everything to do with the person making that statement. What you can do is share how these statements make you feel—judged/timid/uncomfortable/ uncertain—and kindly ask them to stop making these statements. If they continue to do so, please know this is their issue to deal with, not yours; accept them the way they are and love them anyway.

HERE'S A CHEAT SHEET: "Hello, I noticed that you made a comment about how I look and how quickly I'm losing weight. Thank you for your input, you have every right to make a comment. It makes me feel sad and unsupported to hear this from you. Would you mind withholding your comments next time? It would make me feel supported and understood."

UNREALISTIC EXPECTATIONS — STAYING PRESENT

We tend to build mega-plans and create a sea of expectations for how things "should" be. When the painted picture that we made up in our head doesn't meet the expected outcome, we sit in a sea of disappointment. The fastest way to cure an expectation hangover is to face the situation with an open heart and open mind, and ask yourself, "What am I learning?" and "Why is this happening?" It will help you get into a sober mindset about the situation and create a learning experience, instead of another reason to feel disappointed.

PERFECTIONISM — TRUST

With food and fitness, your best effort is your best effort. Withholding food from your body because you can't make a choice or you're stuck in fear of overeating something that's "not clean" is a way to punish your body. Perfectionism over every bite is how we end up being stuck in FOMO, binge eating, and not trusting ourselves around food. Breathe in fear, breathe out trust to make the right decision.

DOUBT — FAITH

At times when you're wrapped in self-doubt, think about this: You wouldn't tell your baby to stop trying to talk if they failed the first time. Well, it's the same on your journey to transformation. If you failed one time, that doesn't mean you stop trying. You keep getting up and keep trying to learn how to walk. Have some faith.

BUSYNESS — GRATITUDE

Next time you feel overwhelmed with your life and daily to-do list, instead of saying, "I have to," start saying, "I choose to." We have so much to be grateful for, but we choose to pay attention to what we lack and what we need more of. The more you find the things, people, situations, lessons you're grateful for, the more you're going to feel at ease.

Practicing gratitude, faith, kindness, trust, compassion, and acceptance toward ourselves are the loudest acts of self-love and the best ways to create brand-new thought patterns on our quest to food freedom and a fulfilled life. As they say, old ways won't open new doors. When we focus on the positive thoughts and beliefs, our actions will follow.

💡 CHAPTER PRACTICE

Every time you catch yourself with any negative thoughts swirling around in your head, bring yourself closer to love-based thinking and forgiveness by saying:

"I forgive this thought, and I choose to release it. I practice (name a positive thought) on my journey to self love."

You'll be amazed at how many times a day you'll catch yourself in a negative space and feeling inadequate. Within seven days, you'll feel a welcome relief from the prison of your own mind and notice yourself feeling happier, more vibrant, and more confident.

If you find yourself feeling stuck in the loop of negative self-talk, the fastest way to get out of that loop is to use Affirmations. Affirmations are sentences aimed to affect the conscious and the subconscious mind. The words comprising the affirmation, automatically and involuntarily, bring related mental images into the mind, which could inspire, energize, and motivate. Repeating affirmations, and the resulting mental images, affect the subconscious mind, which, in turn, influences the behaviors, habits, actions, and reactions.

"I am Sexyfit. I am strong. I believe in me" are great examples of affirmations. Always make sure that your affirmation is positive and avoid NO statements. For example, "I'm NOT fat" is not the most effective. But, "I feel and look great today" does work. You may feel a little cheesy and unauthentic saying it at first, but find those affirmations that you truly believe in, and you'll see how your mood changes instantly when you use them. My best advice is to make sticky notes with positive messages and put them on your bathroom mirror, in your car, and wherever you'll see them. I have one on my fridge that says, "I make choices that influence my energy levels long-term." It keeps me accountable.

Go to www.sexyfit.com/resources page where you can find an eight-minute Positive Affirmation Guided Meditation, which you can use to overcome negative self-talk.

🎙 PODCAST ALERT

Reference the the www.sexyfit.com/resources page to listen to the "How to Deal with Perfectionism" and "How to Heal Expectation Hangover and Attract What You Really Want with Christine Hassler" podcasts.

DEVELOPING EMOTIONAL INTELLIGENCE
AND YOUR RELATIONSHIP WITH YOUR BODY
CHAPTER 7

"She was having a hard time managing her feelings at this point, mostly because she hadn't felt them in so long – they confused her ... After you've been numbed for a while, disorientation is a natural reaction as you come back around. It's like waking up from anesthesia and not knowing exactly where you are."

– Danielle LaPorte

Last year, Facebook announced that it was removing "feeling fat" from its list of status update emoticons after thousands of people signed a petition arguing that it was offensive and promoted negative self-image. I don't know if you remember, but it pictured an emoji with chubby cheeks and a double chin, which petitioners believed reinforced negative body image, and Facebook seemed to agree.

Fat talk has become a social epidemic, a ritual of womanhood, socially acceptable, and even contagious. We've used "feeling fat" as a communication method for years – validation that we do indeed look great, trying to find common ground and filling in conversation gaps, maybe even trying to crack a joke.

IT LOOKS SOMETHING LIKE THIS:
Woman 1: "I feel fat in this dress."
Woman 2: "No, honey you look greatttt!!!!"
Ah, huh. Woman 1 received instant validation and praise that she does look great.

Woman 1 "I feel fat in these pants."
Woman 2: "Yes, meeeee, too. I hate my pants, and I feel like a beached whale."
Bingo, we have commonality and a point of conversation for the next 45 minutes.

LET'S TRY AGAIN:
Woman 1: "I feel so fat, I ate like 10 pounds of cheese last night."
Woman 2 "HA, you fatty!"
Look what we have here — a sarcastic joke, fun, excitement!

Feeling "fat" became a catchphrase for all emotions. It's our go-to to describe feeling disappointment in self; guilt for overeating; lack of self-love; feeling hurt, misunderstood, tired, or run down; or just trying to feel validated and loved. And in a world where we mostly communicate our feelings with an array of colorful emojis, this only moves us further and further away from being in touch with what we feel and why we feel that way, but most importantly how we can feel differently.

I lived fat not happily ever after for many years.

See, we women have become very good at hiding our emotions in the fast-paced, driven world we live in. We're praised for being doers, achievers, go-getters, and working really, really hard. No woman I know has ever been praised for being "so good" at emotions! For being so open and honest in her feminine essence of a nurturing goddess. This sounds like psycho talk to some of us. "Feminine goddess – have you seen me in the morning?" THIS is why we have the emotional intelligence of a kitchen sink when it comes to how WE feel on the inside.

We treat emotions as if they're an inconvenience. Tears? You mean inconvenient body responses of a weak a$$ b***? So, instead of feeling anything, we settle for mushing it all together as " feeling fat" and attempt to find inner peace in the ever-evolving world of "busy," with our never-ending to-do list to prove that we're the "doers, achievers, go-getters." Which is great, and I understand why and how it works because in modern society we need a job and a schedule, an income and a paycheck. I get all that. I, too, go to work and set goals and achieve, and have a to-do list. But here's the deal ...

For as long as I can remember, I overloaded my to do-list with taking as many classes as I could, working as many hours as humanly possible, constantly overgave of myself to my friends and boyfriends at the time. I racked up community work hours, sleeping was for the weak, and not doing something felt like I was completely useless to the world. I was the best at keeping my schedule full and keeping all of the plates spinning in the air at once. People thought I was damn-near superhuman. Which, I thought I was, too! Until all of the plates occasionally spun out of control, crashed on top of my head, and I crashed and burned with them. That's when I would occasionally land in a hospital or my bed with a Xanax prescription because of a mild panic attack.

If you're experiencing any of these, this chapter will change your life in the best ways possible:

- You constantly feel fat, uncomfortable in your clothes.
- You're constantly burned out or stressed.
- You feel like you're running a rat race, and it's just never slowing down.
- It feels like you're giving, giving, giving, and giving to everyone around you.
- You're the last person/thing on your to-do list.
- You feel completely empty by the end of the day.
- Constant anxiety and occasional panic attacks cause an inconvenient paralysis in your schedule when you should be doing things! (usually before big deadlines)
- There's a sense of something always missing, even when things are good.
- Nutrition and fitness are a chore, and the last thing on your agenda.
- You're really good when you have a plan and a purpose, a goal in life, but feel really lost without one.

- You're not sure what you think and how you feel, and oftentimes it's an internal struggle to make a decision — and it's like, "Are there two people living inside my head?"
- You're not sure how you feel at all because you're breezing through your to-do list.
- Your to-do list is nowhere to be found, and you're face deep in a pint of ice cream.
- Buying something, eating something, or otherwise numbing negative emotions is how you find peace.

Welcome to living life as a man in black and white. It feels like a rat race because it is. We — us women — aren't designed to live this way. In the first place, it manifests in our relationship with our body. When it comes to our body, our food choices and our relationship with self, we can't just focus on achieving, planning, goal setting, and "thinking our way into" solutions.

Women — we're highly sensitive beings, that's what makes us different from a man. As my friend Liz Dealto says, "A woman is not a lovelier version of a man." Our inner guidance, our inner voice, our "hunch," intuition, gut feel, or feelings in general, whatever you want to call it, is our internal compass that can never ever steer us the wrong way. When we connect to the emotions, to how we feel, what we feel, and why we feel it, this is how we find all the answers to the simple things, like what to eat for lunch, or even the loaded questions, like what I'm going to be when I grow up.

We have many, many feelings, and FAT is not one of them. We HAVE fat, we have eyeballs, too, but we're not eyeballs.

When we feel fat that means that we're feeling something else. Perhaps, many "something elses." And that something else must be felt, cherished, appreciated, and heard, as this is a way that our body and our intuition are trying to tell us something, to communicate with us, and we must learn to listen.

When I committed to myself to find a solution to my eating disorder that I developed after my bodybuilding career was over, I had no idea where to begin. Per the suggestion of Dr. Something, I went to see a "weight loss coach," thinking that I truly needed to lose weight and all of this "fat" on my body was the root problem of my broken relationship with food and self. By the time I got to her office, I was terrified of food, anything that wasn't a vegetable was considered off-limits, my body was so tired I didn't have the energy to work out, and I had probably purchased most of the buttoned ponchos in every color from Nordstrom to cover myself up. I didn't even believe that it was possible to be "normal" again, where life wouldn't revolve around fear, self-shame, and constant judgment.

In our first session, my coach asked me how I felt. I answered I feel "fine." Turns out "fine" is not a feeling. So she asked me again. I said, "To be honest, I feel fat, and this is why I'm here." Turns out that fat is not a feeling, either, and neither is "busy." All of those are catch-all phrases to NOT feeling anything.

She asked me to keep a journal every time I ate to see how I felt when I did eat. She mentioned something about how this was called intuitive eating, and how it could help me connect with my emotions and let my intuition guide my food choice. All my intuition wanted at the time was a cheeseburger, and I very much doubted how letting my intuition eat it would help anything. Also, at the time, I still had a very strong desire to get back on stage, so she also asked me to go back and connect the dots for WHY I was competing — my desires, reasons, thought patterns behind the need for such rigid, strict, and no-error-allowed environment.

I went home with two homework assignments, both of which sounded kind of absurd because I perceived that none of it would be helpful. But since I'm a very coachable student, I committed myself to doing it HER way.

That night, there I was on my bathroom floor … connecting all of the "dots" and digging deep into the Zlataworld that was carefully sealed off with caution tape for so long. At first, I felt like it was ridiculous to even do it, to connect with my "feeeeelings." I listed every show in bullet points – because bullet points for life! – and how each show made me feel AND what I was looking for in every show and WHY I was looking for it. That's when I first became aware of my tendencies to want to massively control every detail of the outcome and how competing helped me to do exactly that. It was kind of ironic that my need for such tight control got me completely out of control. But what else?

I don't know if at that point the wine kicked in or what, but I remember feeling intense sadness and so alone in the world. The very feeling I tried to avoid for many, many years … since being 15 years old, to be exact. My way of coping with that feeling was to make my body fit a certain standard to feel more included, connected, and a part of something. Whether it was part of a community of orange 16-year-old teenagers backstage at the high school bodybuilding show or 50 overly perfect big-haired pageant queens. The more I was trying to fit in, pun intended, the more I didn't, and more of the comments, replies, and requests to "fix" something about my body came my way. Mostly because I welcomed them so I could fit in better and feel even more accepted. And believe me, there were so many comments:

We all know the fat gut story. And then there were the comments of how I had a "too up-and-down" boyish figure, implying that I didn't have any curves when I was a pageant queen. I was referred to as too thin and as if I should go eat something. Oh, and in bodybuilding – body shaming galore wrapped in a pitch to help myself "improve" — my legs too big, my butt too small, boobs too small, and shoulders weren't ever big enough. Nothing was good enough even if I did win. Then I remember feeling guilty, ashamed, unworthy of love when others noticed I had gained weight after the show. I was called "thick," "built," and "cute for a curvy girl." Label after label. Shaming after shaming. Opinion after opinion.

I was actively putting myself in a situation where my body would be shamed, judged, and compared to others. AND, I was welcoming all of it because I, too, subconsciously spent so much time doing the exact same thing with Pinterest, Instagram, magazines, and friendships that I cultivated in my life.

I sat there on the bathroom floor feeling an enormous amount of guilt for my previously paraded emotional unintelligence masked with my never-ending to-do list. All I wanted all along was to feel certain and in control, and to feel accepted and loved in the lonely world of text message communication, dropped Skype calls with family, and rushed emails.

It didn't need to come to this.

It wasn't the bodybuilding community that was the problem. Neither was it my darling pageant director. Nor my friends. It certainly wasn't the societal pressures or Instagram or Pinterest that was doing that to me.

I was doing it to me.
I was the problem.

I was seeking what I was missing from within myself. I never fully cultivated feeling whole all on my own, where I didn't feel the need to fit in anywhere. I never fully accepted my body for what it was and what it did for me on a daily basis. So there I was. I was stripped naked in front of my bathroom mirror. And for the first time in my life I looked at myself as a whole. Yes, at the time I had cellulite dimples on my stomach, stretch marks on my butt because I gained so much weight so fast, uneven boobs from the first breast surgery, my thighs rubbed together for the first time in eight years.

But it was MY body, and we only get ONE body.

I knew in that moment that I had to start treating my body differently.

I knew in that moment that judgment, compassion, negative talk, shame, perfectionism, and fat shaming would no longer allowed. I had to become my very own best friend.

I was living in what I didn't want to feel like, so I embarked on a journey of what it could feel like.

Walking the recovery journey was like a high school science project. And I obsessively journaled my feelings about food, people, situations, worldly wisdoms. I sat with the feeling of what it felt like to eat a cheeseburger and not purge. What it was like to eat only one cheeseburger and what it feels like to not binge. I started paying attention to what felt good to me when it came to food and started tracking what I ate NOT as a game of calories in, calories out but to see how I felt about it. I got back in the gym and started training to feel better not just to look better, and I tracked how I felt about every training session. At times I'd forget about of all it, get impatient, get the "fuck its," and eat everything in sight because why not. I had to sit with those feelings, too, and accept them as they showed up. In silence, breathing. Breathing a lot.

And it all started to make sense slowly. Before, I lived in a very black-and-white world of "doing," and living in the color of emotions added more depth and meaning to every experience. Not only did I find a best friend within myself, but I started to treat my body as if it were MY one and only secret temple. Which, I should mention, sounded like an absurd yogi quote before.

When our relationship with our body is adverse and anything short of a "temple," we'll do an array of disrespectful things to ourselves. We overeat or forget to eat altogether. We make poor food choices, drink too much alcohol, smoke cigarettes, engage in unsafe sexual encounters, exercise compulsively or not at all. We'll go all day without drinking water. We'll fracture and fragment body parts, and get stuck in the "five more pounds" cycle of not feeling good enough.

The thing is, we only get ONE home, ONE secret temple to live in, and we better get to know it better than anything else in our life. Because at the end of the day it's the only thing that'll be with us until the day we die. Our job, our car, our house, our friends, and everything we worry about FIRST before taking care of ourselves and our body — none of that is constant. We can lose everything tomorrow but our ONE body will always be with us.

Your body is incredible, and with everything it does on a regular basis it damn well deserves to be respected, appreciated, and acknowledged, loved, cherished, understood, heard, and loved as a whole. The key is to cultivate a healthy relationship with ourselves, seeing ourselves as a whole, honoring our body, honoring our body's needs, honoring our self-care, and honoring our emotions to know that it's our foundation. The most important thing we can accomplish in a lifetime is true self-appreciation and self-acceptance, whether or not we see the number we want to on a scale. Until we develop the capacity to love and appreciate ourselves as we are, we'll go through life lost, confused, and seeking something to help us escape ourselves. No matter what external success we achieve, we'll always feel short of true happiness within self.

In the beautiful words of psychotherapist Katherine Woodward Thomas, "Our bodies are the hosts of our great spirits and the home of our grand souls. They house the vastness of the life force that moves in and through us, and grant us the gift of life itself. To relate to them as anything less than this miracle is a distortion of who and what we are."

CHAPTER PRACTICE

WE'RE GOING TO DO WHAT WE CALL "MIRROR WORK"
I ask you to take time out of your schedule today to spend time with your body. Make yourself comfortable in the bathroom or in your room with a mirror. You can light candles if you wish and create a more intimate environment for yourself.

Start your practice with taking off all of your clothes and looking in the mirror for a few seconds. Close your eyes and rest the palms of your hands on your chest. Take 7 deep breaths. Let your body expand and release, and with every breath allow more tension, worry, and stress to release.

When you open your eyes, I ask that you see yourself as though you've seen yourself for the first time. Notice any judgments about yourself right away. What's your attention drawn to? – your thighs? your stomach? I welcome you to connect with every body part you have judgments about in the following steps.

1. Ask that body part to please forgive you for being so hard and unloving toward it.
2. Tell that part of the body something that you can truly appreciate it for.
3. Thank that body part for something.

Go through your entire body, doing this process with each judgment you find. If you have a particularly critical and fractured relationship with your body or one body part, you might wish to do this meditation on a regular basis until all the judgments are neutral and appreciation is restored.

NOTE: This exercise was defined by psychotherapist Katherine Woodward Thomas and appeared in the book "Calling in 'The One.'" I loved it so much, and it perfectly reflects how the recovery to feeling whole in your body should take place.[1]

CULTIVATE STRONGER INNER GUIDANCE IN INTUITION

I ask that you get in the habit of constantly asking yourself how you feel to cultivate stronger inner guidance in intuition. Use the phrase "Does this feel good to me?" as your new compass and your new companion in every situation. If a situation, interaction, or comment about self doesn't feel good to you, ask yourself how you WANT to feel. Taking responsibility for our emotions and how we want to feel in situations gives us the power to shape our experiences and create favorable outcomes.

FOR EXAMPLE: "Does eating this cheeseburger feel good to me?" Yes, it does because I'm traveling in New York City, and this cheeseburger place has 83,743,634 10-star reviews, and this is why I'm here!

"Does eating this fast-food joint cheeseburger feel good to me?" No, because I feel run down, low on energy, don't have time for me, and it's what I want to feel better.

"So, how DO you want to feel?" I want to feel taken care of and energized and rested.

"Will this do it for you? No, I'll go home, take a shower, eat a salad, and go to sleep instead.

This is the ease and level of communication I want you to reach within yourself. Everything you need to know is already inside, and you can let your intuition guide you. Also, it's important to note that nobody is responsible for giving you the emotions that you're looking for; you create the experience based on the emotions you cultivate within self. So if you want to feel taken care of and rested, give that to yourself first before seeking it from someone else. This gets us in a circle of emotional codependence when we're capable of honoring that need within ourselves first. There's nothing wrong with receiving and asking. If anything, PLEASE DO ASK and receive the love from those around you, but don't get hooked on constantly seeking it elsewhere.

UNDERSTANDING THAT SELF-CARE AND SELF-LOVE ARE BASED ON YOUR HABITS AND COMMITMENTS TO SELF

In order for us to cultivate an appreciative, self-accepting, and self-loving relationship, we must look at our list of commitments to ourselves and what habits we have in place to help us feel in tune with our body, our mind, and our life. This is where we get to experience the difference between self-care and self-love. I used to think that taking care of myself and loving myself really meant getting my nails done or taking myself shopping. I was a little better at the perceived self-love "thing" when I was 110 pounds. My body and I would be allowed to go shopping; that would be my reward for all of the hard work. I would dress up more often and spend more money on makeup. We all sort of have a concept of self-care – hair, nails, wax, or for new moms simply an occasional shower. But self-love isn't really taught. There isn't a "SELF-LOVE 101" course you can take in college. Sure, it's something we can Google, but it's usually just a bunch of bad or worse advice about spending a day at a spa, taking a bath, or something along those lines. Usually it seems like a waste of time or money. While taking a bath is a sound piece of advice, there's more to it.

At the core of a great relationship with self and lasting love is a commitment, or a list of commitments. Very much like my first commitment to myself was never to disrespect my body by calling it "fat" again, and to feel whole and at home in my body.

I want you to create a list of 2-5 commitments for yourself that you're going to follow no matter what. These are sacred vows to yourself that you do NOT break. They're non-negotiable, unmovable, unshakable, and unbreakable.

HERE'S MY EXAMPLE:

My Commitment 1 to self is three big meals a day. No matter how busy, if traveling, on an insane schedule, I'm going to eat these three meals, and they're going to be balanced. This is my commitment to my energy levels and taking care of my body.

My Commitment 2 to self is three intense workouts per week. Only three. They can be strength training or a class or crazy HIIT or a run, but they'll happen no matter what. Again, dead, alive, sick, wisdom teeth surgery, I'm going to get these done because this, too, has everything to do with my energy levels that I cannot and will not compromise.

My Commitment 3 to self is housekeeping of mind, body, and life. Every week on Sunday on my DEAD-SET MANDATORY day off, I will sit down and look at myself. I'll take a bath, get my nails done, make sure my hair is colored. I'll check my skin and make a masque at home. I'll check to make sure my eyebrows are done and my laundry is up to date, and I have fresh clothes for next week. I'll call my mom and clean the house while we're catching up. I'll go to the store, buy my groceries, and when I get home I'll prep. I'll do housekeeping in my journal and make sure I'm up to speed on my goals and LIFE. This isn't expensive, neither is it some sort of privileged activity or form of narcissism. This is a necessity. There's the BARE MINIMUM to feeling a sane, happy, excited, content, joyful, kind, caring, smiling self. It's self-love at its finest – basic hygiene, attention to our body, respecting boundaries because we have a day off, and showing ourselves we care so we can SHOW UP for the rest of the world.

Guess what happens when Sundays get taken up by something else? I'm frustrated because I have no food, I feel out of control because my goals list is lost, I feel like a mess with bad hair and chipped nails, and I feel like I have nothing to wear. How do I feel about me? Pretty crappy ...

Once you have your list of commitments, you know what you need to keep your love alive at all times. This is how you consistently stay committed to yourself, to your commitments, and to your goals.

LIST THREE CORE COMMITMENTS TO YOURSELF TO HELP YOU MAKE SUSTAINABLE LIFESTYLE SHIFT

COMMITMENT #1

COMMITMENT #2

COMMITMENT #3

THEN YOU NEED TO MAKE A LIST OF HABITS ...

Habits – make a list of daily habits that can help you reach your goals. 7-9 hours of sleep, 1 gallon of water, 10k steps, planned meals, taking supplements, etc. Make it a point to get to this list every day. What you do every day determines the speed of your success. Without the actual doing, there is no achieving! As many things as you can set on autopilot for yourself the better!

HERE'S MY LIST OF HABITS FOR SUSTAINABLE HEALTH:

- A.M.: wake up to sleep-cycle alarm, 3 gratitudes, shower, take supplements, drink shake, 33 ounces of water, pour free juice powder to go, meditate, make a to-do list, check email. IN THIS ORDER. Notice that my day doesn't start with polluting my mind with social media or email anxiety of other people's agendas.

- P.M.: phone off at 10:30 after bed alarm goes off, read for 15 minutes, hygiene.

You get to create a list of commitments and a list of habits that work for YOU with your schedule, your life, and your capacity right now. I don't expect you to nail down all of these at once. Start slowly with water, or perhaps a gratitude practice for your body. Move into adding one new habit every 30 days. There's no wrong way or right way to create habits, as long as they work with your schedule and they're consistent in such a way that you don't have to think about them. My tip is that if you want to create new habits, create them in existing routines. Like when you brush your teeth at night, drink an extra glass of water afterward.

CREATE A SAMPLE A.M. AND P.M. ROUTINE BASED ON THE HABITS THAT YOU WANT TO CREATE

A.M.:

P.M.:

DISCOVERING YOUR WHY AND CULTIVATING LASTING MOTIVATION
CHAPTER 8

All I need is a little motivation.

I'm looking for motivation to get started!

I was doing so well, and then I lost my motivation.

I don't know what's wrong. I just don't seem to have any motivation.

We treat motivation as something that needs to be found, or can get lost lost or perhaps misplaced like a set of car keys. When we don't have it, we embark on a quest to find it as if we're looking for Waldo. When we DO find it, we ride it as if it were a Magic Mountain roller-coaster. And when it's gone, we pay it a tribute, shove our gym clothes in the back of the closet, and wait until we have the fire to embark on our motivation search again.

If we look at the word motivation as a whole, it's comprised of two parts: "motive," a word you likely know, and "-ation," a suffix that sounds pretty strange on its own.

MOTIVE (noun) — something that causes a person to act in a certain way, do a certain thing, etc.; incentive.

-ATION (suffix) — indicating an action, process, state, condition, or result.

Where does "motive" usually come from? Some of us may find it when we need to get ready for vacation or a wedding or some sort of event. We just can't fathom looking like a "whale" on the beach, and end up telling all of our friends that the diet starts on day X and to not tempt us with food we love until we get back or until after the big event happens. Maybe it comes from when we want to impress people we haven't really cared about in the last 10-20 years at our high school reunion. Or, perhaps we're getting back into the dating scene and want to be in shape so we can appear "datable" and conduct ourselves with confidence. Or, this happens, too: Our girlfriend gets us stoked for the next best diet EVER, starts slinging protein shakes out of the trunk of her car, and together we diet happily ever after. Or, worse, we get a scare from our doctor because of an illness. In my instance, I embarked on a 10-year dieting journey after a silly high school teacher remarked about my "fat gut," and I know many women who start a diet because someone called them names, or made them feel judged and shamed because of their body.

So, let's say we find our momentum, and we jump back on the health horse. When we feel like we're "losing" motivation and need a boost, we embark on a journey down the vicious circle of Pinterest Fitsporations, comparing our body to Instagram models in underpants, and trashing our mind with "No pain, no gain," " team no days off," and "nothing tastes as good as skinny feels" inspirational quotes. Ugh, the waft of a so-called motivational trash can smells a whole lot like judgment, expectation hangovers, a compassion game, perfectionism, self-shaming, and fat talk.

None of "that" is motivating.

All of that is like racing down the fast lane, crashing into a cliff of self-hate.

At the root of WHY we start a new "diet" or sign up for the gym, we're secretly (or openly) looking for ways to punish ourselves out of our "fat" existence and this crappy body we somehow ended up living in. And the whole reason the $8 billion dieting industry (with a B!) is thriving is because it sells you a faster, supercharged version of self-hate packed up in something colorful, enforced, and approved by Dr. Something who promises fast weight loss of seven pounds in seven minutes. Because we want results like "yesterday" regardless of us knowing that all of that doesn't work, we buy it anyway. Don't let anyone take your power away by telling you that your body isn't enough in hopes of reaching their marketing goals. This something-for-nothing game has been keeping scammers and fat-loss wraps in business for years making money on our insecurities.

And it's enough.

Your motive must be bigger than losing 10 pounds or the need to squeeze into a bikini. You can't start from that place again. You can't punish yourself into the body you love. You can't diet your way into food freedom.

So how do we make the shift?

The answer is simple: We must find a WHY for why you want to make this shift. The WHY that's going to help you stick to your goals. The WHY that's going to make it different this time. A strong WHY serves as constant motivation for making healthy choices that are best for us, day in and day out. It helps us in situations when it's hard to find strength and life is stressful. When we have a strong WHY, it's no longer an option; it's the reason behind what we do and a solid foundation for success. When we focus on WHY we want, instead of finding excuses for why we can't do something, we find all of the reasons for WHY we actually CAN achieve the goals we set for ourselves. Our WHY might hurt, might make us emotional, and it has to be so big that there's no other way but to create a great body. Your WHY is different from mine, mine is different from yours. There isn't one universal WHY, but before going any further into the program you absolutely must know yours.

HERE'S THE CATCH: Your WHY must come from a place of self-love.

When you choose the root of your transformation to be self-love, as the foundation, that's when you get to achieve the results for life and experience what it's like to live in food freedom and a body you love. Compassion, gratitude, kindness, acceptance, trust, patience are all here to guide you into that shift.

When you know your WHY, your how is clear. When your WHY is deeply rooted into self-love it's easier to make the right decision for YOU in every situation. Because what's right for you, isn't right for me or might not be right by societal standards, but it's your choice based on your relationship with self and your motivations.

When you know your WHY, your motivation will extend beyond the fast-food version of beauty and fitness, and turn inward to find the many great parts of self that you're yet to fully discover. We must see health and fitness as a foundation for our success, an opportunity to expand ourselves in greater capacity because we live in a body that supports our goals, dreams, and aspirations.

When you know your WHY, your focus shifts to every step in front of you to support your journey, and you get a chance to detach from expectations of fitness as a destination. This will allow you to treat situations a little less seriously, like laughing at yourself when you burn all of your meal prep, forget your socks at home while getting to the gym, almost burn down the house because you forgot to turn off the stove, fall off of a treadmill, or when you let out a mini toot at the gym because the weights are so heavy.

💡 CHAPTER PRACTICE

I'm a firm believer in taking MASSIVE action as soon as possible, I want you to do a quick little mental exercise right now, designed to help you find out WHY you're really here.

Grab a pen and a piece of paper, and start writing ...

1. What's your goal? Where are you going with all of this hard work?

   EXAMPLE: My goal is to lose 10 pounds and feel confident in my skin. I've tried so many programs; I just want one that works.

   Why?
   EXAMPLE: Because I'm tired of starting over.

   Why?
   EXAMPLE: It's frustrating to feel like a failure and that I have no willpower.

   I know there's something in me that will actually make me stick to a program.

   Why?
   EXAMPLE: I want to feel proud of myself and like I'm accomplishing my goals.

   Why?
   EXAMPLE: Because I'm tired of hiding. I want to feel powerful, unstoppable, and like I can achieve anything. I don't want to miss out on opportunities because I don't have the energy or confidence to just go for it.

Okay, now look at what happened there. Pretty quickly, we went from losing 10 pounds to wanting the energy and confidence to achieve goals in life, and take advantage of opportunities.

2. Some mindset shifts take time, some come in an instant when we're fed up with our old ways of being. Some of us might not even know we started diets and exercise programs out of punishment, so we need a guide/a compass to help ourselves in situations.

   Every time you eat, ask yourself: Am I dieting or am I taking care of myself?

   This will help you prevent overeating, undereating, overindulging, and procrastination eating, and will help save you from many forms of mindless eating.

   If the answer is that you're taking care of yourself, go for it. If not, ask yourself WHY you're doing what you're doing to bring more awareness to thought patterns and emotions. This will help you navigate the best course of action to take.

   And for every time you move, ask yourself: Are you moving and training your body, or punishing your body? And if you're skipping the gym and making wine nights a priority instead of fitness, is that helping you take care of you?

If the answer is that you're taking care of yourself, go for it because at times wine nights are good ways to take care of ourselves since we get time to spend with friends. If not, ask yourself WHY you're doing what you're doing to bring more awareness to thought patterns and emotions. This will help you navigate the best course of action to take.

🎙 PODCAST ALERT

Reference the www.sexyfit.com/resources page to listen to the "Why Motivation is BS and What Works Better" and "Dig Deep with Insanity Creator Shaun T" podcasts.

HEART-CENTERED GOALS AND YOUR HEART'S DESIRE
CHAPTER 9

"Direction is more important than speed. Many are going nowhere fast."
— Author Unknown

I waited all the way to the end of the mindset chapter to talk about goals and the art of goal-setting. Mainly because just setting a goal to lose 30 pounds without conscious awareness of our stories, patterns, emotions, and having a solid love-base is bound to be a bogus goal.

All of those elements truly matter and influence how you have set your goals in the past.

If you don't know your fear-based story, you never can set a goal at all.

If you don't know your thought patterns, you'll get stuck in perfectionism, hangover, judgment.

If you aren't emotionally aware and know how to live in balance of masculine and feminine, then no meal plan or workout plan is going to help because emotional intelligence is what drives female fat loss.

If you have no idea what your WHY is, then everything that's sort of inspirational clouds your judgment and you don't have a strong foundation to want to set goals.

If you have set goals in the past and didn't achieve them or you don't set goals, this chapter is hugely important because I'm going to show you how to set heart-centered goals that are going to motivate and inspire you to reach the goals you set. This is a special way that I set goals, and it's very effective. And if you haven't ever set goals before, it's important to set yourself up for success so you know where you're headed.

Having a desire without a goal is like heading to your friend's house that you've never been to before by hopping in the car, and driving across town trying to get "there" but you really have no idea where you're going. But if you have the address, you type it into your GPS, and you get at least 2-3 routes to reach your destination. Clarity is a beautiful thing! And remember, there's no one road to success! You're going to get there as long as you keep moving.

Here's where we fall short: Most of us set bullshit goals.

Why? Because we either never write them down and they remain a wish, or they're unrealistic, they lack certainty, have no time frame, and, most importantly, they lack purpose: a rhyme and reason for why it's important to achieve them.

Here are some examples of crappy fitness goals.

I want to lose "some" weight. I want to fit into my clothes. I just want to feel better.

Cool! Tomorrow you'll lose one pound by not eating all day which will help you kind of fit into your skinny jeans … and, here's a puppy. You feel better, right?

Not really.

What I'm about to share with you has helped me achieve many, many, substantial goals, and it doesn't just apply to fitness. The point of setting a goal is for you to expand and grow in proportion to the goal that you set for yourself. Big goals, big growth — because every new level of your life is going to require a new level of you. Every goal will require parts of you that you never even knew existed to come forward and help you achieve that goal. The point of living is to not stagnate in the same place doing the same thing over and over. The point is the journey to becoming the best version of self as a result of committing to a bigger vision for yourself.

The exact method I'm about to share with you has been vital to my success. This is how I'm able to stay in amazing shape year-round and constantly grow as an athlete to compete in marathons and obstacles races, how I have an amazing relationship with my family and my friends, and how we've grown Sexyfit to be a successful multiple-six-figure business in three short years. You don't need to be a genius. You just need to follow these steps.

I have to mention that my approach has completely changed in the past three years after leaving the competition stage. Because while I was really good at setting goals before, I was always left feeling unhappy because I was running a roller-coaster of achieving, racing to complete my goals. Sure, I was good at goal-setting, but didn't feel very good doing it. I think my eating disorder is proof that not every goal is the best goal. So what I'm about to share with you here is the result of constantly investing in educating myself with the help of the best goal-setting gurus in the world, like Tony Robbins, Brendon Burchard, Darren Hardy, Danielle LaPorte, and many others.

The reason I called my goal-setting strategy heart-centered is because the way I set my goals has switched from what my idea of success looks like to what it feels like. Our goals must be set from an emotional place based on how we feel and how we desire to feel. We as women must default to the emotional outcome and how we want to feel as a result of achieving a goal. Otherwise it'll feel like we're running a heartless rat race of doing "stuff" for the sake of doing.

Many goal-setting strategies focus on what we want to achieve and are typically based on the outside version of what success "should" look like. When we can first connect to the emotions and what we want to feel like, it's easier to break up with the idea of what things should be like and what our path must look like. Remember, our path isn't linear. Our goals are our goals. Our life is our life. When we set the goals from the heart, it's not the world telling us how we want to feel, how we want to feel ourself, and what we're feeling in the world. This is, again, us walking the fine line between the feminine and the masculine, where we honor how we feel and the strategy for how to get there. We want the goals that we set for ourselves to feel good to us. They should inspire us and motivate us to feel a certain way that we desire to feel. If our goals don't feel good to us, we won't feel inspired or connected with the goals, so what's the point? Just because someone else did or we THINK we should do it, doesn't mean we should!

How do you want to feel as the outcome of achieving your goals?

Proud, happy, healthy, energized, excited, peppy? There's not one core feeling. Choose whatever feels best to you and design your goals to produce that emotion every step of the way of your journey. Danielle LaPorte and her incredible book "The Desire Map: A Guide to Creating Goals with Soul" is where I learned this strategy, and it WORKS to insure that you feel fulfilled on your journey to success.[2]

This strategy I'm about to share with you is a result of everything I've learned and exactly how I set my goals every year. Before you even eagerly rush to set your goals, here are some prerequisites I want you to think about: Every goal you have needs to be written down in INK on paper! You can move it on to Google calendar, Evernote, a sticky note, your iPad, or whatever else. But set all of your goals in ink. Period. When you're setting your goals, suspend all reality of what you think is possible for you. If you have never run a mile in your life, it doesn't mean that you can't run a race. If you're not flexible and have 100 pounds to lose, it doesn't mean that you can't do a handstand. You can do absolutely EVERYTHING you set your mind to. I had done a show when I was a chubby overweight Russian kid. I run a successful business, and I didn't have a bed growing up. And I wrote a book when 10 years ago I didn't speak English. You can do it. That said, don't let anyone talk you out of your goals or make you feel silly for setting any goals; and don't let anyone talk you into goals that aren't yours to begin with. I know a lot of people set NO goals for themselves at all and don't understand WHY you need to set goals, and I know a ton of people who are goal-pushers, who will say that you need to run 10 obstacles races with them this year because "it's good for you." Stay the course on the goals you set for YOU, and there's no need to explain yourself. Blinders on and let's go!

I feel like some sort of magician now because I know you can create and achieve ANYTHING you set your mind to if you follow these steps.

Sim sim salabim! ...

1. SET CLEAR GOALS
The key to successful goal-setting and achieving the result you set for yourself, first and foremost, is that your goal needs to have clarity. Clarity gives us focus, strength, purpose, and the power to move in the chosen direction. It illuminates options and helps align with the exact things, activities, beliefs, people, and other resources to help us achieve our goals.

I want you to have clarity. There's a difference between "I want to lose weight" and "I want to lose 15 pounds." This is exactly what clarity looks like: I want to wake up every morning and rate my energy at 10. I want to lose 20 pounds or five inches. I want to get consistent with exercising. I want to run a half marathon. I want to run a mile. I want to squat 50 pounds. I want to take 10,000 steps a day. Etc.

2. KNOW YOUR CAPACITY
I know it's kind of counterintuitive to what I said earlier about thinking that the sky's the limit and you can do anything, but since we're talking about our BODY here, and it's a vessel of its own that IS bound by constraints and what it can physically do at times, we have to respect what our body tells us it needs and appreciate it for what it CAN do. So if

you want to lose 30 pounds in two weeks, that might not be possible or the best course of action to take for your body. Running a marathon in a month if you have never run a mile is downright silly and wouldn't even be within your body's ability, plus the outcome might be devastating and cause long-term injuries. Working out seven days a week for two hours a day to reach a goal when you have three kids, a full-time job, you're going to school, and you're married, well, that might not be realistic or necessary if you don't have the bandwidth to do so. Know your capacity so that you can set goals that are BIG enough to challenge and motivate you, but that aren't too high where you get discouraged or too low where they're not exciting to you.

3. TIME FRAME GOALS
It's essential that goals have a time frame or target date. A commitment to a deadline helps you focus your efforts toward completion of the goal and prevents goals from being overtaken by other unrelated routine tasks that may arise. A time-restrained goal is intended to establish a sense of urgency. Otherwise, there's no sense of urgency, and "someday" is not a day of the week. Set a date!

4. EMOTIONAL OUTCOME
How do you want to feel as a result of achieving this goal—proud, accomplished, sexy, fit, powerful, amazing, massively excited for yourself? I'm going to be very honest and transparent with you: Not every goal is going to be sunshine, rainbows, and butterflies. Some days are going to be hard, some days are going to be really hard, and some days are going to be easy. At times you'll say, "HELL ,YES!" like you're really getting somewhere, and other times you'll find yourself sobbing on the couch because you feel defeated. Attach yourself to the emotional outcome of the goal that you set for yourself. It'll help you connect to the positive emotional state.

At times you have to embrace the suck.

When I ran my first half-marathon in 2014, every time I was training up until race day I was questioning my WHYs, and I felt overtaken by my story of knee pain and that I'm not a runner. My goal was to run a marathon without stopping. At some point when I was setting my goal in the beginning of the year I thought it was a good idea and a good challenge. I was in no way, shape, or form excited to do it, BUT I knew that having a challenge, and expanding above and beyond my story was critical for me. It wasn't even the marathon; it was just my story that I wasn't a runner. On race day, it was a disaster. My socks gave me blisters, my music stopped, it was 90 degrees out, and half of the race track was uphill. It was like the universal challenges kept coming up, going, "What's she gonna do?" "Is she gonna stop?' Nasty thoughts kept creeping up saying, "It's impossible. Too hot. This sucks!"

NO! I remember repeating silly "I am a runner" affirmations to myself the WHOLE time I was running, which, at the time, was at 2:24 minutes.

When I crossed the finish line, I was never MORE proud of myself. I was now a runner, but I was also NOT a quitter. I felt accomplished, proud, excited—crossing that finishing line was me proving to ME that I could do that, and it felt GOOD. Guess what? After that race, running a race is a piece of cake, and I can do it in under two hours because I know exactly how it feels to do it, and I know I CAN do it. Most importantly, I know how to control my MIND and feel my way into the outcome of the goals.

5. RESOURCES/HABITS/COMMITMENTS

You have your goals, time frames, and you know your capacity and emotional outcomes. Now it's time to figure out resources/habits/commitments. What do you NEED in order to achieve your goals? What tools, resources need to be available to you — new shoes, gym membership, new alarm, nutrition tools? You have to know all of the tools you'll need in order to ease your way into your goals. There are so many gadgets available to us — use them. They make life SO much easier, and you don't need to struggle. A silly thing like an iPhone arm strap can make all the difference in the world!

6. CHECKS AND BALANCES

Make sure that you have a system for checks and balances in place that helps you achieve your goals. I recommend setting your BIG goals once per year in 90-day time frames. If you're just starting out, begin with 90-day health, nutrition, and fitness goals, and set one for each category. The best way is to look at your goals as a compound of daily and weekly habits after you set them, and from there on out I want you to sit down weekly and follow up on your goals. It's also important to note that while you're doing your checks and balances, check in with yourself regarding how you FEEL about your journey. Are you connecting to you heart-centered goals or are you running a rat race? If you're off, ask yourself why and journal more on the topics. If you're feeling good, keep up the good work. Watch for more on this in the Accountability chapter.

There's nothing big or intimidating about goal-setting. It's a matter of stepping up to the plate and taking responsibility for the outcome of your effort. It might feel like you're working hard, but you're really just thinking hard about it. This isn't rocket science. This is available to all of us as long as we're willing to keep showing up for ourselves with clear intentions.

💡 CHAPTER PRACTICE

1. This is your time to set your heart-centered goal. First and foremost, instead of thinking your way into a goal right away, I want you to start with a visualization meditation practice. I want to mention that many of us might feel like we're in some way unworthy of a great physical transformation, food freedom, and, ultimately, self-love. I assure you that you're worthy of this and more. Dream big and allow yourself to visualize transformation beyond your mindset borders. To visualize the emotional outcome, sitting with your goals will help you slow down and feel into your goal, and what success feels and looks like to you.

   You can choose to do this practice in silence or with 10-minute meditation music that you can find on sexyfit.com/resources.

   Sit or lie down comfortably and close your eyes.

   Roll your shoulders back, and gently move your neck back and forth. Place your palms upward, relax your face, and eyebrows.

   Take a deep breath in through your stomach and release in a forced fast exhale; repeat three times.

   Reconnect to a normal pace of your breath. If you catch yourself wandering off, gently ask yourself to come back to the present moment and pay attention to your breath.

   Take a moment to connect with your heart-centered goal. Whether you want to run your first mile, or lose 10 pounds or maybe 100. Visualize the emotional outcome of the goal you desire to achieve as if you already have. Honor visions that come to mind.

   Honor any emotion that comes your way. If you feel ready, cultivate that level of enthusiasm so you can reconnect with it at any time and continue to connect with the vision of your goals.

   Breathe deeper and allow your breath to flow smoothly, connecting further into your vision. Let the feeling of your vision and images you see flow though you naturally.

   Flow in this energy comfortably for 10 minutes.

   After you've completed your meditation, grab your journal and allow yourself to journal for 5-10 minutes regarding what you were able to visualize and how you felt.

   I want you to connect with the emotional outcome and the feeling that you desire your goal to bring. Mainly because I want you to know what it feels like when you get there because it's truly the feeling that we long for. Begin to align yourself with that feeling on a daily basis, with every little choice and decision that you make.

2. Now that we know what your goal feels like, it's appropriate to set a clear, timely goal within your capacity and note which resources you need in order to achieve it.

   Follow this goal-setting worksheet on the next page.

HEART-CENTERED GOALS

Set a date on the calendar to revisit your plan in 90 days to set a new goal.

MY WHY	MY GOAL	DATE	ACTION PLAN	HEART-CENTERED FEELING

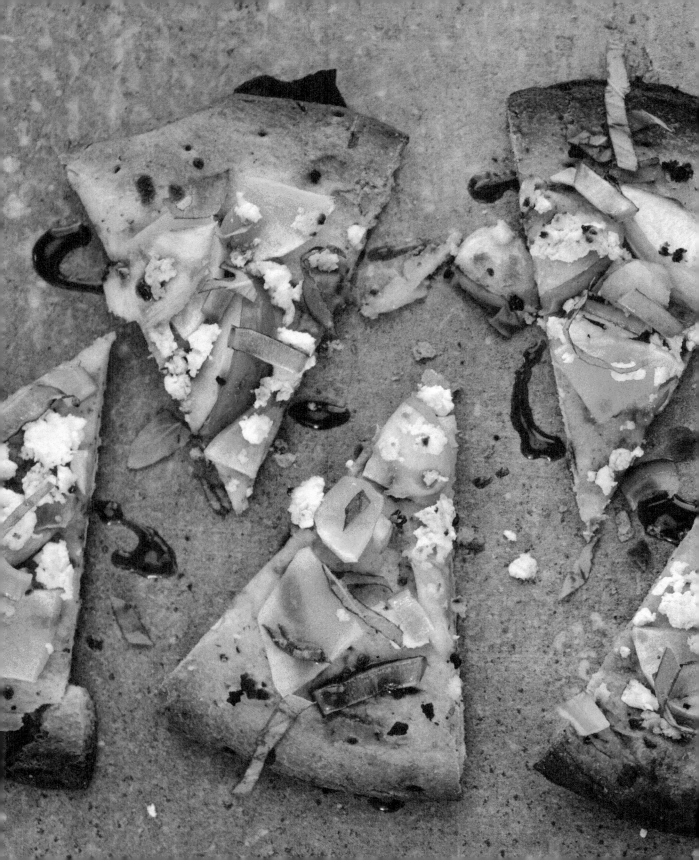

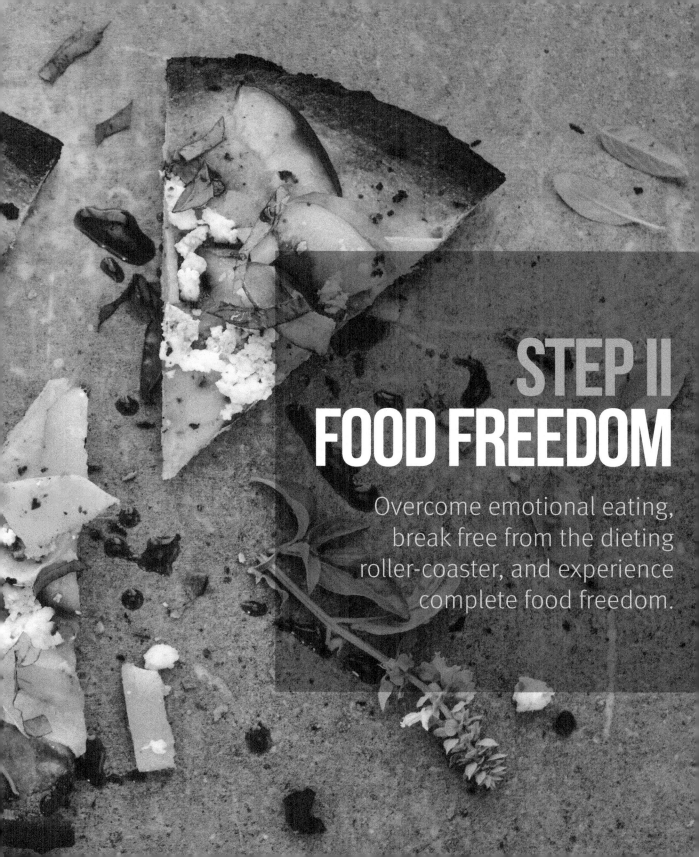

STEP II
FOOD FREEDOM

Overcome emotional eating, break free from the dieting roller-coaster, and experience complete food freedom.

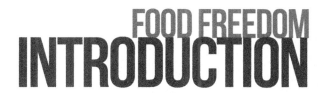

FOOD FREEDOM
INTRODUCTION

"Food is the most widely abused anti-anxiety drug in America,
and exercise is the most underutilized antidepressant."
— Bill Phillips

In the previous section of this book, you had the opportunity to clear your mind from emotional obstacles that have been holding you back from having the body you love. You had the chance to learn a lot of powerful practices that will change your mind, change your body, and, ultimately, change your life for the better.

In this section, I'm going to walk you through the exact nutrition method that has helped hundreds of women just like you lose pounds of body fat, while eating food they love and keeping their results for life. Whether this is your first time reading a nutrition book or you've read a fair share of literature online or otherwise, HOW this section is organized and what I'm about to show you is a method that's a combination of my experience as a fitness professional and spending thousands of hours poring over related materials and interviewing experts in fitness, nutrition, hormonal health, lifestyle, supplementation, herbal medicine, psychology of eating, and years of application in our Sexyfit Community. You may notice that my tone will change a little bit to be more assertive.

This method works because it's not just about "clean eating" or being able to "stick to simple rules." It's about creating a lifestyle that works for you. Please note, I said "creating." This is ultimately what you're doing: You're creating a lifestyle that works with YOUR life, YOUR schedule, and YOUR body. I have no interest in putting you in a box, enforcing strict rules, and cutting out food groups in an attempt to give you fast but unsustainable results. I'm sure you've tried that before, and it didn't lead to sustainable changes. My goal here is to help you create new nutrition habits that will give you energy, confidence in the kitchen and in life, and teach you how to act in every situation.

- We'll understand the difference between fat loss and weight loss, and learn the fundamentals of fat loss for life.
- We'll master the art of the macronutrient lifestyle and how to make it work for you to break free from the restrictive dieting mindset.
- We'll shop, cook, and create meals together so you can experience complete food freedom.

- We'll learn how to take the macronutrient lifestyle and apply it to everyday life, dining out with friends, and traveling.
- We'll determine how lifestyle factors, like sleep, water, stress, and alcohol, influence our progress.

You and I are here to create a lifestyle on your terms with the exact steps and guidelines I'm here to show you. Not rules; guidelines. I often say we have an eating democracy at Sexyfit. I show you the guidelines, you get to make choices on your own and vote on what works for you. If you like to have something laid out for you that's easy to start and follow, I've also included a 21-Day Transformation Plan to jumpstart your Sexyfit journey, as well as 50-plus of my favorite easy-to-make recipes. You get to customize, re-create, or follow as you see fit.

FUEL AND NOURISH
CHAPTER 10

WHY DO WE EAT?

For many of us, me included, food became the fastest shortcut to love, the fastest route to numbing pain, feeling like everything was normal and under control, and moments of euphoria became easier to find with emotionally numbing foods like chocolate and candy.

My personal health and fitness journey spun out of my distorted relationship with food and emotionally eating my way into being close in proximity to my family. Chocolate became the ultimate gateway to time travel, allowing me to have those I love close to me, to comfort me, and to show me love. My quest for happiness blinded me to see that I was rapidly gaining weight and ironically grew unhappier with the reality around me.

It took me years of endless dieting to understand what had happened and what food became for me. Food and strict dieting became my way to control the uncontrollable variables of life around me. Magical number 110 was a way to validate success, and gave a sense of peace and certainty in the fast-paced world around me.

So, why DO we eat?

Well, sister, we eat because food is fuel. The purpose of eating is to get the energy we need to sustain everyday life and to nourish our body. And if our nutrition is dialed in, we'll not only sustain life, but also thrive because we're overflowing with energy and focus.

But we don't necessarily think about food this way, do we?

We eat when we're bored, we eat when we're sad, we eat when we're happy, we eat when we're stressed, we eat when we don't have anything to stress about, we eat together, we eat to belong, we eat for companionship ... there are a thousand reasons why we eat other than the one reason that's the most important of them all: essentially, to feel better, to feel "something."

This is why we have an emotional eating epidemic; food is our remedy, our way to "fix" or control our negative emotions. Food is the fastest way to get that emotion because our brain is a smart cookie (no pun intended) and works fast. Unfortunately, to get safety, love, connection, and acceptance, our brain doesn't ask for kale and a mile run; it goes straight to high-carb, high-fat comfort foods. We're in this pattern because we aren't sure what we feel, but our brain and our body knows that the fastest way to soothe our negative emotions is food.

We can see how that pattern isn't really healthy, and unless we release that pattern we can't get the results we truly want.

Knowing "why" you eat and how you feel while eating are the key steps to creating awareness and mindfulness around the ritual of eating as fuel and nourishment. Once we have awareness, we hold the key to relieving ourself of the toxic patterns of mindless and emotional eating. We simply no longer can knowingly participate in this self-destructive pattern. Once we're aware of our loops and ah-ha moments, we can welcome a change to create new habits and have the opportunity to release the habits that no longer serve.

If you want complete food freedom, to love your body and live your life to the fullest, I welcome you to the first exercise we'll do in this Nutrition chapter to gain awareness around your eating patterns.

💡 CHAPTER PRACTICE

1. I want to make sure you're aware of what and how you're using food in your life right now. Take out your journal and answer the following questions. Once you complete this section, your pattern of using food will be clear to you.

   Food is _____.

   I eat when _____.

   When I'm _____, I eat (what) _____.

   I use food to _____.

   When I feel _____, I do (what) _____.

   When I'm, _____ I eat (where) _____.

2. I want you to carry your journal with you today to create more emotional intelligence around why you eat and how certain foods make you feel. You'll be able to see how your findings from exercise 1 influence your food choices on a regular basis.

   Every time you reach for food, I want you to get in tune with your emotions and ask yourself:

   • How do I feel right now before eating this meal/snack?
   • Why am I eating it?

   And after you're finished with each meal/snack, answer "After eating, I feel _____."

   Please avoid saying I feel "like." Saying "LIKE" is a way to not feel and fill a blank space of emotional doubt.

🎙 PODCAST ALERT

Reference the www.sexyfit.com/resources page to listen to the "Make Peace with Food and Never Diet Again with Mel Wells" and "How to Break Free From Emotional Eating" podcasts.

FAT LOSS vs. WEIGHT LOSS
CHAPTER 11

I propose we start with the basics — calories and the fundamentals of fat loss, and how they support one another. You're probably thinking, here she comes with the calorie-counting talk.

I know it sounds neither exciting nor sexy.

But to get sexy and fit, it's something you really need to know and understand. If this isn't your first rodeo in nutrition, listen even MORE carefully because usually those of us who say "Yeah, yeah, I know all of that" need this info the most. Information overload and our best thinking got us here, so let's talk shop.

What I'm after with you at Sexyfit and what I'm about to share with you is the foundation of sustainable fat loss, and since there's a difference between just weight loss and fat loss, I want to explain both.

Often, when we think about losing weight, the idea of calorie counting immediately pops into our head. It becomes this game of eating less and less, and denying ourselves calorie-dense food choices ... even if they're healthy. It works short-term because weight loss is actually a relatively easy task. Don't eat for a week, or eat way less for a week, and you'll lose weight. It's just that simple. That's why crazy cleanses with cajun peppers work so well — for a short period of time, of course. But what happens a week later when all of the weight comes back, plus some?

Therefore, just weight loss is not what we're after. What we really WANT is sustainable fat loss. When we focus on fat loss, it's no longer a game of eating LESS, working out more, and torturing our body to get quick results. What we want to do is reduce the body fat percentage, balance energy levels, speed up metabolism, and improve body composition and experience complete food freedom.

(Who am I kidding? What we really want is to know how to eat pizza and still look great. I'm getting there! Just hang with me for a bit.)

Take a look at the enormous benefits of focusing on fat loss vs. just weight loss.
At this point, you may wonder if calorie counting is bad and if calories are evil.

FAT LOSS (SEXYFIT) VS. WEIGHT LOSS

FAT-LOSS BENEFITS	WEIGHT-LOSS BENEFITS
• Healthy hormonal composition • Energy balance • Decreased body fat percentage • Increased muscle mass • Increased metabolic rate • Nutrient balance • Healthy relationship with food • Healthy digestion • Restful sleep • Improved mood • Healthy hormonal composition • Shiny nails, hair, skin • Clear skin • Visible muscle/improved muscle composition • Slowed aging	• Quick, short-term results • Energy deficiency • Calorie counting • … and that's about it?

In nutrition and everyday language, calories refer to energy consumption through eating and drinking, and energy usage through physical activity. The primary purpose of calories is to give our body the energy it needs to be nourished. This means that calories aren't evil, terrible monsters that get stuck to our thighs but rather are a way to measure the amount of energy in food.

However, the traditional way of looking at calories and weight loss has been black and white. "A calorie is a calorie—just eat less." We've all heard this before. Except, it's not quite that simple or how it works at all.

The idea that "a calorie is a calorie" comes from a misunderstanding of the laws of thermodynamics in our body. There are two laws of thermodynamics. The first law is a conservation law; it says that the form of energy may change, but the total is always conserved. It's merely a bookkeeping law that tells us that the total energy attributed to work, heat, and changes in chemical composition will be constant; this is how we decided that all calories are created equal. By just following that law, however, we ignore the second very important piece—the dissipation law, which is responsible for the chemical reaction of the calories consumed and explains how certain energy from certain calories will be used.[3]

Different foods go through different metabolic pathways before they're turned into energy, meaning that they digest differently and have different effects on our body.[4]

Protein (made up of amino acids), fats, and carbohydrates are the three sources of energy that are variably stored and assimilated from food each day. The fact that we can carry on our daily lives without thinking about whether to store or mobilize fuels, and which to use, attests to the remarkable efficiency of our body.[5]

We also have to take into consideration that food intake is sporadic. For most of us, it occurs in three to four major sittings per day. Energy expenditure, however, is continuous because we move, breathe, talk on the phone, etc. with variations during the day. Therefore, our body has developed complex systems that direct excess nutrients into storage pools and regulate the mobilization of those nutrients as we need energy.

The situation is analogous to the fuel tank of a car and the throttle that regulates fuel use, except that in a car there's just one fuel source and just one engine.

In humans, the three major nutrients are the three kinds of fuels. Imagine using three different fuels, like diesel, solar, and regular gas, for your car, and it's smart enough to know when to use which fuel. And a variety of tissues and organs may have their own preferences for fuels that varies with time.

Therefore, it's important to know how many calories as total fuel your body needs and how much of each type of fuel it needs to run smoothly throughout the day. At Sexyfit, we all start from learning what macronutrients are, how to properly balance our nutrition plan, how to build a balanced meal plan, and how we can fluidly move through life and make choices throughout the day with macros. We move toward more intuitive eating after 6-12 weeks of tracking macros.

Without understanding this piece and how your body functions from certain nutrients, understanding what nutrients your body craves and how macros support your fitness plan, it will be an endless game of diets, counting points for no reason, and jumping into the next best fad diet trends.

This IS the foundation of sustainable fat loss.

CHAPTER PRACTICE

1. List the benefits of lasting fat loss.

2. What is a calorie?

3. What are the 3 macronutrients to help you create sustainable fat loss and experience complete food freedom?

PODCAST ALERT

Reference the www.sexyfit.com/resources page to listen to the "Fat Loss vs. Weight Loss" podcast.

CHAPTER 12

We're one step closer to food freedom! It's important for us to understand exactly what macros are, what the benefits of each type of macro are, and what the primary food sources of each macro are.

MACRONUTRIENTS (macros, for short) — protein, fats, and carbs — are present in every food. Knowing your macros is essential to knowing your portion sizing and knowing what, when, and how much food to eat to give you the results you want.

PROTEIN (P)

Protein is an important component of every cell in our body. Hair and nails are mostly made of protein. Our body uses protein to build and repair tissues. We also use protein to make enzymes, hormones, and other body chemicals. Protein is an important building block of bones, muscles, cartilage, skin, and blood.[6]

Protein is the number one source of growth and recovery of muscle. If there isn't enough protein, we can't build or maintain the muscle mass we need. When we're looking to decrease body fat percentage and increase our metabolism, as we are with Sexyfit workouts, or any other exercise, our workouts are focused to increase our lean muscle mass. The more muscle we have, the faster our metabolism is. When we undereat protein, our body doesn't have anywhere to source essential amino acids from in order to fuel our metabolism, and give us the muscle mass and strength we need to succeed. Therefore, we're unable to put on the muscle that we need to shape our body and increase metabolic rate. We can't put on muscle, get leaner, lose fat, or have a faster metabolism if our protein macros aren't meeting our athletic requirements.

SOURCES OF PROTEIN: The best sources of protein are lean meats, poultry, eggs, dairy, and protein shakes (powders). Other foods that contain protein are legumes, nuts, and seeds. Even though these foods are often claimed to be good sources of protein, the amount of protein in them is very small. For example, nuts are more than 70% fat and about 14% protein. While nuts are great for us (more about them later), they shouldn't be our primary protein source.

CARBS (C)

The hysterical crusade against carbohydrates has reached an all-time high. Every latest diet trend claims that carbohydrates are like evil little creatures that make us instantly "fat." Hint: the latest war on grains.

In reality, carbohydrates are an essential source of energy that our body needs for life for many different reasons: brain function, liver function, increased muscular endurance, and overall metabolic function.

CARBS ARE ESSENTIAL FOR FAT LOSS.

First, instead of talking about how carbs influence our muscles and metabolism, I want to address how they influence our brain. Because being smart is also really, really sexy.

Our brain is the most selfish organ in our body.

Think of the brain as a metabolic pig—constantly taking energy from the bloodstream and storing none of it for itself. It's no wonder our brain is one of the hungriest organs in our body—more than 80 billion neurons are sending and receiving electrical signals 24 hours a day, creating complex thoughts and emotions. Even when we're asleep, neurons in our brain are busy sending a flurry of electrical signals from one region to the next, consolidating memories and information from the previous day.

To put things into perspective: Our brain occupies only 2% of our body weight, but consumes about 20% of our body's oxygen and up to 50% of our body's glucose.

When it comes to food, our brain acts like a picky child, burning glucose almost exclusively. Glucose is a type of sugar that comes predominantly from starchy foods, like bread, rice, pasta, fruits, and veggies. The body can break down the digestible carbohydrates in these foods into glucose, which is transported in the bloodstream to the brain and other organs for energy.[7]

Our brain cells need glucose to work, but they have no way of storing it, so they rely on a continuous supply via the bloodstream. Our brain is specifically designed to operate on glucose most of our waking life, and when glucose is in short supply the results can be disastrous. If you've ever had the opportunity to experience hypoglycemia (low blood sugar) or if you're diabetic, the symptoms are unmistakable: confusion, lightheadedness, loss of balance, slurred speech, and impaired vision.

In short, if you want to be sharp, witty, and quick on your feet, choose a nutritional approach that allows you to eat enough carbohydrates. Sexyfit is NOT a low-carb diet because I want you to have the energy, focus, and enthusiasm for life. Unfortunately, while low-carb diets may bring quick results, they only leave us slow, dizzy, and dissatisfied.

Also, if you want to be sexy, fit, and lean, carbs are even more important when it comes to muscular endurance and metabolism.

LET ME FILL YOU IN ...

Glycogen is the storage form of glucose and carbohydrates. About 80% of total carbohydrates is stored in skeletal muscle, about 14% is stored in the liver, and about 6% in the blood in the form of glucose. When we're working out, our body uses glycogen stored in the muscles as a main source of energy. Most of us make the typical weight loss mistake where we cut out carbohydrates and increase our activity level. Our body gets depleted of glycogen, and, in turn, we end up bingeing on a crazy amount of carbohydrates to restore those glycogen stores. The more we workout, the more glycogen we need.[8]

Therefore, carbs = glycogen = energy for life and workouts.

OKAY, BUT WHAT ABOUT THE STORY OF INSULIN SPIKES WITH CARBS, YOU ASK?

Our liver is the organ responsible for controlling blood sugar between meals. Much of the carb hate lately has been due to demonizing insulin and making insulin spikes responsible for the "carbs make you fat"-type statements.

In theory, insulin "makes you fat," and carbohydrates "spike insulin." Thus, "carbohydrates make you fat." Sounds so simple, right? Well, yeah, the story is simple ... BUT IT'S FALSE!

So while, yes, it's true that insulin's job is to pull glucose out of the blood and store excess as fat, it's also responsible for driving amino acids into our muscles for protein synthesis and clearing dietary fats out of the blood, as well (which are stored as body fat more efficiently than carbohydrates, I might add).[9] On top of all of that, insulin has a mild anti-catabolic effect[x] (meaning it helps preserve your muscle).[10]

While it's undoubtedly true that eating carbohydrates increases insulin levels, many protein sources also do the same.[11] And, of course, some claim that because your body generally produces more insulin when you eat carbohydrates, this leads to more fat storage. But they're wrong — research has shown that the amount of insulin your body produces in response to eating food (or insulin response, as it's called) doesn't affect the amount of fat stored.[12]

In short, insulin isn't your enemy, and it's certainly not part of a conspiracy between your pancreas and fat cells to ruin your self-image.

LOVE CARBS YET? I LOVE CARBS.

Let's talk more about carbs! Carbs, carbs, carbs! Now that we know that carbs are a primary fuel for our brain function AND they're a primary source of energy for our workouts and our life, carbs also play an important role in our nervous system balance. Because glycogen is tightly connected with the central nervous system as a primary source of fuel, it's not surprising that dramatic reduction of carbs causes additional stress on our body. Research reveals that lack of carbohydrate intake and a high level of stress are among the main reasons for adrenal fatigue and "burnout."

The more I do research, the more my body amazes me every day. Everything is connected! Eat your carbs. Here are the types of carbs and sources.

- **SIMPLE CARBS** are made of just one or two sugar molecules, and they're digested very quickly, which makes them the quickest form of energy.

  SOURCES OF SIMPLE CARBS: ALL types of sugar (white, brown, agave syrup, honey, molasses, corn and maple syrups, and others); jams and jellies; fruit drinks, including juices; soda; candy; and the majority of processed foods you see on a shelf at any store.

- **COMPLEX CARBOHYDRATES** are referred to as dietary starch and are made of sugar molecules strung together like a necklace. They're usually rich in fiber, which makes them satisfying and promotes slower digestion.

  SOURCES OF COMPLEX CARBS: green vegetables; whole grains and foods made from them, like oatmeal; whole-grain breads and pastas; starchy vegetables, like sweet potatoes, corn, and pumpkin; legumes (beans, lentils, and peas); brown rice; quinoa; buckwheat; millet; and others.

FATS (F)

Onto another macronutrient that has been demonized for years. "You eat fat, you get fat." This is the notion we've been living with since the '80s. We're finally out of the demonizing fat craze and the times of "fat-free" gimmicks, as well as the "low-fat" obsession. Hopefully? Are we? I think we are. Because carbs are getting most of the negative attention these days. If you still have any doubt about how amazing fats are for you, I'm about to break it down as to why you and I both MUST LOVE fats.

WHY DO WE NEED FATS?

Virtually all natural foods contain some fat. It's in food because both plants and animals use fats as the most economical way to store energy. It's needed for their growth, development, and function when there's a shortage of food supply (or a shortage of sunlight in the case of plants).

Certain specific dietary fats have other essential functions. We're much like other animals, so we do actually need some fat in our diet to survive. And while in general, as with most things, too much fat is bad, a certain amount is perfectly compatible with good health.

WHAT ARE FATS FOR?
- A source of energy—our body uses the fat we eat, and fats we make from other nutrients in our body, to provide the energy for most of our life functions.
- Energy store—the extra calories that we consume, but don't need to use immediately, are stored for future use in special fat cells (adipose tissue).
- Essential fatty acids—dietary fats that are essential for growth development and cell functions, but can't be made by our body's processes.
- Proper functioning of nerves and brain—fats are part of myelin, a fatty material that wraps around our nerve cells so that they can send electrical messages; our brains contain large amounts of essential fats.
- Maintaining healthy skin and other tissues—all of our body's cells need to contain some fats as essential parts of cell membranes, controlling what goes in and out of our cells.
- Transporting fat-soluble vitamins A, D, E, and K through the bloodstream to where they're needed.
- Forming steroid hormones needed to regulate many bodily processes.

SOURCES OF FAT
There are three sources of fat: monounsaturated, polyunsaturated, and trans.[13]

MONOUNSATURATED FATS
The main source of fat is monounsaturated fats (MUFAs). Liquid at room temperature, they turn solid when they're chilled. Common sources of MUFAs are olive oil, avocados, and nuts.

Research shows that diets with healthy amounts of monounsaturated fats have a host of amazing health benefits, such as decreased risk for breast cancer. A study of women in Sweden found that those with diets higher in monounsaturated fats (as opposed to polyunsaturated fats) resulted in less frequent incidence of breast cancer, and lower risk for heart disease and stroke. Diets with monounsaturated fats correlate with healthy hearts and fewer strokes, and reduced belly fat. A study published by the American Diabetes Association found that diets with monounsaturated fats could improve the loss of belly fat better than high-carbohydrate diets.[X]

MAKE THE MOST OF MUFAs WITH THESE FOODS
Great sources of monounsaturated fats are:
- Olive oil
- Avocados
- Tea seed oil
- Almonds, cashews, and pecans
- Macadamia nuts

POLYUNSATURATED FATS

These are mostly found in plant foods, such as nuts, seeds, and vegetable oils, and in cold-blooded seafoods. In natural foods, they come protected with antioxidant vitamins. There are two main classes of polyunsaturated fatty acids: omega-3 and omega-6. These include the essential fatty acids. Oily fish (e.g., herring, salmon, and mackerel) is a good source of omega-3, while omega-6 is mainly found in plant foods, such as sunflower oil and grapeseed oil.

TRANS FATS

This type of fat can be natural or artificial. They're mostly artificially created through a process known as hydrogenation (which involves heating and chemical structure change). Artificial trans fats are mostly found in fast foods, fried foods, and commercial baked products, such as cookies, and are the most unhealthy fats (even worse than saturated fats!). Natural trans fats can be found in small amounts of milk and beef, and in quite a large concentration in cheese.

To summarize, ALL FOOD CONTAINS MACRONUTRIENTS LIKE PROTEINS, FATS, AND CARBS. All macronutrients in each category can be swapped with one another in the same macronutrient family.

EXAMPLE:
PROTEIN: chicken = turkey = cod = steak = shrimp, etc.
CARBS: rice = quinoa = buckwheat = oatmeal = potato
CARBS (VEGETABLES): kale = spinach = romaine lettuce = cucumbers
CARBS (FRUIT): apple = pear = grapes = peach
FATS: almonds = walnuts = cashews

NOTE: While the macros per each food differ, they can be substituted for one another.

WHY IS THIS IMPORTANT TO UNDERSTAND?
All foods within their macronutrient category are swappable.
Protein doesn't swap with vegetables, and it doesn't swap with fats.
They only swap within their category.

Therefore, when you're looking at any recipes provided in the meal plan, or any recipe for that matter, you know that even though it calls for chicken you can use turkey instead. I get this question a lot: I'm allergic to walnuts. Okay, but you're most likely not allergic to cashews, too, so use that instead. Maybe you're allergic to tomatoes; so, okay, then eat cucumbers instead because essentially they're the same macronutrient and will process similarly in your system.

This also works extremely well for us picky eaters. We don't like certain foods and maybe recipes call for those foods that we don't like. Now you and I can both substitute macros without feeling the frustration of not being able to follow the recipe to a T.

Macros and calories are not mutually exclusive.
Macros and calories are not mutually exclusive.
Macros and calories are not mutually exclusive.

I felt the need to say that three times since we tend to get confused.

Each macro holds a certain amount of energy, meaning each macro contains a certain amount of calories.

The calorie values for each macronutrient are:

1 gram of protein = 4 calories
1 gram of carbohydrate = 4 calories
1 gram of fat = 9 calories

SO WHAT WILL YOU BE EATING ON THE SEXYFIT METHOD?

- Chicken — yes
- Lettuce — yes
- Cupcake — yes
- Pancake — yes
- Maple syrup — yes
- Taco — yes
- Pizza — yes
- Protein shake — yes
- Blueberries — yes
- Yogurt — yes
- Rice — yes
- Ice cream — yes
- Hummus — yes
- Salt — yes
- Ketchup — yes
- Fries — yes

Wait, does this mean we can eat whatever we want, when we want, and how much we want?

In a nutshell, YES! As long as it fits YOUR macros. As promised, complete food freedom and results.

But first, look at this example:

A cupcake I bought from Vons had somewhere around 280 calories, containing 1 gram of protein, 16 grams of fat, and 34 grams of carbs (with 24 grams of added sugar).

A meal made with 4 ounces of grilled chicken, a half cup of brown rice, and fresh vegetables has about the same amount of calories, but the macros breakdown is completely different: about 35 grams of protein, 5 grams of fat, and 30 grams of carbs, with no added sugars at all.

SO WHICH ONE IS BETTER, AND WHICH ONE "FITS" BEST?
While these two foods have about the same amount of calories, the macronutrient breakdowns are completely different. The cupcake has almost no protein, a lot of fat, and a lot of simple carbs, while the chicken meal is high in protein, low in fat, and has a good amount of complex carbs. Eating the same amount of calories has different effects on your body. The chicken meal will provide you with a great amount of energy and will keep you full longer to avoid cravings, while the cupcake won't satisfy the hunger and instead will spike your insulin levels that will shortly crash, causing you to crave more simple carbs (a.k.a. sugars). It will, however, satisfy your sweet tooth and can fit your macronutrient breakdown for the day if you're smart about what you spend your macros on.

WHICH IS IT? CHICKEN OR CUPCAKES?

The answer is both or either, if it fits your macros.

Yes. It's okay to eat a cupcake. Donuts are okay, too. So are salads. If you want a burger, go get one. NOT one PARTICULAR FOOD makes us gain weight. That's just science, I'm not hypothesizing. Sure, some foods hold more nutritional value than others, but not one food has the evil properties to make us "fat."

Restricting the foods we love to eat will only lead to more deprivation and a long-term disorderly way of looking at food. We've been doing this for years, saying "fat" makes us "fat" or ice cream is unhealthy, and pointing out that whoever is too thin "should eat a burger." I skipped my birthday cake for seven years in a row while competing because I thought one slice would make me "fat" and completely derail my progress. So not true. Think of all the recent diets that came out, always telling us to say NO to something. No sugar, no pizza, no grains, no rice, no fruit, no whole yogurt, no dairy, no gluten = NO LIFE!

I have three words — WTF! Why?

Isn't it nice to hear YES for a change?

It's enough of this madness. We've created a very rigid, restrictive approach to dieting over the years. So much food confusion has caused us to want to fit within these "rules" and has given us anxiety over trying to make a choice. Having the freedom to eat pizza or a cupcake once in awhile is so freeing for many of us.

However, if no one food makes us gain, what does? The primary reason we do gain weight is because of energy overage (a.k.a. caloric overage), or if we eat way too little for a long period of time and our metabolism has slowed down due to extreme caloric restriction.

WAIT, BUT WHAT ABOUT "CLEAN EATING." ISN'T THAT SUPPOSED TO BE GOOD FOR ME?

I stand behind natural unprocessed food 100%. Yes, "clean eating" is certainly the aim of any healthy, balanced nutrition plan IF "clean eating" refers to eating natural unprocessed foods. Unfortunately, "clean eating" doesn't mean the same thing for everyone. For many, it has become an association with a 1,200-calorie diet myth. At the end of the day, "clean eating" sounds to me like another way to label certain foods in an attempt to restrict our eating habits.

I'm not behind naming a nutrition approach or any food "clean."

What I do suggest is that 90% of your daily intake does come from natural unprocessed foods within 6-12 weeks of practicing macros. See, while we have macronutrients, our body also requires micronutrients, which are minerals and vitamins that we mostly get from natural foods that once grew, swam, flew, or walked the earth. Those are important, too.

If you're just starting out and you have a lot of processed foods in your diet, choose healthier options gradually. Apply the principle of addition and not subtraction. There's enough struggle in this world. Make it easy for yourself. Add healthy foods slowly; subtract what you can give up over time. Pay attention to how certain foods make you feel. It's better to apply the compound effect of adding up small changes and choices than attempting a complete overhaul and feeling overwhelmed.

You'll have a period of adjustment learning what's IN your food and how much food you should be eating, not to mention the slow transition away from sugars and highly processed food. After you go through that transition, you'll go down the route of becoming an ingredient snob and really start to pay attention to the quality of the food that you're eating. The truth is, it's not easier than ever to find healthier alternatives for the over-processed foods we love; we just have to care and pay attention. You'll notice that over time you'll tend to make better choices based on how those foods make YOU feel. It's a natural transition.

I could write an entire separate book on inflammation, the influence of gluten on our hormonal system and the high inflammatory effects of lactose, and the side-effects of both on our digestive system. I could talk endlessly about food allergies, GMOs, MSGs, and the dangers of corn and lack of integrity in farming, or the high use of antibiotics in beef and poultry. But I won't. I want you to be able to make those choices and listen to your body. Not because I told you NOT to eat gluten or dairy or because I scared you with the latest GMO research, but because you made the decision to figure out how you'll feel as a result. It's worth trying when you're ready and open to do it. But get the basics down first! Because no matter how many new non-inflammatory, gluten-free diets you start, the basics will still be the basics. So start there.

If you're already eating healthy and are mostly eating unprocessed foods, the benefits for you are that you can finally get more in tune with your body and hunger cues, and finally eat enough for your weight and height. Most of our clients start here and realize that while they've been attempting to eat very healthy, they missed the label-reading process or have been undereating all of these years due to the "clean eating" myth or wild propaganda of 1,200-calorie diets.

If you're a crazy perfectionist like I once was, and you have a load of guilt over eating certain foods, or if having a slice of pizza at your kid's birthday party throws you into a panic, you'll find yourself loving this approach because it allows you to integrate certain foods, and navigate around everyday situations and trust your body to tell you what it needs.

WITH MACROS, YOU GET TO DECIDE

I know how you feel and I know what you'll be going through because I've been there myself.

I've been through quite a few of those transitions. From sugar addiction to learning the rigid clean eating approach. That took a lot of time and effort. And then later from extreme clean eating to no-rules eating back to the world of balanced eating on macros. There's no one right way to do this. Even for me, the hardest transition was going from the extreme clean eating mindset while going through food bingeing to balanced nutrition. So I went through the journey of incorporating unhealthy food into my nutrition on purpose so I could overcome my developed fear of food. My mental state was more important to me at the time because it was the foundation of my success. Gradually I listened to my body and realized that certain processed foods didn't make me feel well. Others I was okay with. I also became 99% lactose-free; I completely eliminate sugar; I eat very little gluten on a daily basis; and I don't eat beef, pork, or eggs unless they're organically sourced. I switched to Kosher chicken and started paying attention to what brands of healthy foods made me feel better.

If you're wondering what I actually DO eat, well, that'd be everything that you'll see in the 21-Day Transformation Plan. I do love a good pizza once in awhile, and I love wings during football season #GoChargers. "Everything in moderation" is my motto now, but it took willingness and the desire to learn. I got here with macros, releasing old patterns of restrictive dieting, and trusting my body.

The macronutrient approach might seem a bit confusing at first, but it's the way to get back to the basics and fundamentals of how our body works and what it needs. You get to determine how much you need to eat to thrive in life, tap into your inner wisdom of what you feel like eating (vs following a strict plan) and make food choices that you both enjoy and benefit your body. The more you apply this method, the more you get to notice how your body responds to certain foods. You'll able to clearly see patterns. AND, most importantly, you'll get to choose what you want to eat and what feels best to you. It becomes your lifestyle on your terms and your gateway to complete food freedom.

CHAPTER PRACTICE

Take out your journal and answer the questions listed below. The point of this exercise is to help you remember what each nutrient does and how it benefits you. We've become so food-phobic over the years that right now we need to remember that each nutrient nurtures our body in its own way. I want to make sure this information sticks and you can easily navigate around macros in your daily life.

- What are the 3 main macronutrients?
- What are the benefits of healthy fats?
- What is glycogen, and why do we need it?
- What certain foods/food groups do you fear?
- How can you integrate it once per week to overcome that food fear?

PODCAST ALERT

Reference the www.sexyfit.com/resources page to listen to the "How to Jump Start Your Life and Transform Your Body with Natalie Jill" and "Stop The Food Obsession, Hack Your Diet, Conquer Your Life with Betty Rocker" podcasts.

YOUR MACROS YOUR WAY
CHAPTER 13

You're one step closer to complete food freedom! At this point, it's important to understand that every nutrient has a purpose: protein, carbs, and fat are each unique and have a very important job in our system. I can't stress this enough. This is why cutting out food groups only works short-term. Our body needs fuel from all of the nutrients and will eventually work its magic to get us to eat it.

We're all familiar with the saying "Heart wants what heart wants." Well, body wants what body wants.

In this chapter, you get to calculate your own unique set of macros and understand how much energy your body needs on a regular basis. Each one of us has a unique set of macros based on our weight, height, and age. This is why every single one of us is going to end up with a unique set of numbers. I'm going to help you do this in three simple steps. Or really one simple step if you want to go to sexyfit.com/countmymacros to get your macros for free.

Even though you can easily get your macros online, I do think it's important for you to know where your macros come from. Here are the three variables that we take into consideration:

STEP 1: CALCULATE YOUR TDEE
TDEE stands for: total daily energy expenditure, i.e., the amount of energy we burn every day when we're just walking around, standing, watching Netflix, or running around town picking up our kids or slaying our work day. If we work out or keep active, we burn more calories. If we sit at a desk and have a fairly sedentary lifestyle, we burn fewer.

An average woman who's 5'-4," weighs 145 pounds, and is around 30 years old burns upwards of 2,100 calories per day. This means that in order to maintain her current weight, she could eat up to 2,100 calories per day and not worry about weight gain if she has a healthy metabolism.

What happens if we continuously undereat? Our metabolism slows down to a halt, our digestive system suffers, and we constantly lack energy and feel fatigued. When we do eat, we feel bloated, constipated, and just not right.

You MUST eat and way more then any average diet propaganda will make you believe.

I'm not sure where the 1,200-calorie myth propaganda came from. You know that whole myth about eating only 1,200 calories per day in order to lose weight? Somehow this is magically the universal number if we want to get "thin"?

WHO?!
WHY?!
HOW?!

In the world is this still a thing?

No.
No.
And NO!

Can you tell I'm outraged about this?

There's no way! This is so wrong. Why would a woman who's 5'-5" and 200 pounds who's trying to lose weight use the same calorie amount to lose weight as a woman who's 5'-2" and 130 pounds? Both of those women are a different weight and height, and most likely a different age. It's time to put the 1,200 calories or LESS myth to rest and fuel our body properly, build up our metabolism, and nourish OUR body.

Your TDEE will allow you to see how many calories you need to eat at maintenance to remain the same weight you are now.

STEP 2: CALCULATE MACROS
Based on our TDEE, we get to see how many calories from each nutrient we need in order to thrive in our body and achieve the results we're looking for. Our macros are going to look something like this:

145 protein
145 carbs
45 fat

Or, 145 P, 145 C, 45 F

Remember, each macro holds a certain number of calories, so we'll still have calories to count. Macros and calories aren't independent of each other. Here's the formula we'll need to count calories:

P = 4 calories
C = 4 calories
F = 9 cal ories

NOTE: Fat is a dense nutrient, so it yields more calories.

STEP 3: SET UP A DEFICIT
Yes, we need to eat in deficit in order to lose body fat. The higher the deficit, in theory the faster the fat loss, however certain considerations apply. I would never recommend for anyone to eat a 50% deficit, as most women do, by just eating nothing or eating fewer than 1,200 calories. That's torturous, silly, and doesn't work long-term. I recommend that you start with a conservative deficit of 10-20%. I know some of us will crave fast results, but I consider consistent results that stick to be the "fastest" since you actually get to keep them.

EXAMPLES OF DEFICIT:

15-20% below maintenance calories = conservative deficit
20-25% below maintenance calories = moderate deficit
25-30% below maintenance calories = aggressive deficit (risky)
31-40% below maintenance calories = very aggressive deficit (dangerous and unhealthy)
50%+ below maintenance calories = semi-starvation/starvation

So those were the three steps to understanding your macros and all the variables of macros. Head over to sexyfit.com/countmymacros to get your numbers.

THE SLOW PLUS METHOD

For those of us who have been dieting for quite some time, we've experienced metabolic slowdown. After we see our macros, eating so much food per day might not be sustainable for our digestive system and overall well-being. Drastic caloric increase comes as a shock that would cause confusion within our system, leading to the storage of body fat. For those women who have been dieting for a long time, I recommend the "slow plus" method.

Meaning, if your TDEE is around 2,000 calories and your macros are 160 grams of protein, 145 grams of carbs, and 60 grams of fat, and the entire time before Sexyfit you've only eaten 1,000-1,300 calories, it can come as a shock to your body to eat so much. Therefore, start slowly with the current amount of calories or your BMR (whichever you choose), calculate your macros based on that number, and week by week add calories until you reach your TDEE.

WHY DOES THIS WORK?

We slowly build our metabolism back up to normal speed and create an optimal state for our body to be able to burn calories and have a healthy metabolism. We're basically tricking our body out of the adaptive thermogenesis and giving it a reason to burn more calories on a regular basis. Most of our Sexyfit clients whom we work with one on one have tried the "slow plus" formula and absolutely love it. Here's how this method works ...

Slowly increase your caloric intake by 150 calories over seven days until you reach your TDEE. It'll take you around four weeks to get your calories up to maintenance, but in the process you'll experience an increase in energy, actual fat loss because your body isn't scared of food anymore, improved digestion, and more strength in your workouts. I suggest the following plan:

Weeks 1-2: INCREASE your protein intake by 100 calories per week.
Weeks 2-3: INCREASE your carbohydrates intake by 100 calories per week.
Weeks 4-5: INCREASE your fats intake by 100 calories per week.

🔅 CHAPTER PRACTICE

Visit sexyfit.com/countmymacros and get your macronutrient set. Remember what your macros are, since you're going to need them in the next chapter. If you're feeling a bit overwhelmed, allow yourself some time to review the chapter again. Some of this information might be dense and you'll need to take a look at everything one more time. Move away from feeling overwhelmed by taking a moment to breathe, and reconnect with your goals and your why. If you're feeling excited and ready to go, let's go!

📡 PODCAST ALERT

Reference the www.sexyfit.com/resources page to listen to the "Why 'Clean Eating' Failed You and What Actually Works" podcast.

HOW TO MEASURE AND COUNT YOUR MACROS
CHAPTER 14

Check you out, sister, you're a macro nutrient PRO! You know WHY you need macros, you know what they do, and you have your own set of macros. Now that you know your macros, I'm going to walk you through the step-by-step process of how to find macros in food, how to measure macros, and how to track macros.

I want to make sure you have all the tools and strategies you need.

ALL MACROS IN A FOOD CAN BE FOUND ON A NUTRITION LABEL OR ON THE CHARTS IN THE FOLLOWING PAGES.

Now we know that all macros are okay to substitute within each macro category. We also know how to measure them. Next, it's important to figure out where the macros can be found.

Macros can be found two ways …

1. ON A NUTRITION LABEL
The first place to look is on the nutrition label. But what are we looking for?

First, look for protein, total carbohydrates, and total fat. You know that protein-packed foods are going to be higher in protein. Kind of a given. But at times, when they're highly processed, they'll also be higher in fat, plus have added carbs.

At times, you'll look for the carb source on a label and see that it's through the roof relative to all of the other nutrients. While there might not be anything wrong with that, it's something we must pay attention to.

After you know the macronutrient breakdown of the food you chose, take a look at the serving size and number of servings per container. This is important and very relevant because for highly processed foods a lot of the serving sizes will be noted as ⅛ of a cup. Have you ever eaten ⅛ of a cup of ice cream? Yeah … me either. Food marketers are incredibly smart. I still buy into some brands thinking the portion sizes are bigger. ALWAYS read the serving size!

The third—and very important—thing to look at is the sugar content. What's up, Sugaaa?! (OMG, I really couldn't help myself but to say that.) Okay, so, sugar.

Brace yourself for a Zlata-rant.

ALTERNATE NAMES FOR SUGAR

Agave (or agave nectar)
Barbados Sugar
Barley Malt (or syrup)
Beet Sugar
Brown Rice Syrup
Brown Sugar
Buttered Syrup
Cane Crystals
Cane Juice (or sugar)
Caramel
Carob Syrup
Castor Sugar
Coconut Sugar
Coconut Palm Sugar
Confectioner's Sugar
Corn Syrup (or solids)
Crystaline Fructose
Date Sugar
Dehydrated Cane Juice
Demerara Sugar
Dextrin
Dextrose
Diastatic Malt
Evaporated Cane Juice
Fructose
Fruit Juice (or concentrate)
Galactose
Glucose (or glucose solids)
Golden Syrup
Grape Sugar
High Fructose Corn Syrup
Honey
Icing Sugar
Invert Sugar
Jaggery
Lactose
Malt Syrup
Maltodextrin
Maltose
Mannose
Maple Syrup
Molasses
Monk Fruit / Luo Han Guo
Muscovado Sugar
Palm Sugar
Panela
Panocha
Rapadura
Raw Cane Sugar
Refiner's Syrup
Rice Syrup (or bran syrup)
Saccharose
Sorghum Syrup
Sucanat
Sucrose
Sugar (granulated)
Tapioca Syrup
Treacle
Turbinado Sugar
Yellow Sugar

Sugar is claimed to be as addictive as cocaine (wow, that myth really stuck). Everyone seems to blame the obesity epidemic on sugar itself. Sugar is the enemy of our time.

Why's everyone freaking out about sugar? Should you freak out, too?

The answer is yes. And no. I don't have an issue with sugar. Eat your sugar, Sugar. Well, let me rephrase that. Eat up to 30 grams of natural sugar per day. I'll explain why ...

Many nutritionists and fitness gurus say that fruit isn't allowed while trying to lose fat. I have to disagree with them wholeheartedly on that argument but regardless, I'm going to get on the excess sugar hating train with everyone else. Call me hypocritical in a way because I've already established that I'm not here to tell you to give up donuts and cookies. But I am here to show you how to put together a sensible plan that you can enjoy and stick to for life, even with cookies.

So to do my due diligence, let me share with you when sugar actually becomes dangerously physiologically addictive, downright scary, and, quite frankly, ridiculous.

When sugar is present in every single food we're eating throughout the day... even the "healthy" kind, it sends our body on a blood sugar roller-coaster. We've all heard of the sugar crash, right?

"The struggle is real" when we intentionally eat a cookie or something that contains a high amount of carbohydrates. But the thing is, many of our Sexyfit clients unknowingly consume close to 70 grams of sugar per day thinking that they "don't eat that much sugar." That's almost 18 tablespoons of the sweet stuff per day. And three times more than the recommended amount of sugar.

If you drink soda, one can has around 43 grams of sugar, which is approximately 12 teaspoons of sugar.

It's downright ridiculous and dangerous that a lot of processed foods, even if they're labeled as "healthy"— whether sweet or savory—have added sugar. Let me repeat again, sweet OR savory processed foods have sugar. Whether you love chips or you love cookies, it's a very similar thing because food marketers these days are trying to make you like their products by manipulating the flavors with sugar.

And it doesn't really stop there, sister. Once food companies realized that you and I were smart enough to figure out what the sugar content on the label is, they started putting it on the label under a variety of names. A shocking amount, actually. Take a look at this list ...

Some of these sugars have recently been advertised and promoted as healthy. Agave is a shining example of such propaganda. Sugar is sugar, Sugar.

Research shows that eating a high amount of sugar produces changes in the brain, and, as a result, we create addictive behavior patterns toward sugar. Due to a high consumption of sugar, our body (our brain, specifically) gets the feeling of pleasure and satisfaction due to the increased release of dopamine. Dopamine receptors are all over our brain. Heck, doing a drug like heroin brings on a deluge of dopamine. Too much sugar too often can steer the brain into overdrive, and that kickstarts a series of "unfortunate events" — loss of control, cravings, and increased tolerance to sugar. All of those effects can be physically and psychologically taxing over time, leading to weight gain and dependence.

ANOTHER FUN FACT: Since our digestive system has a ton of neurons, and it's tightly connected with the nervous system, it's no surprise that we eat foods with a high sugar content to help us deal with our emotional problems and out of stress to help us cope. I know all about this tricky endeavour after using beloved Snickers® to medicate myself for missing my family and separation depression.

But there's hope for all of us, Snickers and sugar lovers included. The less sugar we eat, the less sugar we crave.

Why do I say 30 grams of sugar per day?

First and foremost, according to research by the American Heart Association, 30 grams of sugar per day is the suggested amount.[14] And also in our experience with many Sexyfit clients, this seems to be the "sweet spot" that doesn't cut out sugar completely yet allows us to indulge in any sweets, as well as our favorite savory foods.

Okay, try 30 grams of sugar a day, look at label and watch out for sugar and fake sugars like a hawk. Rant over.

On to the next thing ...

2. MOST OF THE FOODS THAT DON'T HAVE A LABEL ARE UNPROCESSED FOODS
This means that when we buy sweet potatoes or a bag of grapes at the store we won't necessarily find a label. Since we're mostly relying on unprocessed foods as a source of energy, this might present a minor problem. I provided you with a measurement and macros breakdown for most of the foods without a label in the table on the following page.

At first it might seem tedious, but, sister, this knowledge comes with time. It's only a matter of a short period of time until you know the macros breakdown for 99% of the food that you'll eat on a regular basis.

TIP: If you're using MyFitnessPal,® you can enter "Sexyfit" in front of the name of the food and it will give you the correct measurements from the chart at right. For example, "Sexyfit Zucchini" will give you the proper measurements in the proper units.

Natural foods, like fruits, veggies, etc., aren't going to be on a label, so I broke them down for you here, including how to measure them.

HOW TO MEASURE FOOD AND FOOD MEASUREMENTS
Most of the food you'll be eating will need to be measured at first. Yes, measured. It's impossible to eyeball your food in the beginning and know what 4 ounces of chicken and ½ cup of rice looks like. It took me years to master this, and still to this day I measure foods.

PROTEINS

FOOD	SERVING SIZE	CALORIES	PROTEINS	CARBS	FATS
Bass	4 ozs	140	26	0	3
Chicken Breast, boneless/skinless	5 ozs	233.75	44	0	5
Cod	4 ozs	119	26	0	1
Crab	4 ozs	111	23	1.5	1
Fat-Free Cottage Cheese	1/2 cup	70	15	5	0
Egg, whites only	4 each	68	14	1	0
Flounder	4 ozs	132	28	0	0
Haddock	4 ozs	127	28	0	0
Halibut	4 ozs	159	30	0	4
Orange Roughy	4 ozs	101	21	0	1
Perch	4 ozs	133	28	0	1
Red Snapper	4 ozs	145	23	0	2
Tilapia	3.5 ozs	96	20.1	0	1.7
Tuna, solid albacore	4 ozs	140	30	0	3
Turkey, breast	4 ozs	153	34	0	0.8

FRUITS

FOOD	SERVING SIZE	CALORIES	PROTEINS	CARBS	FATS
Apples, medium	1 Apple	81	0	21	0
Banana, medium	1 Banana	105	1	27	1
Grapefruit	1/2 Grapefruit	46	1	12	0
Oranges, medium	1 Orange	69	1	17	0.3
Papaya, medium	1 Papaya	119	2	30	0.4
Peaches, medium	1 Peach	37	1	10	0.1
Pears, medium	1 Pear	98	1	25	0
Pineapple, fresh	8 ozs	130	0	30	0
Raspberries	8 ozs	60	1	14	1
Strawberries	8 ozs	45	1	11	1
Watermelon	8 ozs	50	1	11	1

VEGGIES

FOOD	SERVING SIZE	CALORIES	PROTEINS	CARBS	FATS
Asparagus	1 cup	27	3	5	0
Broccoli	1 cup	31	3	6	0
Cabbage	1 cup	22	1	5	0
Cauliflower	1 cup	25	2	5	0
Celery	1 cup	16	1	3	0
Cucumber, slices	1 cup	16	1	3	0
Garden Salad	1 medium	73.5	2	14	0
Green Beans, uncooked	1 cup	34	2	8	0
Romaine Lettuce	1 cup	8	1	2	0
Mushrooms	1 cup	37	3	6	0
Onions, chopped	1 cup	64	2	15	0
Peppers, Green or Red	1 cup	30	1	7	0
Spinach	1 cup	33	3	6	0
Squash, Summer (cooked)	1 cup	36	2	8	1
Tomatoes (raw)	1 cup	25	2	5	0
Zucchini	1 cup	20	2	4	0

STARCHES & GRAINS: A.K.A. CARBS

FOOD	SERVING SIZE	CALORIES	PROTEINS	CARBS	FATS
Brown rice, cooked	1 cup	220	4	46	0
Wild rice, cooked	1 cup	166	7	35	1
Grits, Quaker, uncooked	1/2 cup	289	7	62	1
Oatmeal, Quaker, uncooked	1/2 cup	140	5	26	3
Cream of rice	1/2 cup	320	5.5	71.5	0.5
Quinoa	1/2 cup	313	12	54.5	5
Oat bran hot cereal	1/2 cup	150	7	25	3
Corn tortilla, 7" diameter	1 tortilla	55	1	11	0.75
Yam, baked or boiled	5 ozs	150	4	35	0
Black beans, cooked	1 cup	227	15	41	1
Rice cakes	1 each	35	1.6	7	0

FATS

FOOD	SERVING SIZE	CALORIES	PROTEINS	CARBS	FATS
Raw almonds	1 ozs	163	6	6	14
Raw cashews	1 ozs	155	5	9	12
Raw walnuts	1 ozs	183	4	4	18
All-Natural peanut butter	1 tablespoon	94	4	3	8
All -Natural cashew butter	1 tablespoon	94	3	4	8
All-Natural almond butter	1 tablespoon	101	2	3	9
Extra-Virgin olive oil	1 tablespoon	119	0	0	14
Avocado	1 ozs	47	1	2	4

You're going to need a digital food scale to measure proteins, and fats like nuts and sweet potato. The Fitlosophy Digital Food Scale is certainly the best of the best. It has four units to measure and will take the measure back to zero in a click of a button when you want to add ingredients to the same dish ... perfect for smoothies and salads.

This brings me to an important chat about the units of measurement for food ...

PROTEIN — Measure protein in ounces. All protein is measured cooked.

CARBS — Measure grains in cups. All grains are measured cooked. Potatoes are pretty much the only vegetable to be measured uncooked, and they're tracked in ounces. All green vegetables are measured in cups and uncooked. Fruit is measured in cups and uncooked, as well.

FATS — Measure nut butters in tablespoons. Measure oils in tablespoons, as well. When it comes to nuts and avocado, as well as seeds, measure them in ounces.

DO NOT EYEBALL your food unless you're eating at a restaurant! Don't make eyeballing a habit during the first three months of using this plan. It won't serve you in the long run. You'll only be cheating yourself out of an opportunity to get this right.

About the only thing you don't really need to measure are leafy greens like kale, arugula, spinach, or mixed greens. I've never in my life heard of anyone overeating kale. Feel free to eat unlimited amounts and enjoy your salads.

ALL MACROS MUST BE TRACKED IN A FITNESS TRACKER

All macros are counted in grams. Have I said this before?

Not pie charts, percentages, red or green dots, or whatever else. Grams. There are lots of tracking applications available. My favorite app is MyFitnessPal. It helps me and our clients keep our macros on point at all times. However, because it's a community-based tool, sometimes the information can be incorrect when it comes to food measurements. If you're not sure that the macros of the food you entered are correct, add "Sexyfit" before the name of your food in the search tab (Sexyfit Zucchini, for example) — our macros are always correct!

Track all of the food you're currently eating without any negativity or judgment as to if it's "good" or "bad" in your opinion. When tracking your food, track everything you put into your mouth. From sauces to ketchup to mayo, to an extra bite of this here and there. And by "everything," I mean EVERYTHING.

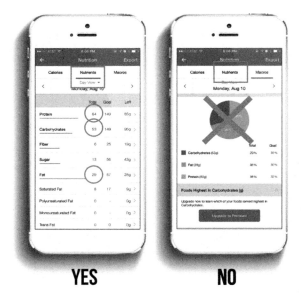

YES   **NO**

You'll see that your macros are going to be shown in protein, carbs, and fats in whatever nutritional tracking app you choose to use. And you're only looking at grams!

Again, don't look at pie charts, yellow or green lines, butterflies, or ANYTHING else. This is an example of the MyFitnessPal macros breakdown. I'm in the Nutrients section — not the Macros section — because it's easier to see this way. I previously entered my target macros, therefore the program shows me how many macros I have left based on my preset needs. You should do this, too. NEVER let MyFitnessPal set YOUR numbers for you. ONLY preset your own macros after calculating them. MFP is not your coach, and it's not you. It's a tool with basic knowledge and math skills.

Here's an example of what I'm talking about ...

The longer you use the app, the better it knows your mealtimes, recent food choices, and specific macros recipes you preset for yourself. At first it might seem confusing, overwhelming, and frustrating. My best suggestion is to treat it as a game, so it's not a place that discourages you but allows you to create awareness in a fun, exciting way.

I want you to commit to macros for the duration of the 21-Day Transformation Plan, with no exceptions. With consistent tracking, you should be able to see patterns, and how you feel when you have more or less of the nutrients you need. You should be able to know exactly what makes you feel good, what makes you energized, and what foods are not necessarily working for you. Most of our clients go through a six-month tracking period. To this day, I track my macros when I feel like I need to get a little more control over my plan or I'm starting a new training program. What you can measure you can improve.

💡 CHAPTER PRACTICE

Get a digital food scale right now. Immediately. This is the first step. Order one on Amazon if you need to.

In order to start tracking your macros, take out your phone or set up your new tracking app on your desktop. Go into settings and adjust your macros to the ones we gave you at Sexyfit. Adjust as closely as possible. Usually it will ask you for total calories first, and then ask to adjust for grams or percentages. Remember, we count everything in grams! Don't let the application set your macros for you, or it will be confusing. You adjust your macros based on the macros we gave you. Your app doesn't know you!

Track everything that you ate today and yesterday. Even if you need to guess portion sizes. After you're done, take a look at the total nutrient breakdown. Where's your protein at? How many carbs did you have? What nutrients are you low or high on? Bringing awareness to your current macros intake gives you a solid place to start and know what you need to work on.

🎙️ PODCAST ALERT

Reference the www.sexyfit.com/resources page to listen to the "How to Read a Label" and "Top 6 Apps and Gadgets I Can't Live Without" podcasts.

HOW TO CREATE A
BALANCED MEAL
CHAPTER 15

Wow, sister, you're almost a pro at the macros counting! You know how to calculate your macros, you know how to measure them, and how to track them. Check you out right now!

Now you and I are going to work on building a meal, and shopping for your new lifestyle and beyond. While the grocery list, recipes, and other tools to make this easier are already included, to ensure long-term success, I want to make sure I cover all of the bases when it comes to the Sexyfit nutrition approach.

First and foremost, I want to show you how to create a macro-friendly meal.

HEADS UP: The most common comment about this type of approach is that the protein number is quite high, and lots of women aren't used to hitting their protein macros at first. Another typical comment is that right off the bat women don't know how to create a meal that's going to help them nail their macros.

The first step in all meal planning is to include protein. Your protein essentially serves as the foundation for your creation.

As an example, I propose that we pick chicken as our foundation protein. You're welcome to choose any protein source you like, which is what makes this lifestyle so flexible.

After you pick your protein, it's time to add the next most vital set of ingredients. Your next best choices are non-starchy or starchy vegetables.

So we'll add sweet potato fries or sweet potato, as well as some steamed cauliflower with red peppers.

Sounds yummy, right?

If this were a salad, we could add leafy greens, like kale, and more veggies, like cucumbers, radishes, or mushrooms.

Now you have a solid foundation of protein and carbohydrates.

To complete your meal, add healthy fats like avocado, nuts, olive oil, etc.

So now we can add a creamy mustard dressing to our sweet potato fries or sweet potato. Or in the case of a salad, you can add seeds and balsamic vinaigrette dressing, salt and pepper, and have a delicious salad ready in 10 minutes or less. Voilà, your meal is dressed up, accessorized, and ready to go!

It's very simple. Let's try the same strategy with a protein smoothie.

Pick your protein powder base — you can choose from the variety of protein powder types available — whey, casein, egg white, plant-based or collagen protein.

Dress it up with fresh blueberries and raspberries.

Accessorize with dark chocolate shreds.

See, its really easy.

What's also worth mentioning is how you treat your meal time. If food for you is a constant race of shoving it in your mouth between meetings, you'll never feel fully happy and satisfied. This might show up as overeating at parties or dinner because "you never eat this way." I do realize not every meal is going to be a Michelin restaurant-like experience, but practicing mindfulness during your meal time is equally as important as simply eating. Remember the feminine and masculine side? It shows up here in the best way. Sure I've eaten my fair share of meals out of plastic food storage containers with a plastic fork. Did I look great? Yes. Was I ever truly satisfied with a meal? NO.

You masculine energy is very much focused on the macros, meal planning and meal prepping, and knowing what meal comes next. It's natural for the masculine side of us to think this way. Our feminine side will come into play when we need to plate a meal, add spices, make it beautiful, and make it a bit festive. To be very honest and transparent, this is something I hadn't really started practicing until recently, but it really made all the difference in the world with how satisfied and happy and full I was after my meals. I got so inspired by our photoshoot food stylist (yes, that's a real job!), and how carefully she assembled every meal with love and care. She was the ultimate feminine food inspo for me. I rarely ever eat out of food storage containers anymore if I'm at home and have taken my on-the-go food approach to a minimum. It has changed my entire experience with food, and it's by far the best habit I could create.

I urge you to create an experience for yourself where you set the table, grab a white napkin, chew your food, and connect with the flavor of what you're eating. How it looks matters as much as what it taste likes and as much as what it does. This way your brain knows you're eating and not talking on the phone, driving, or staring at the computer. Our brain needs a cue that it might need to turn on our digestive system. This is why if we eat at our desk, our tummy might hurt. Or if we constantly eat on the go, we're never full or satisfied.

Enjoy creating a relationship with your food, and set yourself up for a mindful and joyful experience of self-love with your food.

CHAPTER PRACTICE

1. Build every meal today in the steps as mentioned in this chapter. Train your mind to go to protein first, veggies second, and then play dress-up. Make sure your meals are colorful and actually look attractive.

2. Today, create an experience out of at least one of your meals. Set up the table, light a candle, grab a white napkin, and feel the experience. Journal about the meal you created and how it made you feel.

IT ALL STARTS AT HOME
CHAPTER 16

Your nutrition starts with what's in your pantry and in your fridge. It's about the law of proximity in this case. What food you have at home is what you'll eat, what you'll bring to work with you as lunch, and what you'll have for dinner.

The situation in our fridge and pantry can go two ways.

It's either a total ghost town, or it looks like you're preparing for WWIII. Either way, let's figure it out. I know you'll have an urge to get organized and ready to go with your new lifestyle, so I want to make it easy for you.

START WITH YOUR FRIDGE:

1. Open your freezer and toss everything. I'm just kidding but maybe not. Your food is a source of nutrients and energy. As much as I'm pro-flexible dieting and no restrictions, certain food — such as frozen meals, pre-made mozzarella sticks, and frozen burritos — that stuff I can't get on board with. Ideally, the only food in your freezer is vegetables, proteins, and some pre-made meals you froze yourself during meal prep.

2. Check expiration dates on everything. If it has been in your fridge since 1991, you can probably toss it.

3. If you have food that has been in there for more than a month, I don't think it's good for you, so let's toss that, too.

4. You're looking to organize your fridge in such a way that you can easily find all of the foods you need for meal prep and leave yourself room for pre-made meals in food storage containers.

5. Top shelf — It's the warmest part of the fridge compartment and best for pre-prepared foods, such as yogurt, cheese, and sauces. Store cooked meat and leftovers in sealed containers on the shelves underneath.

6. Fridge door — The temperature in the door racks can fluctuate because they're exposed to the warm air of the kitchen when the door is opened. The door racks are a good place for condiments, jams, and dressings. (Oh, I have such incredible recipes for you!) A lidded compartment is ideal for keeping butter and margarine extra cold.

7. Bottom drawers — Use one for food and veggies, and a second one for meat and poultry. Line the bottom of your refrigerator's crisper drawer with paper towels. They'll absorb the excess moisture that causes veggies to rot. Note on lettuce: Lettuce needs moisture to stay fresh and will quickly wilt if it dehydrates. Wrap lettuce in damp paper towels and store in a plastic bag. If salad greens begin to wilt, soak them in ice water to crisp them up before fixing a salad. Prevent mushrooms from getting slimy by wrapping them in paper towels before refrigerating. Store avocados unbagged in the refrigerator. And apples away from other foods. Apples give off ethylene gas, which can cause foods to spoil. If they get too soft, just cook them. The rest of the fruits and veggies can live together quite nicely.

8. Bottom shelf — When you store meat and poultry in the bottom drawers, it doesn't drip and contaminate other foods.

9. Before you go to the grocery store, rotate older foods forward so you know what you need to use first.

10. If you want to take it to the next level, you can put a lazy susan in your fridge to help you stay organized.

Now that we're wrapped up with the fridge, let's move on to the pantry. Other processed food (I use "food" as a relative term) that I can't get on board with are boxed pasta meals and instant mashed potatoes. We can hardly call them food because they're modified to look and taste like food, but indeed are NOT food.

The more nutrient-rich food you eat, the better you're going to feel. Imagine making fresh mashed potatoes with butter. Doesn't that sound much better than instant mashed potatoes out of a bag? I thought so.

HERE'S A LIST OF FOOD TO KEEP IN YOUR PANTRY:
- Whole wheat pasta
- Quinoa pasta
- Rice, brown rice
- Buckwheat
- Oats
- Legumes
- Flour (whole wheat, coconut, oat, brown rice, etc.)
- Honey
- Coffee, tea, spices, dry herbs
- Canned fish or chicken (check ingredients on these always)
- Raw or roasted nuts
- Nut butters

FEEL FREE TO SAY GOOD-BYE TO:
- Chips, pretzels, any nightly snacks you feel like you have no control over
- Bleached all-purpose flour
- White sugar
- Mac 'n' cheese or anything that has so many ingredients; you could cook that food faster than reading all of the processed ingredients out loud. Again, these aren't nourishing foods for your body.

CHAPTER PRACTICE

It's cleaning time! I find cleaning very therapeutic; fingers crossed that you do, too. After you complete this chapter, please bravely rush over to your fridge and pantry. This is the time to clean, organize, toss, and create space for the new healthier foods. If you have a lot of processed food in your fridge, and you're willing and ready to let it go, feel free to donate it to the nearest charity or a homeless shelter. There's nothing like making someone else's day with your generosity.

PODCAST ALERT

Reference the www.sexyfit.com/resources page to listen to the "Food Storing Tips" podcast.

GROCERY SHOPPING FOR YOUR SEXYFIT LIFESTYLE
CHAPTER 17

Here comes the fun part!

Think of grocery shopping like shopping for an outfit for a business meeting. We need a skirt, blazer, blouse, and nice shoes. But if we don't go off of a list of what we need, we end up with a sports bra, Crocs,™ and a nightgown. None of those pieces of the outfit go together. And neither do a bunch of groceries we buy without planning our meals.

Therefore, grocery shopping is actually a two-step process.

First, its planning your meals and knowing what ingredients we need to get. It's going to be really easy with the 21-Day Transformation Plan to know exactly what we need to get because I laid out the grocery plan and meal plan for you. In the future, make it a habit once per week to quickly jot down what meals you want to make and then head to the store. Each week you do this, it's going to take less and less time. The more you practice, the easier it gets.

After you plan your meals, break down your grocery list into PCF (protein, carbs, and fats). Starting with your foundation, which is protein, shop for fruit and veggies after that. If something is on sale, swap some of your ingredients for cheaper ones. After you're done, move to the aisle where you can find the healthy fats.

The key is to keep your eyes on the prize and move along the perimeter of the store. Ideally, you don't even need to go down the aisles unless you need tea or peanut butter. The more detailed your list, the faster you'll get in and out of the grocery store. Shop for a week so that you don't have to come back to the store every night. We don't have this kind of time. The better your list, the less time you're going to spend in the grocery store throughout the week. Not to mention, shopping once per week saves you lots of money!

Saving money and saving time? Who doesn't love that?

I always suggest that you have at least a few easy emergency meals that you can put in a pan or microwave, like frozen rice in bags or frozen chicken strips that are easy to make in case you get home and you're pressed for time.

If you choose to get chocolate, chips, crackers, mayo, ketchup, wraps, or other foods to fill up your macros, make the most sensible choice based on ingredients. Stay mindful when shopping, and, for the love of Snickers,® please don't shop hungry.

Here's a basic food shopping list ...

PROTEINS
- Chicken breast
- Chicken thigh (no skin)
- Turkey breast
- Fish fllets
- Lean beef (4 grams of fat per serving, top roast and steak)
- Lean pork (sirloin or anything that ends with "loin")
- Ground meats (less Than 10% fat)
- Fat-free Greek Yogurt
- Low-fat or Fat-free cottage cheese
- Beans (if canned, no salt added)
- Edamame beans
- Egg whites and whole Eggs

FATS
- Nuts of any kind and nut butters (only nuts in the ingredients)
- Seeds
- Olive oil or sunflower oil for salads
- Grapeseed oil or coconut oil for cooking
- Avocado
- Fatty fish (salmon, mackerel, sardines)
- Grass-fed butter
- Cheese (low-fat mozzarella, fresh mozzarella, goat cheese)

CARBS
- Quinoa
- Brown rice, black rice, wild rice, red rice
- Rolled oats
- Protein granola
- Buckwheat
- Millet
- Whole wheat pasta, quinoa pasta, or brown rice pasta
- All vegetables
- All fruits

💡 CHAPTER PRACTICE

Next time you go to the grocery store, make a list of groceries you need in P, C, F columns on a piece of paper or in your cell phone's notes.

Head over to the store and only buy items from your list. Track the amount of time it takes you. I bet it will half as long because you are not lollygagging around the story trying to think what "sounds good."

MEAL PREP STRATEGIES
CHAPTER 18

Having meals ready to go is what makes all the difference on our journey. Once again, it's the law of proximity. If we have healthy meals on the go with us, we're more likely going to eat the meals that we've prepared.

Love it or hate it, meal prep is the only way to sustainable transformation.

And since you'll have to do your meal prep almost every week, or sometimes twice per week, I would say that loving it is probably the best way to go. When you create the right environment, and change your state of mind about the actions you take, you'll soon find the joy and pleasure in meal prep.

Not only do you get to save money, save time, and rid yourself of food anxiety, hAnger, and escaping the doubtful question of "what's for lunch?", but you'll get to connect with your food and the joy of cooking. If you've never spent time in the kitchen, cooking doesn't sound like much fun right now, but cooking is natural to us. It's the most feminine thing we can possibly do. Remember the dance between the masculine and the feminine I talked about in the first section of the book? — meal plans, macros, understanding the science behind food — these are inherently masculine energy tasks that use the right side of our brain. In the kitchen, we get to create, connect, nurture, and love. It's the peak meditative state ... of course, if you allow it to be.

Have your friends over, listen to a podcast, watch a movie, talk to your kids, talk to yourself, reconnect with old friends on the phone, listen to music. Create an environment you enjoy because you can't escape this process. Cooking is therapy that lets you connect with the most feminine side of you.

If you treat it as a rigid task of batch cooking, sigh over dishes, and hate every minute of it, of course you're not going to be motivated to do it. Sure, not every meal prep is going to be a pleasurable three-hour ordeal. Some are going to be short and sweet; other times you get to spend more time with your food. Either way, make it a joyous experience.

HERE ARE MY TOP MEAL PREP TIPS:

1. Sundays are usually an awesome day to dedicate to meal prep. I also suggest an additional mid-week day to make sure that your meals are fresh and fun. The key is to not move the date and to stay consistent with meal prepping. You'll notice how skipping one hour of meal prep is going to accumulate to wasting time throughout the week in delis, Starbucks, and wishing you actually did it. When you cook twice per week, you never run out of food, and you never get bored with your meals.

2. After you dedicate your time to meal prep, make sure that you're cooking meals you actually LOVE and will want to eat. A common complaint about meal prep is that our meals don't look good, and we actually don't want to eat them. Macros are here to give you the food freedom and the flexibility to eat the foods you LOVE, so make them count. Remember, you eat with your eyes first. It has to look appealing, otherwise when you open the container, it's like, "Yuck, I don't want that." Put your protein and carbs on top of roasted vegetables. Dress it up with spices and greens.

Your food has to look sexy! Like YOU!

3. If you fear getting bored with the same food over and over, alternate your proteins. Meaning, one day cook chicken and turkey for lunch and dinner, and the next time cook fish and steak, and after that prep chicken and fish. There are so many healthy sources of protein to go around. I don't want you to just eat chicken and chicken with chicken on top. The same actually goes for your grains and your vegetables. There are so many choices to choose from that it's virtually unlimited.

THERE ARE A COUPLE OF WAYS YOU CAN DO YOUR MEAL PREP …

One way is to purchase all of the food at once, cook all of the food at once, and distribute it in meals by containers. This works best if you're going to eat most of the meals on the go and away from the house. I suggest that you plan your dinner meals to make warm and fresh, but if you choose to put them in containers, awesome. This way you aren't tempted to swing by the drive-though for something easy on the way home, or you avoid coming home and eating half of the pantry.

Another way is to cook only lunches and snacks ahead of time if you choose to do your breakfasts and dinners at home. Making breakfast at home provides an opportunity to sit down and start your day with mindfulness about your food. I love this because it allows me to take the time to sit and really enjoy the food. I also take my sweet time sipping coffee or tea, while relaxing with my planner to get organized. If you don't have the luxury of a quiet morning, you can always freeze your protein shake ingredients and throw them in a blender in the morning. Again, this leaves you making dinners at home every night. I pre-cut all of the vegetables, so take this opportunity to put them in a frying pan or bake them with my choice of protein. This again adds the element of mindfulness to my day of cooking, and really takes care of my body and my mind.

If you spend most of your time at home with the kids, or work from home and you don't mind all of the cooking throughout the day, you can always pre-cut all of your vegetables, pre-cook your protein, and then just make all of your meals at home one at a time.

BONUS TIP: I also suggest that you plan accordingly and have easy snacks in your car, your purse, or as a last resort at the office. Meetings run late, traffic happens, we forget meals at home, we oversleep. Grab single-serving nuts, natural protein bars, natural beef jerky, or a piece of fruit for easy on-the-go snack options.

MEAL PREP KITCHEN ESSENTIALS:

GLASS FOOD-STORAGE CONTAINERS

Healthy eating can be made a lot easier if you cook your meals in advance. To do this, you're going to need a lot of glass food-storage containers. We recommend Rubbermaid containers, as they resist stains, are BPA free, and are stackable.

COLLAPSIBLE MEASURING CUPS

Along with the need for the previously mentioned digital food scale, you're going to want to get measuring cups to add spices to dishes, to add almond or coconut milk to smoothies, or to measure out grains. Good Cook has a great set of collapsible silicone measuring cups to save space in your drawers.

TINFOIL

Your new healthy diet will more than likely include a lot of roasting because it's one of the healthier cooking methods. Because of this, you're going to often need good quality tinfoil so juices don't run onto the oven tray and foods don't stick to the pan.

SPIRALIZER

Love oodles of noodles and can't live without your favorite Italian-inspired recipe? I have a solution for carb lovers like you and me. A spiralizer is a totally awesome tool when it comes to cooking your favorite pasta dishes and making them healthy. Especially great for zucchini or yellow squash.

COUNTERTOP BLENDER

The NutriBullet Blender/Mixer System by Magic Bullet is portable, safe for kids, easy to use, and effortlessly pulverizes fruits, vegetables, superfoods, and protein shakes into a delicious, smooth texture. If you want to make an amazing, easy, on-the-go protein shake, this is the number-one tool to have. What I love about it is that you can interchange lids, and take it with you to drink in the car or at work.

SLOW COOKER

Possibly the most talked about cost-saving gadget, the slow cooker gets rave reviews because it uses a small amount of energy over a long period of time and, therefore, much less electricity than a traditional oven. But it saves money in other ways, too. Slow cooking means you can use cheaper cuts of meat (which become meltingly tender after a full day of cooking at a low temperature) and you'll relinquish takeout, since you'll have a lovely home-cooked meal waiting when you arrive.

TIMER

Sister, I've set off my smoke alarm more times than I care to admit because I forgot to use my food timer. This innocent mistake caused my fair share of funny Pinterest food fails and hundreds of dollars of wasted ingredients. Don't make the same mistake.

MUFFIN PAN

Single-handedly one of the best inventions of humankind when it comes to kitchen gadgets. WHY? Because you can make just about anything in a small portion that's easy to grab on the go. Mini-quiches. You got it. Breakfast muffins? Nailed it. Turkey meatloaf muffins? SOLD! Sister, I'm telling you, a muffin pan is a must.

💡 CHAPTER PRACTICE

To set yourself up for success, organize the tools you'll need for successful meal prep before heading out to the grocery store. Make a list if you're missing any of the tools you need.

Write down 3 ideas for how to make meal prep a fun activity and execute one tonight.

1.

2.

3.

🎙 PODCAST ALERT

Reference the www.sexyfit.com/resources page to listen to the "The Meal Prep" podcast.

YOUR ULTIMATE DINING OUT GUIDE
CHAPTER 19

Dining out and macros, easy! Sure, at times, it might be complex, but it'll teach you a lot of valuable skills. First and foremost, learning to ask what's in your food.

Yes, I'm that annoying friend who's going to ask how the food is prepped: Do they use butter? What kind of sauce is it? I'm also most likely going to say no to bread, ask for dressing on the side, swap veggies, and get an extra serving of protein.

My food, MY way.

You, sister, feel free to do the same.

If you decide to venture out, make sure that you ask about the recipe if you're unclear about the ingredients. In the moment, set aside what people might be thinking of you. It doesn't matter, and they're probably not even thinking anything. The only person at the dinner table you're responsible to make happy is you, so go ahead and ask, sister. I know a lot of us get a bit timid and confused, and don't want to be a pain. At the end of the day, it's your body, you get to choose what to eat and how much to eat. Your waiter doesn't mind; neither does the chef. This isn't a big deal, and it's what they do. Therefore, ask away.

The second skill is how to eat on macros in every situation. Coffee date? Dinner? Date night? Night out with friends? Forgot your food? Business meeting? Traveling?Life happens, macros work.

Previously when you used old dieting techniques it may have felt like you were held prisoner to a meal plan or some diet restriction that was imposed on you. Oftentimes, we get less social because we don't know how to resist temptation or are afraid of overeating at parties. No more. You get to choose and you get to play and you get to LIVE to the fullest.

I often get asked how we can track macros on the food when we're eating out. My recommendation is to stick to the type of meal that we'd typically be having at that time. If it's lunch, what do you usually have for lunch? So as to not send yourself on a roller-coaster, find something similar on the menu to order.

And this right here is an absolute NO-NO! Please don't make a habit out of "I'm eating out today, so infinity macros it is because I don't know what's in there and tomorrow is a new day." That's bogus! If you feel the need to overeat, feel like you've been missing out all of this time on "good food," take a look at how you treat and indulge in food every day. If you never eat good food, you can plan your meal accordingly. If you feel like you're missing out on something, cook better meals for yourself. Dining out is NOT a reason to check out.

TIP: To help you stay within your macros, you can use my favorite **ONE CARB RULE**. Usually when we go out, we have a choice of alcoholic beverage, carbs as a side dish or main dish, bread on the table, and dessert later. All four of those choices together are bound to put you over on your macros. But you can compromise by picking just one carb that you're going to stick to eating at that time. This way you're being sensible with your new plan, and you're able to stay on track with your macros.

I also suggest looking up a menu before going to the restaurant so you can plan your day based on the dinner you might want to have.

If you're going out, this is the only time you can eyeball your macros. THE. ONLY. TIME!

I'm including a cheat sheet for how you can easily eyeball measurements when you're going out. You can find it on the next page. Take a picture of it with your phone and save it for easy reference. After you're done with the meal, after you leave the restaurant, track your macros and move on with the night.

NOTE: After you master the macros approach—about six months to a year later—you can actually start to eyeball your food; until then, measure everything.

ATTENTION:

- DO NOT bring a food scale with you to the restaurant!!!!!
- DO NOT bring your OWN food to the restaurant, either. It doesn't have to be that hard! While it will be accurate, yes, is that really necessary? The answer is NO! You can always ask what the measurement size is for certain dishes on your plate, but please DO NOT bring food with you or bust out a food scale in the middle of a date.

If you eat out a LOT, start making some meals, like breakfast and snacks, at home. Afterward, you can start making lunches, if necessary. You must have some sort of food at home to come back to and eat frequent steady meals at home. You health and your wallet will thank me later.

💡 CHAPTER PRACTICE

Next time you have a dining out experience, purposely ask how the meal is cooked or the ingredients of the meal, just to get in the habit of asking for help when you need it.

On purpose, ask to alter, add, take out an ingredient to fit your macros better. For example, if you're out and order a spinach walnut salad, ask for dressing on the side and to bring walnuts on the side, as well. Yes, it might sound absurd right now, but I just want you to get in the habit of asking for what you need.

📡 PODCAST ALERT

Reference the www.sexyfit.com/resources page to listen to the "Dating Dining Out Survival Trick" podcast.

EVERYDAY OBJECTS AND PORTION SIZES

SIZE MATTERS! What you eat is equally important to how much you eat. Here are some common everyday objects that you can use as visuals to properly estimate portion sizes.

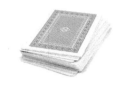

RED MEAT
3 ozs

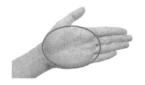

POULTRY
4 ozs

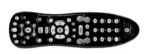

FISH
4 ozs

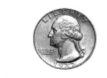

OIL
1 Tablespoon

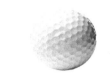

NUT BUTTER
1 Tablespoon

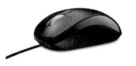

SWEET POTATO
3 ozs

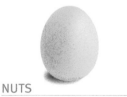

NUTS
¼ cup/1 oz

SALAD DRESSING
2 ozs

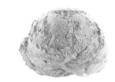

BEANS
½ cup

FRUIT
1 cup

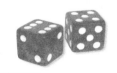

CHEESE
1.5 ozs

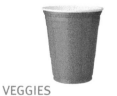

VEGGIES
20 ozs

RICE & GRAINS
½ cup

DARK CHOCOLATE
1.5 ozs

BUTTER
1 teaspoon

WHAT ABOUT TRAVELING?
CHAPTER 20

Whether you travel for work or travel for fun, eating on macros is easy! Just a side note: I love to travel! I actually studied abroad in Vienna, and have traveled most of Europe and the Middle East. I even had a chance to travel to Jerusalem! So cool!

And not only am I a big travel buff, but I also worked internationally and managed to handle my macronutrient lifestyle like a boss—even though it wasn't always easy in places like Milan or Hong Kong! But where there's a will, there's a way. AND, it will require some thinking and some planning.

HERE ARE MY SIMPLE TIPS FOR HOW TO MAKE TRAVEL A FUN EXPERIENCE!

1. ALWAYS TRACK YOUR FOOD
When you're traveling, it's easy to get sidetracked and find excuses for having a bad day with your diet. It's important to be honest with yourself and keep your motivation up by actually doing what you said you would do instead of beating yourself up. Tracking your food while traveling will also make you feel in control.

2. PRE-PURCHASE BARS AND PRE-PACK SHAKES FOR THE DAYS YOU'LL BE TRAVELING
You won't always know what kind of food will be available to you. At times you'll have no idea if there's going to be food available at all. The toughest kinds of macros to find when you're traveling are proteins. To save yourself time and set yourself up for success, take along single-packet protein powder or protein bars. I also provide more options in the following tips.

3. PRE-PLAN YOUR BREAKFASTS
If you're grabbing lunch or dinner at places you're not used to eating at, you may have some digestion and bloating issues. That's why my pre-planned breakfasts always include a green juice. If a standard continental breakfast is served at a hotel, a hard-boiled egg and a piece of toast with butter would be a good solution. You can also research breakfast places so you can plan ahead when you go on vacation. Or you can have pre-prepped hard-boiled eggs and individual packs of plain oatmeal in your room.

4. LOOK UP RESTAURANT OPTIONS BEFORE YOU GO
If you're traveling with co-workers or your family, there will always be a question of where to eat. If you already have that information available, they'll love you because you made a decision for them, and you'll know what you can grab on the go.

5. MAKE A COMMITMENT TO YOURSELF THAT YOU'LL STAY ON TRACK

This is a decision you're making meal by meal, choice by choice, day in and day out. Healthy eating, a healthy lifestyle, and the Sexyfit lifestyle isn't something that you do on "normal" days and then lose it if you're traveling. Vacation time isn't a free-for-all when you get to be naughty, eat everything in sight, and shun nutrient-rich foods.

CHAPTER PRACTICE

Next time you're traveling, keep these foods in mind. You can take this list with you when you're going grocery shopping.

PROTEIN:
- Hard boiled eggs
- Beef jerky (check ingredients to not include sugar)
- Pre-cooked shrimp
- Pre-cooked chicken
- Collagen protein
- Protein bars (6 ingredients or less)

CARBS:
- Veggies, like carrots, celery, cucumbers, peppers, snap peas all travel very well
- Kale chips
- Jicama
- Apples, pears, peaches, bananas, or any other fruit
- Applesauce
- Oatmeal packets
- One-minute rice

FATS:
- Nuts, seeds, nut butters
- Avocado
- Canned olives

TIP: The toughest source of macro to find while traveling is protein, so always have your ready-to-go items ready to go.

PODCAST ALERT

Reference the www.sexyfit.com/resources page to listen to the "Travel Tips to Stay Sexy and Fit" podcast.

CHAPTER 21

WATER

Think of what you need to survive, really just survive. Food? Water? Air? Facebook?

Let's start with water first.

Water is of major importance to all living things; in some organisms, up to 90% of their body weight comes from water. Up to 60% of the human adult body is water. According to H.H. Mitchell, Journal of Biological Chemistry 158, the brain and heart are comprised of 73% water, and the lungs are about 83% water. The skin contains 64% water, muscles and kidneys are 79%, and even the bones are watery at 31%.

WATER SERVES A NUMBER OF ESSENTIAL FUNCTIONS TO KEEP US GOING:

- A vital nutrient to the life of every cell; acts first as a building material
- Regulates our internal body temperature by sweating and respiration
- Carbohydrates and proteins that our bodies use as food are metabolized and transported by water in the bloodstream
- Assists in flushing waste mainly through urination
- Acts as a shock absorber for brain, spinal cord, and fetus
- Forms saliva
- Lubricates joints

I typically recommend that you drink anywhere between ¾ to one gallon DAILY.

Otherwise your body gets dehydrated, especially when you work out regularly. It's essential that you have enough water in your body to improve hydration and fitness performance, and decrease hunger levels.

I also recommend adding electrolytes to your water because your body gets rid of potassium via sweating. The fastest way to restore the level of potassium your body needs is to drink water with electrolytes. They come in handy little packets that you can get at any pharmacy.

One important thing to remember: watch out for sweet drinks. They leave you more hungry and may even make you feel bloated. If you add Crystal Light to your water to make it more flavorful, and you feel like you're bloated for no reason, it's very likely that you're bloated from drinking those flavorful, colorful water drinks. If you don't like drinking plain water and want to add more flavor to it, add lemon, strawberries, or fresh mint to it. It's fresh, has no added sweeteners, and you can improvise and try different flavors knowing that this water is healthy and will help you with hydration.

WAYS TO INCREASE YOUR WATER INTAKE:
- Drink a cup of water right when you wake up (keep a glass of water next to the bed)
- Drink another cup of water when you get to the kitchen
- Fill up a water bottle and drink on your way to work
- Keep a half-gallon bottle of water with you throughout the day, making sure you actually drink it
- At night, drink one cup of water right before going to bed
- If you have a desk job, keep a half-gallon at your desk and drink it throughout the day

SLEEP

We live in a culture where we glorify the absence of sleep as a measure of success.

"I'll sleep when I'm dead."

However, this line of thinking is absolutely detrimental to our fat loss.

One way to think about the function of sleep is to compare it to another of our life-sustaining activities: eating. Hunger is a protective mechanism that has evolved to ensure that we consume the nutrients our bodies require to grow, repair tissues, and function properly. And although it's relatively easy to grasp the role that eating serves — given that it involves physically consuming the substances our bodies need — eating and sleeping are not as different as they might seem, since both are regulated by powerful internal drives.

What's really interesting when it comes to fat loss, cravings, and overall energy levels is that when we're sleep-deprived our body's hormones are off balance. Take leptin and ghrelin, for example. (Don't these hormones sound like "Lord of the Rings" characters?)

Leptin is a hormone that's responsible for how satisfied we are after a meal. When we're sleep-depraved, our body releases LESS leptin, therefore, we're less satisfied with our meals.

Ghrelin, on the other hand, is a hormone that's responsible for our hunger cues. When we lack sleep, our body releases higher amount of ghrelin. As a result, we feel more hungry throughout the day.

Interesting, right?

When we lack sleep, our body produces more hunger-stimulating hormones and LESS of the hormones that make us feel satisfied after a meal.[15]

Insulin and sleep is also something to pay attention to. Within just one night of sleep-deprivation, our body's ability to properly use insulin (the master storage hormone) becomes completely disrupted. In fact, University of Chicago researchers found that insulin sensitivity dropped by more than 30%.

Here's why that's bad: When our insulin is functioning well, fat cells remove fatty acids and lipids from our bloodstream and prevent storage. When we become more insulin-resistant, fats (lipids) circulate in our blood and pump out more insulin. Eventually, this excess insulin ends up storing fat in all of the wrong places, such as tissues like our liver. And this is exactly how we become fat and suffer from diseases like diabetes.

That said, you need to sleep.

HOW MUCH IS OPTIMAL?

Between 7-8 hours is optimal, at times between 9-10 if you're spending a lot of time at the gym. Your body needs to recover and the most efficient recovery typically happens during your much needed snooze time.

ALCOHOL

Alcohol is the centerpiece of any dieting discussion: Can I drink? If so, how much can I drink without hurting my fat-loss progress?

My main concern with alcohol consumption is that when we drink beer, wine, or any spirits, our body gives priority to processing alcohol. Meaning it stops doing pretty much anything else and does this instead:

Ethanol › Acetaldehyde › Acetate › Acetyl-CoA

As the alcohol begins to digest, it splits into two compounds: fat and acetate. The fat is taken through the bloodstream and is stored wherever we tend to deposit fat. The acetate is taken into the bloodstream and used as our primary energy fuel.[16]

This means that rather than burning protein, carbohydrates, or fat as a fuel, our body relies on the acetate for energy. It completely stops burning anything else. Suddenly, we have a surplus of protein, carbs, and fat circulating in our body with nowhere to go.

Contrary to popular belief, however, alcohol is not easily converted to fat. That process is too costly. But all that acetate and acetyl-CoA showing up in the cells does signal to the body that no sugar or fat needs to be burned. So rather than a fat storer, alcohol is more of a fat-burning suppressor. Alcohol also seems to impact brain chemistry, which is known to impact hunger and cravings. It raises dopamine and lowers serotonin. Dopamine is associated with desire and reward. It raises adrenaline and also lowers melatonin. This can negatively impact sleep, which is highly correlated with increased hunger and cravings.

FUN FACT: Red wine contains histamine, which raises cortisol, which increases our appetite. Cortisol causes the body to break down muscle and suppresses recovery from exercise, while low testosterone, which is also a result of drinking alcohol, makes the body less likely to build lean muscle or to burn fat as a fuel. Bad news for us wine lovers.

Alcohol is a non-nutritive calorie source, and it's valued at 7 calories per gram. It'll drain your levels of B vitamins, zinc, magnesium, and others. This can put you at risk for what's known as long-latency diseases or issues. This is when the metabolism suffers slowly over time due to poor nutrition.[16]

Not to mention the excess calories when we're drinking. One glass of wine equals approximately 100 calories. Have you ever just had one glass? Not to mention the sugary cocktails that can run upwards of 400-600 empty calories. Here's my conclusion: Alcohol suppresses fat burning, robs the body of nutrients, releases more cortisol in some instances, racks up empty calories, increases appetite, and decreases the ability to recover from hard workouts.

I would suggest avoiding alcohol completely during the 21-Day Transformation Plan and then only drink up to one to two times per week thereafter. Stick to vodka or gin, since they have the lowest toxicity and caloric intake of all the alcohols.

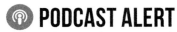 **PODCAST ALERT**

Reference the www.sexyfit.com/resources page to listen to the "Drinking and Fat Loss" and "Why is Water Important" podcasts.

THREE EASY STEPS TO EASE INTO YOUR NEW LIFESTYLE
CHAPTER 22

READY, SET, SEXYFIT!

Okay, sister! You're ready to rock 'n' roll!

Now that you're all ready to go, if you want to give macros a shot and jump into this new lifestyle, START HERE. It'll make the entire process a whole lot easier and stress-free.

STEP 1: SEE WHAT YOU GOT
After tracking for one day, take a look at your macros, based on numbers in grams. You're only looking at protein, carbohydrates, and fats. In this instance, you also want to pay attention to sugar because it'll shoot your carbs really high if a lot of foods you're eating have added sugar.

STEP 2: SWAP 'EM
Swap the food you're already used to eating with unprocessed alternatives. For example, if you're accustomed to enjoying certain sausages with your eggs in the morning, check out the ingredients label. How many ingredients does it have? If it's less than six, no sugar added, and you can pronounce most of the ingredients, keep it. If it has 3,948,579,034,875,390,872 ingredients, other than chicken/pork/beef or whatever it's supposed to have, swap it for a healthier alternative. Everyone is happy. You get to keep your favorite sausages, and your body is happy because it has to process less ingredients.

Another example is yogurt. I'm pro-yogurt if you're not allergic to lactose and if you like your yogurt kinda sour. Yogurt it up, eat it, enjoy it. BUT, your yogurt can't contain 15 food colorings, added jam with five kinds of sugar, and granola made out of wood chips (true story). You aren't going to be any less happy with Greek yogurt to which you added walnuts and berries yourself, and maybe some stevia drops for sweetness. It's still the same meal, just 10 times healthier for you. Note that yogurt is lactose and will always have some sugar, but it shouldn't contain added sugar.

Nutrition isn't about taking everything away and completely disturbing your current habits. It's about first substituting what you're already doing, to make the transition easier and less frustrating.

You can also find the food swap table on the next page. We made it easier for you to swap all of your favorite brands to healthier alternatives.

PROCESSED FOODS AND THEIR REPLACEMENTS

INSTEAD OF:	TRY:
Peanut butter that contains oils, sugars, etc.	Any nut butter with nuts as the only ingredient (salt is also okay)
Sliced, store-bought bread	Homemade or store-bought with 5 ingredients maximum
Cereal	Homemade granola (or protein granola) with minimum ingredients
Frozen, microwave meals	Pre-make and freeze your own meals
Pancake syrup	Real maple syrup
Processed cheese products	Mozzarella or goat cheese
Canned soups	Make your own and freeze
Flavored yogurts	Plain yogurt and add fresh berries
Granola and protein bars	Homemade or store-bought with 5 ingredients maximum
Candy bars	Dark chocolate

STEP 3: ADD IT UP

You're all swapped up and got sugar down to a minimum. At this point, you're probably amazed at how much sugar there was in your daily food choices. NOW it's time to add more food to your daily intake to hit your macros. Most of the women we work with have the hardest time with protein, so consider adding a protein shake or making your protein portions larger in every sitting. All of us are going to end up with a different meal frequency because of our lifestyle, work situation, and family arrangements.

At first, three meals and one snack seems to work best. But you can later break it down into three meals and two snacks, or three meals and three snacks, if you wish. There isn't science to support that if we eat small meals throughout the day the fat loss is far better. However, I'll tell you in my experience of coaching hundreds of women that this seems to be the best way when it comes to managing hunger and preventing sudden lows in blood sugar, which leads to loss of energy and feeling angry at the world. Eating more frequently helps us manage our mood and prevents overeating during the times we actually get to eat.

We've all had those times in our life where we came home and ate half the pantry because we didn't get to eat all day. That's like throwing a giant rock down your digestive system when your body wasn't prepared to digest all of THAT food quite yet.

No matter where you're starting, the above three steps are going to help you MASTER your macros. You'll start to notice over time that your taste buds are changing since you're choosing different foods because you've become more in tune with your hunger cues and what kind of nutrients satisfy you more.

MACROS AND INTUITIVE EATING
CHAPTER 23

Sister, I'm so thrilled and grateful that I'm able to share my strategies with you. The macronutrient style of eating has helped me overcome my challenges with the traditional dieter's mindset, helped cure my eating disorder, and, ultimately, allowed me to return to a place of peace with food and myself. I know that you're probably wondering, "Am I going to have to track macros for the rest of my life?"

The answer is "Yes" and "NO." This style of eating is a tool for you to use in many different situations – when you want to achieve a transformation, simply learn to nourish your body with enough nutrients, become a runner, or put on more muscle mass. My goal with writing this book was to educate you, and show you the exact steps to help you transform your relationship with your body and your food, AND achieve total food freedom.

Yes you'll need to track your macros for at least six weeks to fully help your body adjust to the amount of food your it needs to have a healthy metabolism, for your energy levels to drastically improve, and to see dramatic results in how your body looks and feels. I suggest 12 weeks of daily macros tracking for full benefits, and to also see your patterns and recurring gaps.

After 12 weeks, you'll have learned what your portion sizes are, how your body responds to nutrients, which food combos work best for you, how to fuel YOUR body for success, and you'll have created solid habits around meal planning and meal prepping. Feel free to retire MyFitnessPal and see how your new habits stick. You can start to eyeball portion sizes (I attached a table), count in your head what nutrients you need to fill your macros, and overall stay mindful of all of the habits that you've learned.

Nutrition is an effort task that's so simple and yet we've made it so complex. Based on the hundreds of women we coach, 12 weeks is a sufficient amount of time to reap all of the benefits that macros provide for you, and you can be set free to make your own decisions based on what you know about yourself.

I, too, rarely track macros now. Only when I feel off with my energy levels, or I feel like I'm eating way too little or way too much (holidays). Feel free to use it loosely for a week or two if you're feeling off or if you're starting a new fitness program.

Macros are easy and fun if you allow them to be. Learn what works for you. Listen to your body, and you're now set free.

NUTRITION FAQ'S

WHAT ARE MACROS?
Macros are macronutrients—the nutrients our bodies need in larger quantities. Those are: protein, carbohydrates, and fats, measured in grams.

DO I NEED TO "EAT CLEAN?"
No, you don't have to eat "clean." Weight loss majorly depends on the type of calories in vs. calories out, but there are other factors, as well, such as vitamins, minerals that micronutrients give you, and hormones that regulate our bodies. Eat a majority of things that are healthy, yes, but also eat what you ENJOY—if that's tilapia and veggies, great! As long as by the end of the night you're hitting your calorie and macro targets, that's what matters for weight and body composition—but the composition of your macros DOES matter, as well.

WILL I ALWAYS HAVE TO COUNT MACROS?
We recommend that you stick to counting macros for at least 21 days per the transformation plan. Ideally, you want to track macros for 12 weeks to see your patterns, understand what nutrients your body craves, and to help you understand how your body works. After that, you get to practice a more intuitive eating approach to nutrition.

I CRAVE CHOCOLATE ALL OF THE TIME.
IS THIS NORMAL?
If you crave chocolate, you're most likely deficient in magnesium. Start a magnesium supplement in the form of a powder or pill.

WILL CARBS OR FAT MAKE ME FAT?
No.

DO I NEED TO EAT EXTRA CALORIES IF I'M BREASTFEEDING?
First of all, congratulations on your baby! If you're breastfeeding, you may want to add somewhere between 200-500 extra calories, but it's going to depend on the level of your activity and your starting stats. An average breastfeeding woman who wants to lose weight should eat between 1,500-1,800 calories, but it can vary. Please always consult your doctor first.

CAN I STILL DRINK ALCOHOL?
Alcohol is metabolized by the body in a slightly different manner than any other macronutrient. It has 7 calories per gram and should be tracked. Excessive consumption may stall progress (because your liver is processing the alcohol and slowing the other processes down), but in moderation—and by moderation I mean 1-2 drinks per week MAX (tracked)—it's fine.

DO I NEED TO CHANGE MY MACROS ON REST DAYS?
No. Rest days are already factored in, so just stay consistent!

SHOULD I TRACK MY VITAMINS/SUPPLEMENTS/ FISH OIL/GUM/SPICES?
Most supplements aren't caloric, but if you want to keep track of your micronutrients as well, then yes, track the supplements, too. The only one we do recommend always tracking is fish oil; since it's pure fat, it adds up.

HOW OFTEN SHOULD I CHANGE MY MACROS?

You should change them if your goal changes or if progress stalls for more than two to three weeks.

DO I NEED SUPPLEMENTS?

Supplements are just that: supplementary. However, you should always consult your doctor and ask for a FULL blood work panel to find out if you're in need of certain vitamins or minerals. Protein powder is great if it helps you hit your protein goals, but it is by no means required — just personal preference.

DOES IT MATTER WHEN I EAT? HOW MANY MEALS I EAT? CAN I EAT CARBS/PROTEIN, CARBS/FAT, PROTEIN/FAT TOGETHER?

Meal timing, frequency, and composition have very little bearing on body weight and body composition as long as you hit your macro and calorie targets by the end of the day.

WHAT ABOUT INTERMITTENT FASTING?

This is fine to do but is purely personal preference concerning meal timing, and won't help you hit your goals any faster or better. A lot of women notice that they do have more energy during a workout and perform better when they eat something before exercising.

SHOULD I COUNT NET CARBS OR TOTAL CARBS?

We always count total carbs. That ALREADY includes sugar and fiber.

DOES MY SUGAR INTAKE MATTER?

We recommend you eat no more than 25 grams of added sugar per day and also limit fruits with a high glycemic index.

HOW SHOULD I WEIGH THINGS? DO I NEED TO WEIGH EVERYTHING?

Yes, you need to weigh everything — on a digital kitchen scale in grams. Do you need to weigh everything forever, no. But you do need to learn.

I'M STUFFED AND CAN'T EAT ANY MORE, BUT STILL HAVE CALORIES LEFT. HELP!

There's no need to force-feed yourself, but try not to be too much under! Try to eat bigger meals during the first part of the day, so you won't be left with 800 calories to eat at 8 p.m.

HOW CLOSE DO I NEED TO BE TO MY MACROS?

Try to stay within +/- 5 grams of fats and +/- 10 grams of protein and carbs every day.

I WENT WAY OVER ON ONE MACRO BUT STILL HAVE CALORIES/MACROS LEFT. HELP!

Carbs and protein have 4 calories/gram, fat has 9 calories/gram. So, for instance, if you went over on fat by 4 grams, that's 36 calories, so subtract 36 calories ideally from carbs first = 9 grams. Try to hit protein and fat first, and if you come under on anything, let it be carbs. Carbs have no required minimum by the body, but protein and fat do.

HOW MUCH WATER SHOULD I DRINK?

At least .66 ounces/body weight in pounds per day. If you're 100 pounds, that'd be 66 ounces/day. If you're severely overweight, it can be less.

SHOULD I WEIGH MY MEATS/VEGGIES/WHATEVER ON ELSE ON EARTH RAW OR COOKED?

Raw will always be more accurate, but here's the general rule: If you weigh it raw, then log it in MyFitnessPal, etc. as raw. For example: "Raw Chicken Breast, Boneless/Skinless — 400 grams"; OR, if you weigh it cooked, then log it as cooked: "Cooked Chicken Breast, Boneless/Skinless — 400 grams."

WAIT, GUM AND CINNAMON AND NO-STICK COOKING SPRAY REALLY HAVE CALORIES?!

Yes, everything has calories in it.

WHAT SCALE SHOULD I GET?!

Any digital kitchen scale that measures IN GRAMS and has a "tare" button is great. (A tare button resets the zero of the scale display when an empty container is placed on the weighing platform.)

I'M HUNGRY. IS THAT NORMAL?
You're eating on a calorie deficit, so, yes, being hungry sometimes while your body is adjusting is normal.

CAN MY BODY ONLY DEAL WITH SO MUCH PROTEIN AT A TIME?
We absorb all of the protein we eat, but, depending on what we're doing with our time, how old we are, how large or small we are, how active we are, how much we're lifting, and how much stress we're under, we use the protein we absorb in different ways and proportions. It's safe to consume up to 50 grams of protein at once.[17]

SHOULD I BE TAKING A FAT BURNER?
No. No. No. It's useless and a waste of money. Caffeine will do the same thing in giving you energy. The BEST and ONLY effective fat burner is a calorie deficit and exercise.

SHOULD I BE TAKING BCAAs?
If you take a protein powder regularly, taking BCAAs separately is unnecessary. Protein powder already contains these branched chain amino acids.

SHOULD I BE TAKING CLA?
You can. There are studies that prove that taking a certain dose of CLA can help you reduce body fat.[18]

CAN I DRINK COFFEE?
Sure, why not? One to two cups of coffee daily is a safe amount to drink.

CAN I CHEW GUM?
Yes, you can.

HOW DO I CARB CYCLE?
Carb cycling is eating more carbohydrates on some days (High Carb days) to help promote muscle growth and eating less carbohydrates on other days (Low Carb days) to help minimize fat gain and even promote fat loss. You alternate High Carb days on intense workout days with Low Carb days on easy workout/rest days. I don't recommend carb cycling to start with. This topic could be a whole other book, so get the basics down first.

WHAT'S YOUR TAKE ON CARB LOADING?
Carb loading is known for helping to prepare for a race/long and intense workout that's at least 90 minutes long. However, studies have shown that higher glycogen levels don't necessarily occur after classical carbohydrate-loading procedures, so carb loading is unnecessary.[19] Again, get the basics down first.

DO I HAVE TO TRACK EVERYTHING I EAT?
Yes, you do. A lot of times mindless snacking causes us to overeat, and sometimes we can consume up to 500 calories in taking bites of food throughout the day—a bite of pizza, bite of candy bar, eating our child's chicken nuggets leftovers. So it's best to stick to actual meals and tracking everything.

DO I FOLLOW CALORIES OR MACROS ON MYFITNESSPAL? I HIT MY MACROS, BUT I'M OVER/UNDER ON CALORIES!
Follow macros (in grams; don't look at the pie chart, unless you're done with your macros for the day). Sometimes the macros are rounded up, sometimes the nutritional labels are wrong, so macros don't always add up in MFP.

I HAVE ____ GRAMS OF PROTEIN/CARBS/FAT LEFT … WHAT DO I EAT?!
It's really up to you. As long as the food you eat has the macros you're short of and is minimally processed.

WHAT ABOUT GREEN JUICE REPLACEMENTS?
Fresh foods are always best, but if you need a little green boost on days you can't eat enough vegetables, you can definitely add a green juice supplement.

HOW DO I COUNT GREEN JUICE?
It's nearly impossible to say exactly how many calories are in green juice, but we can make a close approximation. Simply measure out how many ounces (there are 8 ounces in a cup) of each ingredient is contained in the juice. Then add it up to get the final number.

I'M NEVER HUNGRY AND CAN'T EAT ALL OF MY MACROS. NOW WHAT?

Most likely the reason you're never hungry is because your metabolism slowed down due to frequent dieting and restricting of foods/limiting to low calorie numbers. Start eating small 200-300 calorie meals every three to four hours, and in no time you'll find it a lot easier to fill your macros.

I WORK LONG DAYS AND DON'T ALWAYS GET TO EAT. DO I HAVE TO EAT SIX TIMES A DAY?

You absolutely don't have to eat six times a day. You need to make a routine that works for you. If it's six meals, great; if it's four, great, as well. The goal is to fill your macros by having balanced meals (that have all three macros in them) and to never be hungry.

I DON'T EAT BREAKFAST. WHAT DO I DO?

If you aren't hungry in the morning, it's most likely due to a life-long habit of not having breakfast. Start with having something small in the morning, like half of a banana or half of a piece of toast with avocado, and see how it feels. Having breakfast or not is entirely up to you.

I'M HUNGRY ALL OF THE TIME. IT'S SO ANNOYING! HELP!

There are usually two reasons for being hungry. First, your activity level is higher than the amount of food you consume, so in this case you need to reevaluate your macros. Second, you don't balance your meals, which causes your insulin levels to spike and then crash, which in turn will make you feel hungry all of the time. To prevent this from happening, make sure you have all three macros at every meal. This will make your meals balanced and will keep you fuller longer.

THAT'S TOO MUCH PROTEIN!

If you're struggling to reach your daily protein goals, make sure your breakfast has at least 25-30 grams of protein; make sure you have protein at every meal; and start adding high-protein foods to your diet, such as egg whites, edamame beans, black bean pasta, and others.

THAT'S TOO MUCH FAT!

If you're struggling to reach your daily fat goals, there's an easy fix. Add more healthy fats into your diet, such as nuts and seeds, avocado, coconut milk, and, of course, nut butters.

I REMEMBER READING SOMEWHERE ABOUT THE TESTING THAT ZLATA RECOMMENDS TO GET DONE AT A NATUROPATH. COULD YOU REFERENCE THE FILE? I'M SETTING UP AN APPOINTMENT, AND I WANT TO KNOW WHAT TO ASK FOR.

You need t4, t3, and Cortisol tests to be done, and I also always suggest that you know what your food allergies are, as well. Reference the www.sexyfit.com/resources page to listen to the "Adrenal Fatigue | How To Recover Naturally" and "Overcoming Adrenal Fatigue and Feeling Like Yourself Again with Dr. Andrea Maxim" podcasts.

I EAT A LOT OF VEGGIES THROUGHOUT THE DAY, AND THEY'RE KILLING MY CARBS MACRO.

Foods like cucumbers, leafy greens, zucchini — no. Eat all you want. Veggies like tomatoes, bell peppers, and such have sugars and, therefore, are higher in carbs. Count those for sure. Check MyFitnessPal for macros. Veggies like broccoli, Brussels sprouts, etc. will have carbs in them.

DO WE HAVE TO FOLLOW THE MEAL PLAN OR IS IT MORE IMPORTANT TO FOLLOW OUR MACROS? I'M HAVING A HARD TIME EATING THE AMOUNT OF CALORIES I'M SUPPOSED TO AND ALSO STAYING WITHIN CLOSE RANGE OF MY MACROS.

Follow the macros count to the T. Not "within" macros but "to the T" macros. That meal plan is a general outline of what you can eat, but you make it fit your macros count. Which is why there's no macros count/portions on the meal plan. Sorta kinda following the program isn't following it at all.

21-DAY TRANSFORMATION MEAL PLAN

SISTER, WE ARE READY TO GO!

Now it's time to dive into the 21-Day Transformation Sample Meal Plan and the 40-plus simple recipes that our Sexyfit team has created for this book. Every recipe that you see here was carefully thought through to make sure it's packed with flavor, easy to make, and fits your budget. You'll see that we use similar ingredients in many recipes because eating healthy doesn't have to be expensive. We created these recipes in a way that you don't have to spend hours in the kitchen, prepping, sorting, or trying to chase down a weird ingredient that's only sold at a store across town.

You have a few options for yummy, easy breakfasts: Best Avocado Toast Ever and Soulful Sunday Pancakes are my absolute favorites. What I love about having pancakes on Sunday is that you can make a large batch and freeze them to eat throughout the week for breakfast or a snack. It saves so much time! Other recipes include Tutti Frutti Muffin Cups and Green and Lean Quiche. What I love about these two meals is that they're very easy to take along with you if you'd like to eat breakfast at work or if you're in a hurry to leave the house. Not to mention, they're delish! All of the oatmeal options here are real time-savers. Remember, you're not limited on your topping options and what you choose to mix into your oatmeal – it's completely up to you as long as it fits your macros.

For lunches, you'll see that you have a few different options, as well. We added carbohydrates in lunches for those days when you have a lighter breakfast. That way, by the time lunch comes around, you'll be ready to eat all of your yummy carbs. We also planned the lunch recipes in such a way that you can reuse the protein source you had the night before in a new dish. This way, healthy eating never gets boring because it doesn't have to be — and it's delicious and super simple. Wait until you try the Tuna Salad recipe or my mom's special Salmon Tartare.

For dinners, we wanted to make sure that you and your whole family can enjoy these meals together. If you have company, they don't have to eat "diet" food with you.

What about sauces and dressings? I'm SO glad you asked. Sauces and dressings are a common issue when we start our journey, mainly because ketchup and ranch are delicious. But, unfortunately, many of the options you see in the supermarket are just … ahem, garbage. We made sure that in this book you have your favorite recipes done the Sexyfit way, and we're sure you'll love them.

You'll also notice that you have flex options for your snacks. You can either choose from the snack recipes we provided, or have simpler options, like an apple and almonds/almond butter or carrots and hummus. The 21-Day Transformation Sample Meal Plan is created around having three big meals a day and one small snack. If you choose to have five to six meals per day, just make sure to track your portion sizes accordingly. It's whatever fits your macros, sister.

Oh, oh, oh, and because I know you love chocolate, brownies, and other delicious sweet treats, keep flipping pages because the recipes included here are to die for. I seriously could do a princess twirl about how excited I am for you to try these recipes, test out this meal plan, and sit back and go, "THIS IS SO EASY and SO DELICIOUS!"

You don't have to follow this plan to the T but stick as closely to it as a possible. We gave you two weeks' worth of meal plans to follow, and you get to create the third week all on your own — it's all about being hands-on and learning how to eat for YOU.

If you like certain recipes, and like to eat the same foods over and over until you want to switch to something else, pick the recipes you like and go for it. If you like a good variety, this should be an easy plan for you. If you've never set foot in the kitchen and have no idea how it all works, I'm not a trained chef who went to Le Cordon Bleu to be able to make these recipes, either. If I can do it, you can do it, and if hundreds of women could do it, you can manage, too. Continue to show up for yourself, and remember that cooking is so easy and so natural to us. It's the most feminine and soulful thing we can do ... well, after shoe shopping, but you know what I mean. Every woman CAN cook. If the meal doesn't quite look like the picture right away, give yourself a break. I'm going to tell you the truth here: It took a team of prop stylists, food stylists, and incredibly talented photographers and designers to make these recipes look sooooo delicious. Do your best and forget the rest; eventually you'll get there. If you've been cooking for quite some time, feel free to tweak, change ingredients, and alter the recipes as you wish — but just make sure they fit your macros.

Remember that you can substitute macros within each category.

If you see a chicken recipe, it can be made with turkey or likewise. If you don't like zucchini, use cauliflower or any other vegetable instead. If you don't like veggies, use any of the sauces that are provided in the end of the recipe chapter to spice things up before you get used to the taste. Your taste buds do and will change. If you're allergic to nuts or anything else on the menu, substitute with foods you aren't allergic to within the same category.

And what if you're going out with friends or craving something?

If you're going out with friends, order a meal that's closest to the provided meal plan or a dish that sounds good to you at the time. Track your macros and make it fit. If you have cravings or want to fit in any of the yummy desserts in section four, make room in your macros by adjusting what you have planned. If you want a piece of cake that someone brought into the break room, look at your MFP and plan accordingly. If it doesn't fit, IT DOESN'T fix. It doesn't mean, oh, whatever, it's macros, it sorta fits; if it doesn't fit, it doesn't fix. This is flexible enough to where you aren't missing out on anything. Dreams don't work unless you do. Make it fit.

NOTE: All the provided macros are approximate. You have to adjust your portion sizes based on YOUR macros. The more you do this, the more you know how much and what to eat. Use this as a sample and work in some your favorite recipes as you go!

SAMPLE MEAL PLAN: 4 MEALS PER DAY

	SU	M	TU	W	TH	F	SA

WEEK 1

	SU	M	TU	W	TH	F	SA
BREAKFAST	Soulful Sunday Pancakes	Best Avocado Toast Ever	Nutty and Nice Overnight Oats	Not Your Mama's Omelette	Best Avocado Toast Ever	Nutty and Nice Overnight Oats	Not Your Mama's Omelette
LUNCH	Hometown Teryaki Salmon Bolw	Tuna Salad You'll Actually Like	Hometown Teryaki Salmon Bowl	Caliente Chicken Tacos	Tuna Salad You'll Actually Like	Hometown Teryaki Salmon Bowl	Caliente Chicken Tacos
SNACK	Any Snack Option	Any Snack Option	Any Snack Option	Any Snack Option	Any Snack Option	Any Snack Option	Any Snack Option
DINNER	For The Love of Peaches Pizza or Dancing Shrimp Avocado Salad + Dessert	One Pan Salmon	Dancing Shrimp Avocado Salad	One Pan Salmon	One Pan Chicken	Dancing Shrimp Avocado Salad	Three Best Friends: Sweet Slide, Zucchini Mini, Pinapple Man Mini Burgers

WEEK 2

	SU	M	TU	W	TH	F	SA
BREAKFAST	Take Me For A Spinich Waffles	Life Is A Peach Oatmeal Bowl	Tutti Frutti Muffin Cups	Tutti Frutti Muffin Cups	Nutty and Nice Overnight Oats	Green and Lean Quiche	Green and Lean Quiche
LUNCH	Not Your Average Chang's Lettuce Wraps	Chicken Oodle Noodle	Colorful 'N' Lean Shrimp Pasta	Fajita Mamacita Salad	Fajita Mamacita Salad	Svetlana's Salmon Tartar	Not Your Average Chang's Lettuce Wraps
SNACK	Any Snack Option	Any Snack Option	Any Snack Option	Any Snack Option	Any Snack Option	Any Snack Option	Any Snack Option
DINNER	For The Love of Peaches Pizza	Dancing Shrimp Avocado Salad	Sweet Shashlik Kebabs	Sexyfit Style Chicken Nuggets	Raw and Real Salmon Salad	Turkey 'Shroomburger	Three Best Friends: Sweet Slide, Zucchini Mini, Pinapple Man Mini Burgers

SAMPLE MEAL PLAN: 4 MEALS PER DAY

	SU	M	TU	W	TH	F	SA
WEEK 3							
BREAKFAST							
LUNCH							
SNACK							
DINNER							

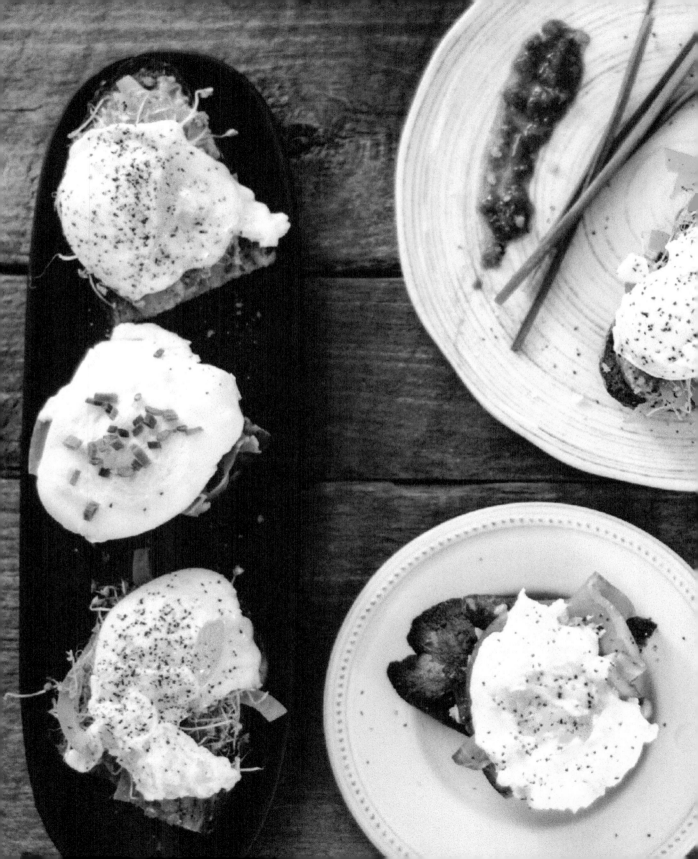

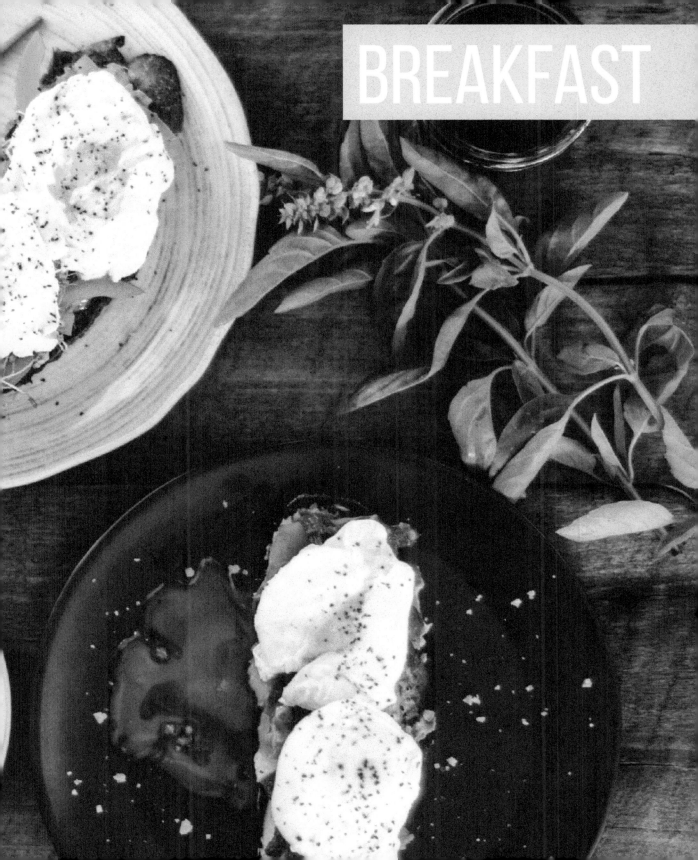

BREAKFAST

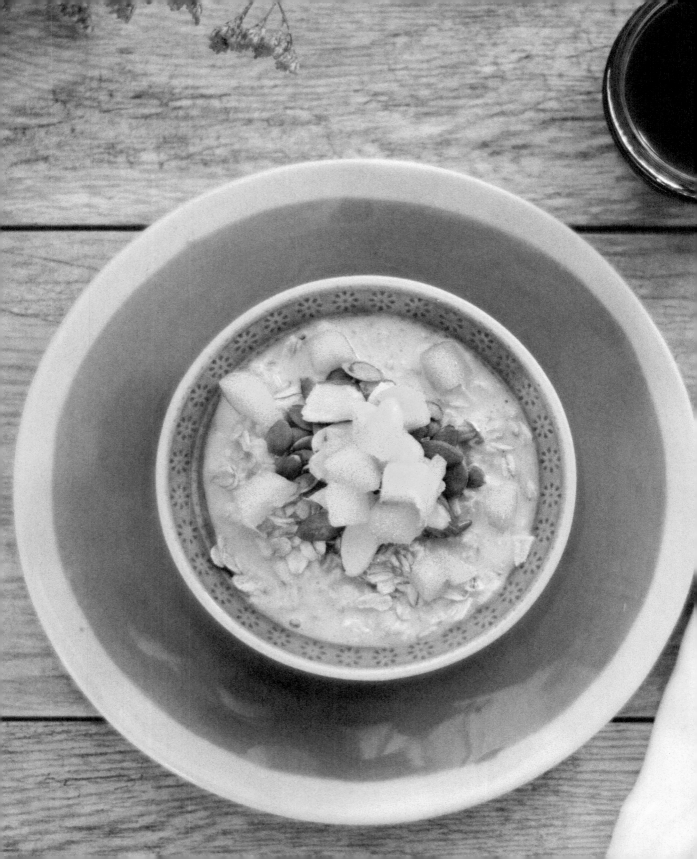

LIFE IS A PEACH OATMEAL BOWL

SERVES 2 | CALORIES PER SERVING 239

INGREDIENTS

½ C Steel cut oats
1 C Coconut milk – light
1 scoop Vanilla protein powder
1½ tsp Chia seeds
1 T Pumpkin seeds
1 T Slivered almonds
1 Peach

MACROS

Protein 16.9 g
Carbs 22 g
Fat 9.9 g

DIRECTIONS

> Cook oats according to the directions on the package, using coconut milk in place of water. Stir in the protein powder right before taking the oats off the stove.
> Cut peach into small cubes.
> Add the chia and pumpkin seeds, almonds, and peach to the bowl.

CHEF'S TIP:

All seeds are beneficial for your health, as they're high in omega-3 fatty acids. You can substitute chia and pumpkin seeds with flax seeds, sunflower seeds, or hemp seeds.

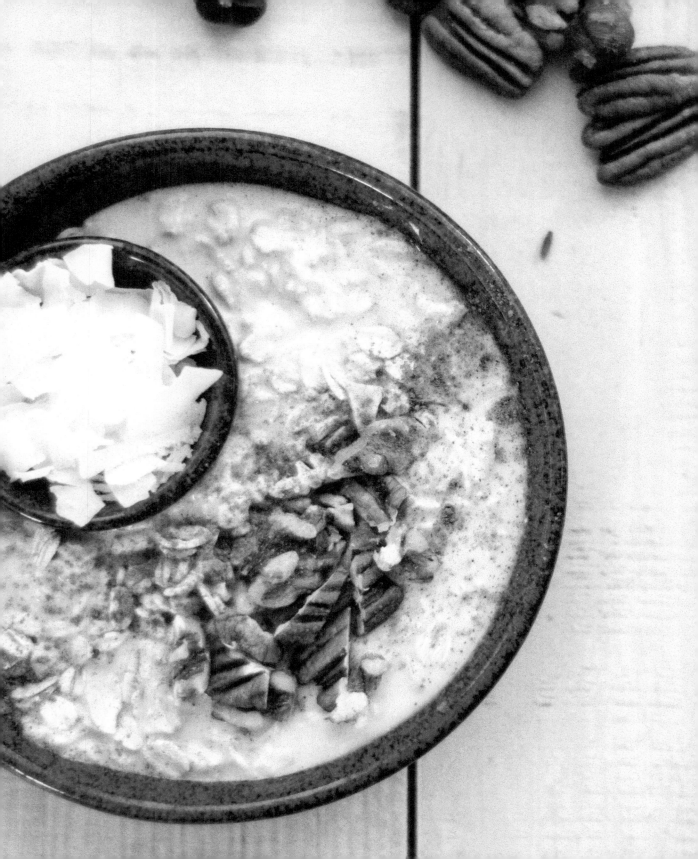

NUTTY AND NICE OVERNIGHT OATS

SERVES 2 | CALORIES PER SERVING 219

INGREDIENTS

½ C Steel cut oats
1 C Coconut milk – light
1 scoop Protein powder – vanilla
6 Hazelnuts – whole
1 T Walnuts – chopped
1 T Coconut – unsweetened,
(shaved)
Cinnamon – ground

MACROS

Protein 15.9 g
Carbs 15.3 g
Fat 11.1 g

DIRECTIONS

> Add dry oats, coconut milk, and protein powder into a container. Mix well and place in the refrigerator overnight.

> Mix well again and pour into a bowl. Add hazelnuts, walnuts, and coconut, and sprinkle with cinnamon.

CHEF'S TIP:

If you choose to add berries, do so when you're ready to eat in the morning. They always taste better fresh.

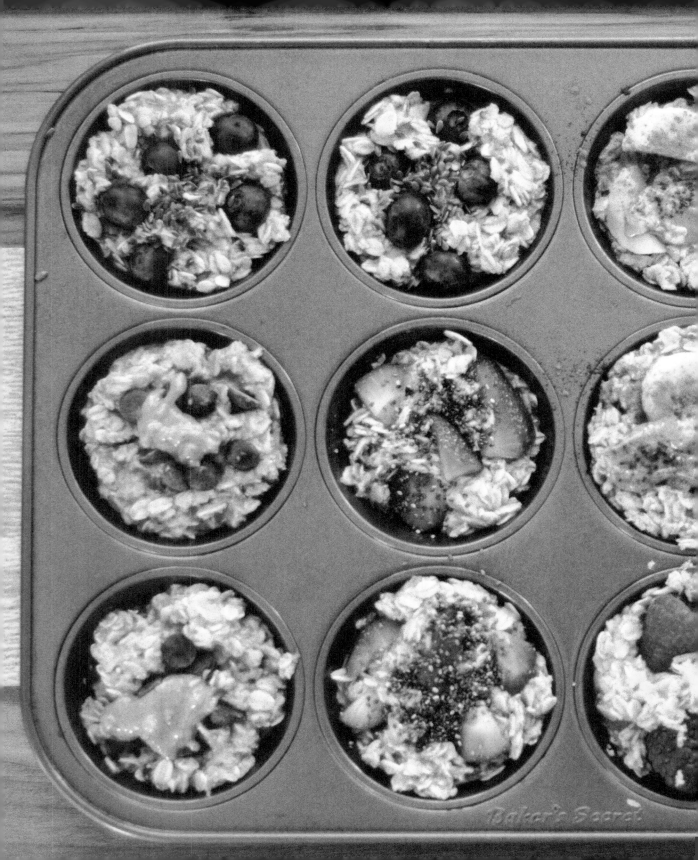

TUTTI FRUTTI MUFFIN CUPS

SERVES 9 (1 MUFFIN PER SERVING) | CALORIES PER SERVING SEE BELOW

INGREDIENTS

3 C Old-fashioned rolled oats
(not quick)
¼ C Maple syrup
2 scoops Protein powder – vanilla
2 tsp Cinnamon – ground
2 tsp Baking powder
1 tsp Salt
¾ C Almond milk
2 eggs
½ C Applesauce
2 tsp Vanilla extract

DIRECTIONS

> Preheat oven to 375° F.
> Beat the eggs and add all liquid ingredients.
> In a separate bowl, mix together all dry ingredients.
> Add the egg mixture to the bowl with the dry ingredients and mix well.
> Divide the oats mixture between 9 muffin cups.
> Add the toppings of choice, squeezing them into the oats mixture.
> Bake for 30-40 minutes, or until the top becomes golden and an inserted toothpick comes out clean.

TOPPING IDEAS WITH MACROS BREAKDOWNS (PER EACH MUFFIN)

> 5 Blueberries and ½ T Flaxseed
Calories 150, Protein 4.5 g, Carbs 27.5 g, Fat 3.1 g

> 5 Chocolate chips and ½ T Peanut butter
Calories 154, Protein 4.6 g, Carbs 27.1 g, Fat 3.7 g

> 1½ Strawberries and ½ T Chia seeds
Calories 149, Protein 4.5 g, Carbs 27.2 g, Fat 3.1 g

> ¼ Banana, ½ T Almond butter, and Cinnamon sprinkles
Calories 156, Protein 4.5 g, Carbs 28 g, Fat 3.6 g

> 4 Raspberries and ½ tsp Lemon zest
Calories 142, Protein 4.2 g, Carbs 26.6 g, Fat 2.7 g

CHEF'S TIP:

To increase the protein content, add 3 T of protein powder. You can use unflavored powder or vanilla flavored to make your muffins sweeter.

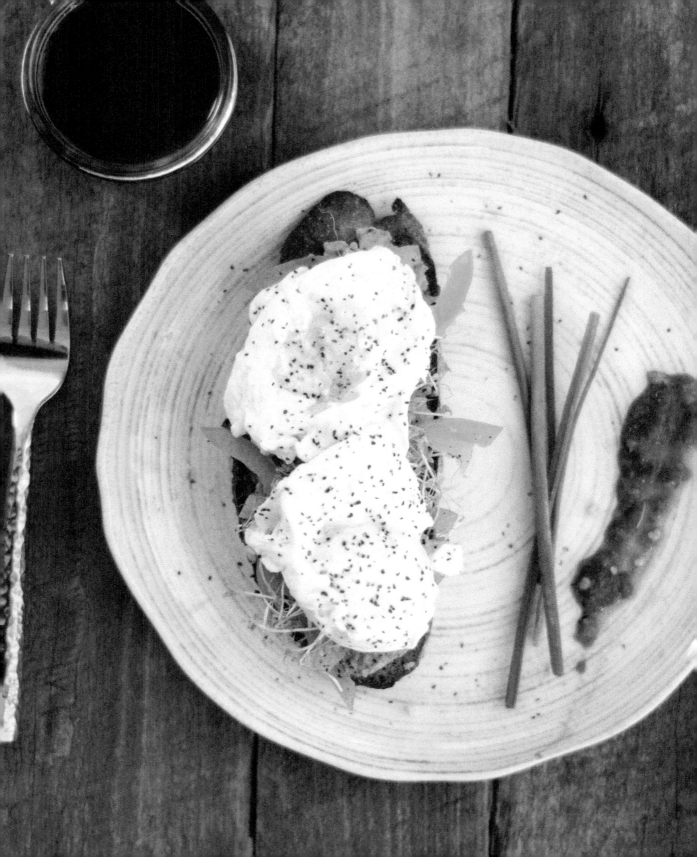

BEST AVOCADO TOAST EVER

SERVES 1 | CALORIES PER SERVING 126*

INGREDIENTS

1 slice of Artisan
whole wheat bread
1 oz Avocado
¼ Bell pepper – orange
Egg (poached, fried, or boiled)
⅓ C Sprouts

MACROS

Protein 2.8 g
Carbs 3.7 g
Fat 8.8 g

*NOTE: This value will depend
on the type of bread you're
using, so the macros are
for the toppings only – add
the macros from your bread
to the macros above.

DIRECTIONS

> Toast a slice of bread in the toaster or toaster oven.
> Spread avocado on the toast.
> Arrange bell peppers and sprouts.
> Add the egg on top.

CHEF'S TIP:

A poached egg adds more flavor to Avocado Toast. If you don't know how to poach an egg, search for videos on YouTube. After a couple of times, you'll be a pro!

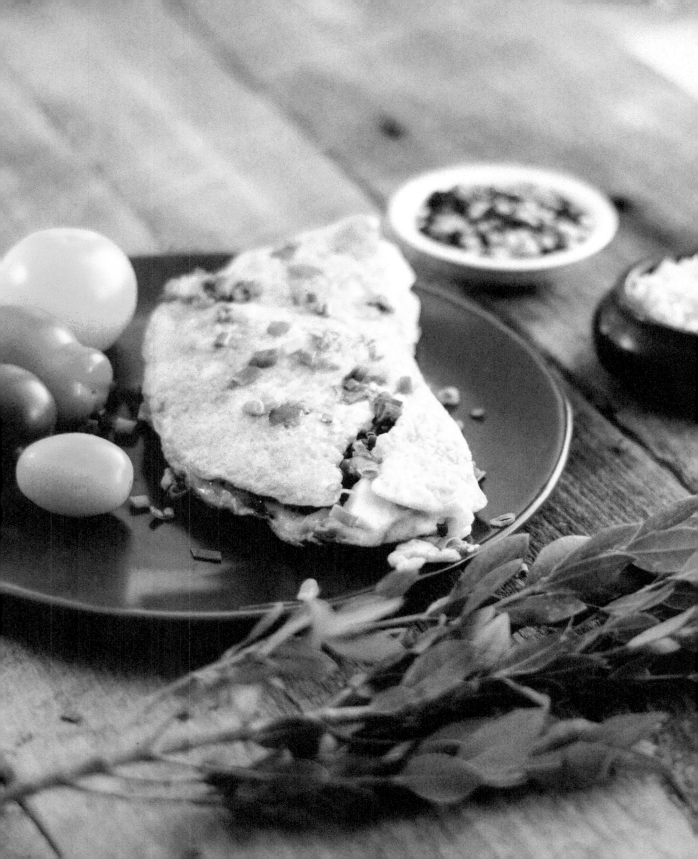

NOT YOUR MAMA'S OMELETTE

SERVES 1 | CALORIES PER SERVING 249

INGREDIENTS

3 Artichokes hearts
3 Mushrooms – sliced
½ Tomato – chopped
1 oz Feta cheese – crumbled
1 Egg
6 T Egg whites
Green onions – chopped

MACROS

Protein 29.1 g
Carbs 19.4 g
Fat 9.8 g

DIRECTIONS

› Preheat a nonstick pan on medium heat.
› Beat the egg and egg whites together, and pour mixture into the pan.
› Add artichokes, mushrooms, tomato, green onions, and feta cheese.
› Stir once, then turn to low heat and cover the pan with a lid.
  Cook for about 5 minutes until eggs are firm.

CHEF'S TIP:

Always choose brown mushrooms, such as crimini or baby bella.
They have more potassium than white mushrooms, and are more
flavorful and have a better texture.

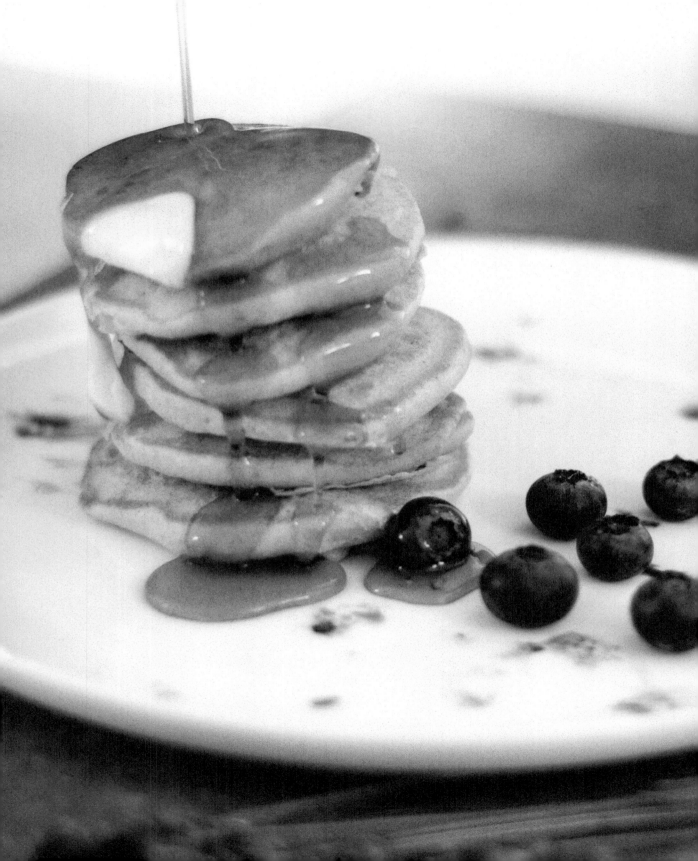

SOULFUL SUNDAY PANCAKES

SERVES 12 | CALORIES PER ONE SMALL PANCAKE 51

INGREDIENTS

1 C Kodiak waffle mix
1 Egg
1 C Egg whites
¼ C Blueberries

MACROS

Protein 5.2 g
Carbs 5.9 g
Fat 0.7 g

DIRECTIONS

› Preheat a nonstick pan on medium heat.
› Blend the waffle mix with the egg and egg whites.
› Pour the mixture into the pan and place 3 blueberries on top of each pancake.
› Cook 2 minutes on each side.

CHEF'S TIP:

I use Kodiak waffle mix because it's quick and has great ingredients, but you can make your own protein pancake mix by mixing dry ingredients and adding unflavored protein powder. Keep it in a dry place in an airtight container. To increase the protein-to-carbs ratio, I use egg whites in place of water or milk.

This recipe makes 12 small pancakes or 3 large ones.

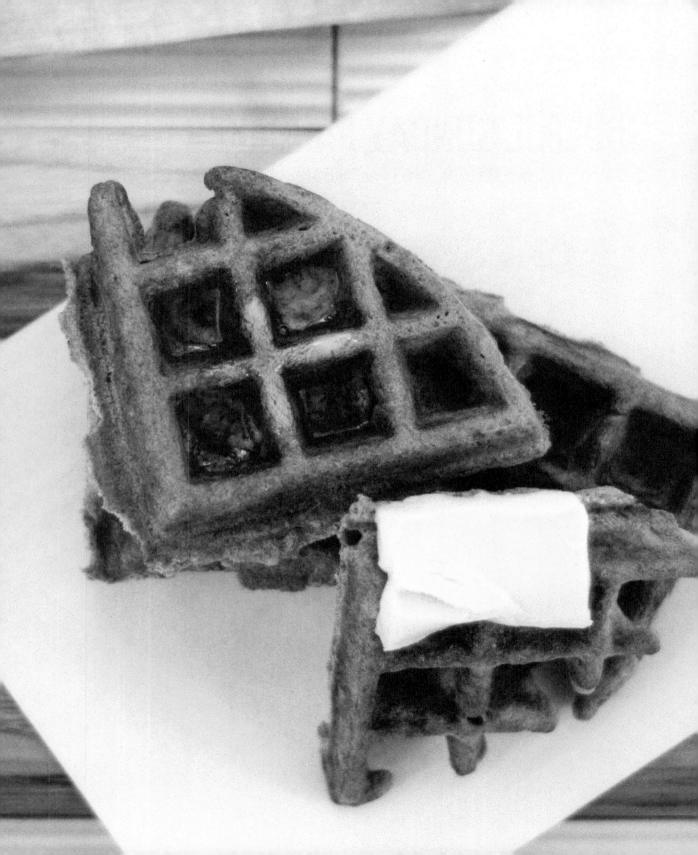

TAKE ME FOR A SPINACH WAFFLES

SERVES 1 | CALORIES PER SERVING 197

INGREDIENTS

1 C Kodiak waffle mix
2 Eggs
1 C Egg whites
1 C Spinach

MACROS

Protein 20.6 g
Carbs 20.5 g
Fat 3 g

DIRECTIONS

> Preheat the waffle maker.
> Add all ingredients to a blender and blend until the spinach is completely mixed in.
> Follow your waffle maker instructions to cook the waffles.
> Serve with a topping of choice.

CHEF'S TIP:

I use Kodiak waffle mix because it's quick and has great ingredients. To increase the protein-to-carbs ratio, I use egg whites in place of water or milk. If using syrup, choose a pure maple syrup. Compared to a highly processed pancake syrup that has high fructose corn syrup, pure maple syrup only has one ingredient and has more than 63 antioxidants. In addition, it features high levels of zinc and manganese which may help keep your heart healthy and boost your immunity system.

This recipe makes 3 medium-size round waffles.

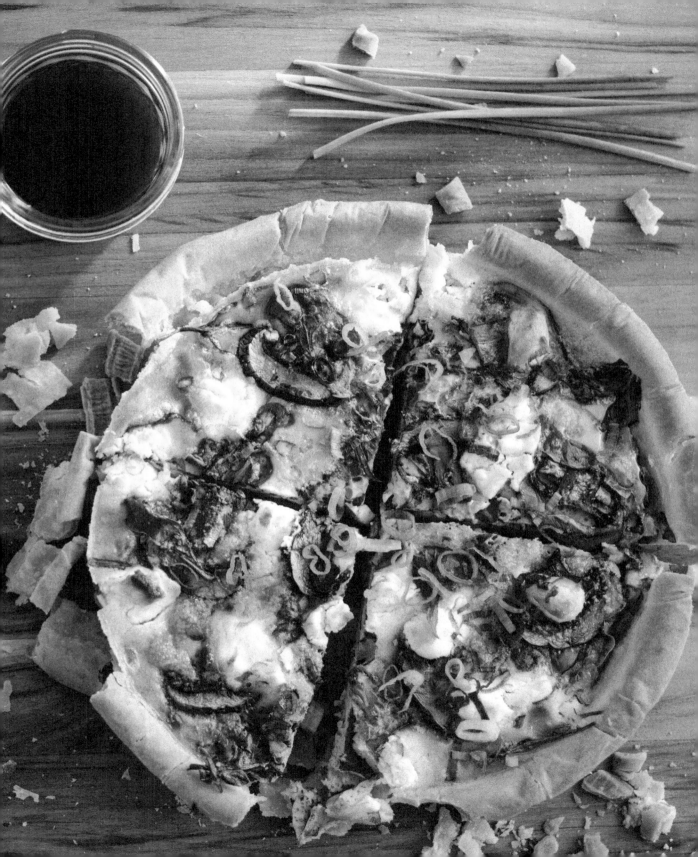

GREEN AND LEAN QUICHE

SERVES 12 | CALORIES PER SERVING 152

INGREDIENTS

1 Quiche crust
(store-bought or follow the
gluten-free recipe below)
6 Heirloom cherry
tomatoes – halved
3 Mushrooms – sliced
⅓ C Green onions – chopped
2 ozs Goat cheese
2 Eggs
12 T Egg whites

MACROS

Protein 6.3 g
Carbs 3.5 g
Fat 13.1 g

DIRECTIONS

> Add tomatoes, mushrooms, and goat cheese to the quiche crust.
> In a large bowl, combine the eggs and egg whites. Add salt and pepper to taste.
> Pour into crust. Add the green onions.
> Put pie pan on a baking sheet to avoid spills. Bake on the middle rack of the oven for 30-35 minutes or until edges are slightly browned.
> Let the quiche cool for 30 minutes before serving.

INGREDIENTS AND DIRECTIONS FOR GLUTEN-FREE CRUST

1½ C Almond flour
½ tsp Salt
½ tsp Baking soda
¼ C Coconut oil
1 T Water

> Preheat oven to 350° F.
> In a large bowl, combine almond flour, salt, and baking soda. Stir the wet ingredients into the dry ingredients until thoroughly combined. Press the dough into a 9½" pie pan.
> Bake for 15 minutes or until golden brown. Remove from the oven and let cool completely before filling.

CHEF'S TIP:

You can make 3-4 quiche crusts at once and freeze them for up to 6 weeks to make a quick and easy breakfast for the whole family. Please note that gluten-free crusts are usually higher in fat.

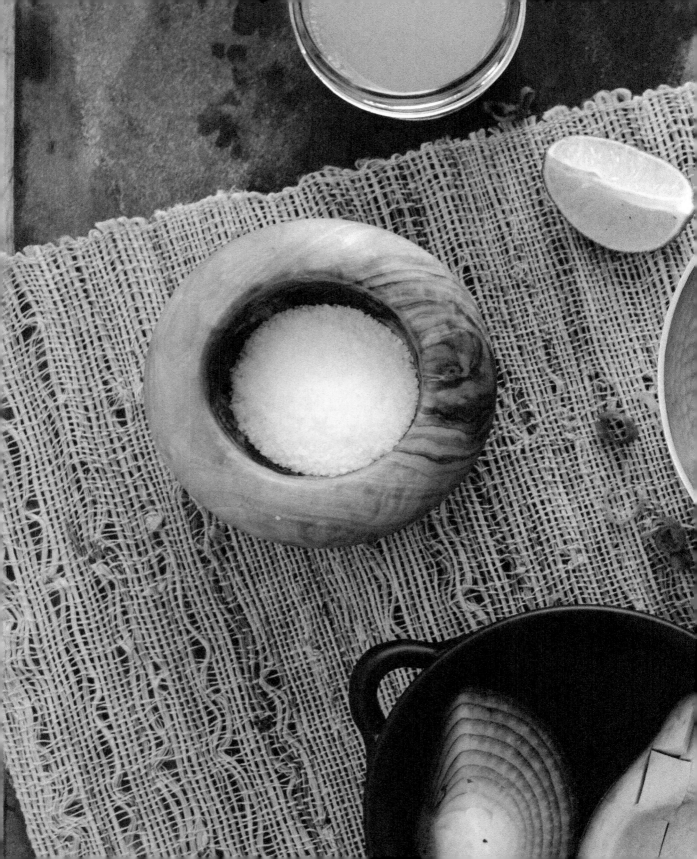

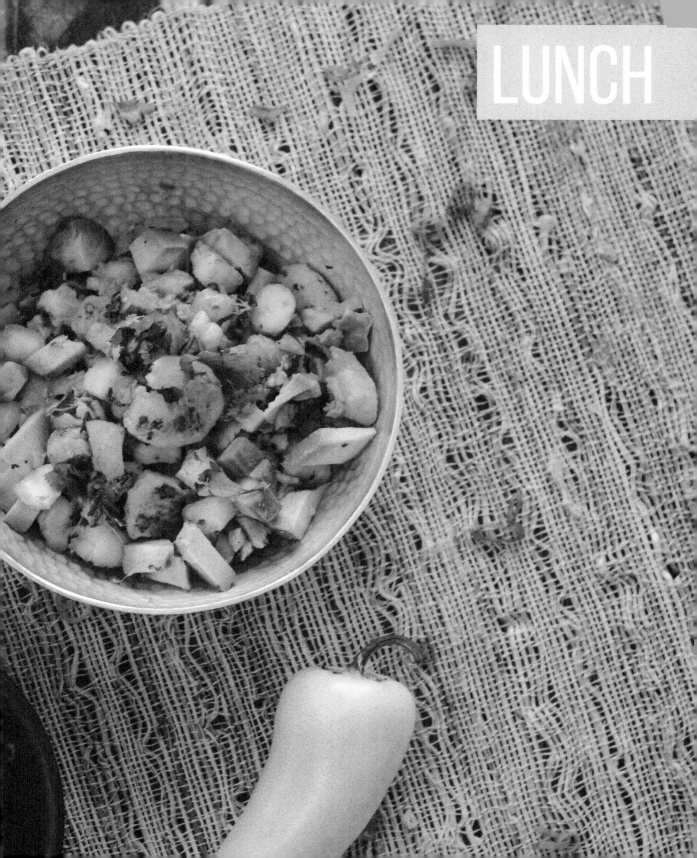

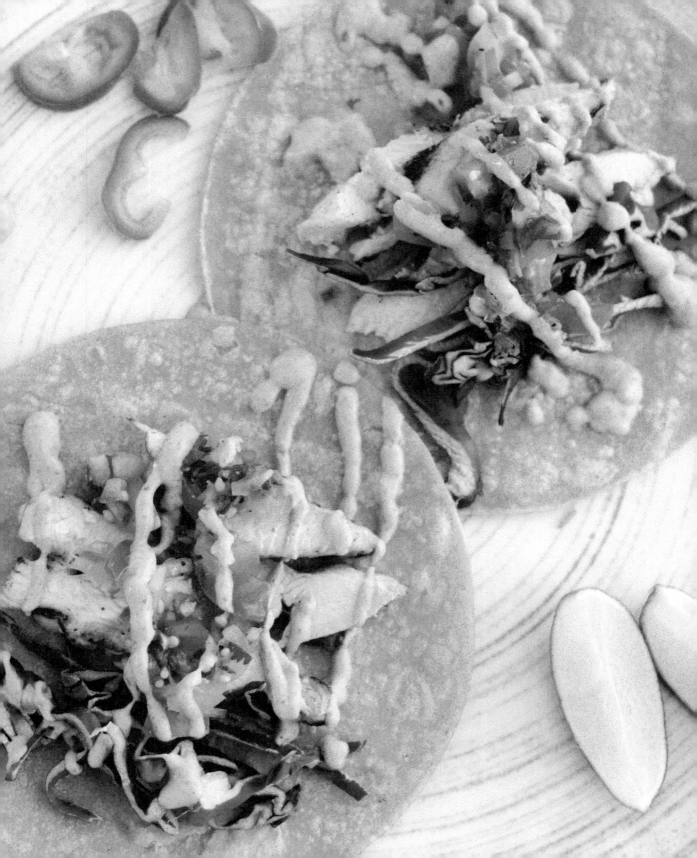

CALIENTE CHICKEN TACOS

SERVES 1 | CALORIES PER SERVING 283 (3 TACOS)

INGREDIENTS

3 ozs Chicken – sliced
½ C Purple cabbage – sliced
3 Tortillas (I use La Tortilla
organic yellow corn tortillas)
Salt and pepper
Pico de Gallo (see Page 217)
Creamy Avocado and Cilantro
Dressing (see Page 207)
Sundried Tomato Guacamole
(see Page 215)

MACROS

Protein 32 g
Carbs 34 g
Fat 12 g

DIRECTIONS

> Make the three sauces.
> Cook the chicken in a nonstick skillet over high heat for 13 minutes, and season with salt and pepper.
> Heat tortillas in a nonstick skillet on medium heat for 1 minute on each side.
> Add chicken, cabbage, and 1 serving of Pico de Gallo on top of the tortilla, and add 1 serving of Avocado Cilantro Dressing.
> Serve with 1 serving of Sundried Tomato Guacamole.

CHEF'S TIP:

If you don't have any tortillas on hand but have 20 minutes of spare time and some whole wheat flour, you can easily make your own. Just mix 1 C whole wheat flour, ½ C oat flour (if you don't have it, just process regular rolled oats in a blender until they become flour), 2 T olive oil, 1 C water (more or less, the dough shouldn't be sticky), and 1 tsp salt. Knead, roll, and heat in a pan for 2 minutes on each side. Makes 20 small taco tortillas.

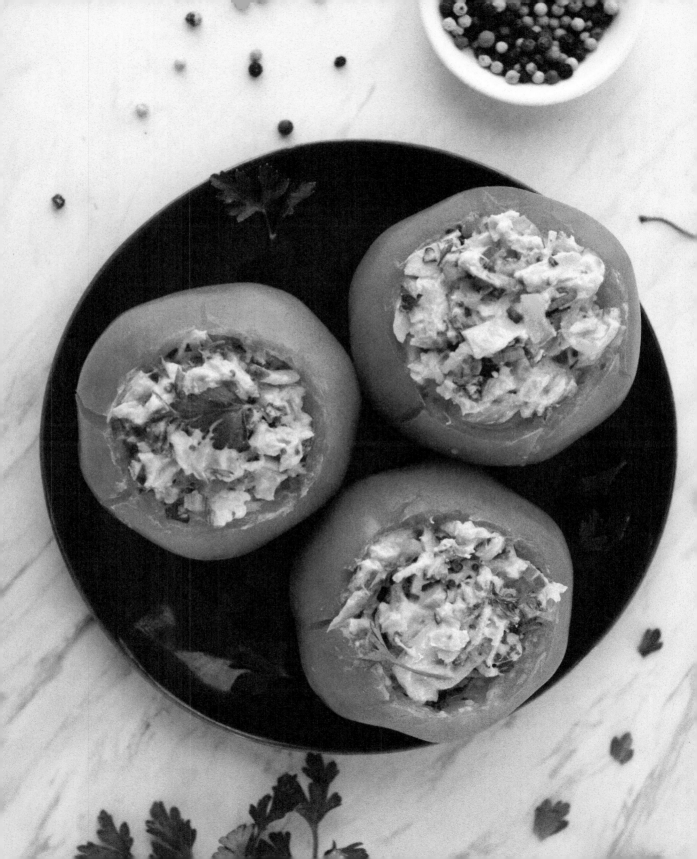

TUNA SALAD YOU'LL ACTUALLY LIKE

SERVES 1 | CALORIES PER ONE STUFFED TOMATO 157*

INGREDIENTS

SALAD

1 can Tuna in water
½ Cucumber – cubed
¼ Red onion – diced
½ Tomato – cubed
⅓ Yellow bell pepper – diced
¼ C Walnuts – chopped
Parsley – chopped
3 medium Tomatoes

DRESSING

2 T Honey
2 T Mustard
1 T Greek yogurt

MACROS

Protein 7.2 g
Carbs 11.1 g
Fat 11.6 g

*NOTE: This value will depend on the size and weight of your tomato, so the macros are for the tuna salad only – weigh your tomatoes and add the macros to the macros above.

DIRECTIONS

› Prep the vegetables.
› Add the tuna, vegetables, walnuts, and parsley to a bowl. Add the dressing, salt and pepper to taste, and mix well.
› Scoop out the middle of the medium tomatoes.
› Divide the tuna salad between three tomatoes.

CHEF'S TIP:

To lower the fat content and increase protein content, skip the walnuts and add another can of tuna.

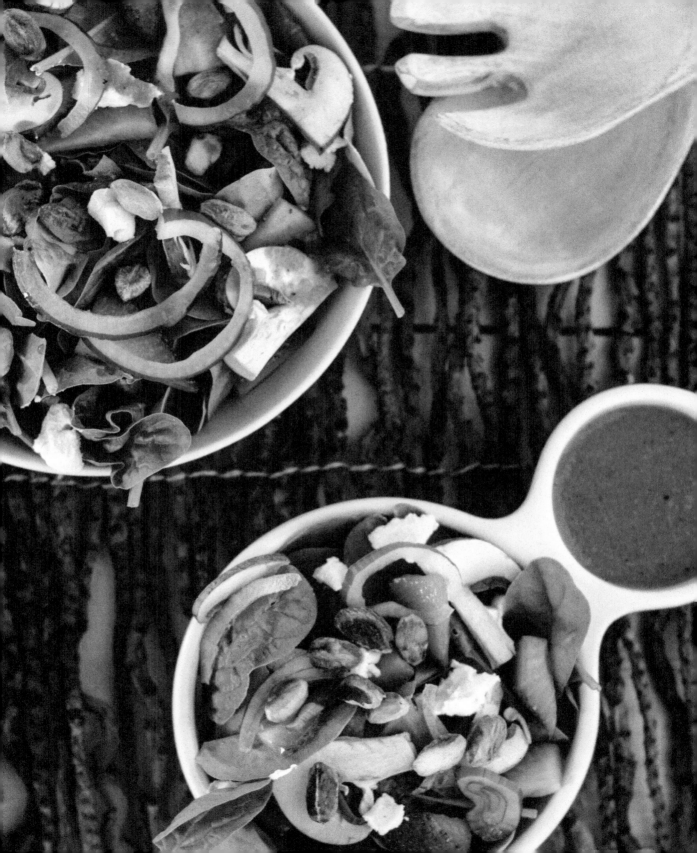

FITSPO SPINACH SALAD

SERVES 1 | CALORIES PER SERVING 179

INGREDIENTS

½ C Spinach
2 Strawberries – sliced
8 Cranberries
¼ Apple – sliced
1 T Walnuts – chopped
1 T Pistachios – chopped
¼ Red onion – diced
1 T Pomegranate Dressing
(see Page 211)

MACROS

Protein 3 g
Carbs 27.2 g
Fat 8 g

DIRECTIONS

> Make the Pomegranate Dressing.
> Add all ingredients to a bowl, and salt and pepper to taste.
> Serve with Pomegranate Dressing.

CHEF'S TIP:

You can caramelize the onions with the strawberries for a more distinct flavor.

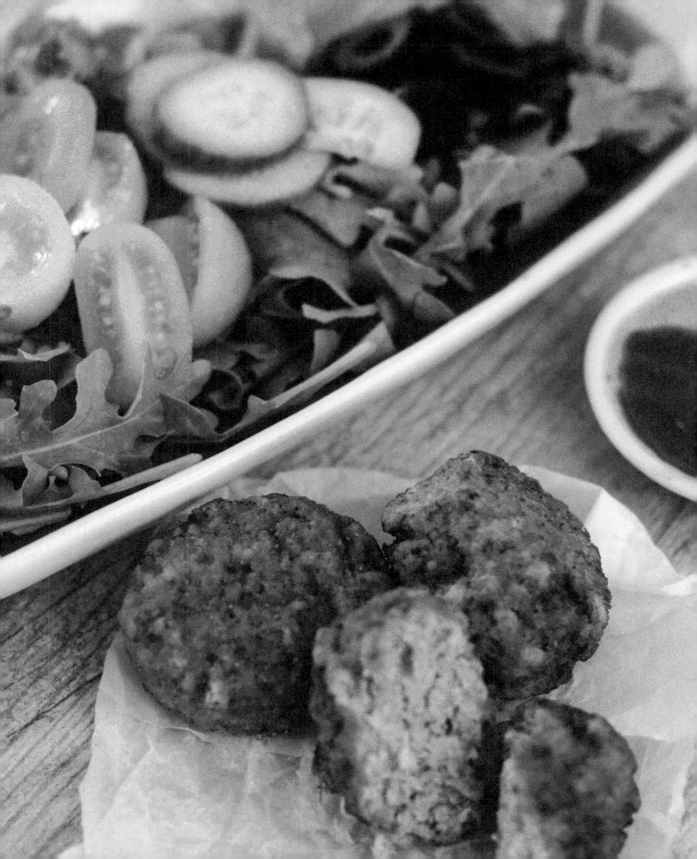

FANCY FALAFEL SALAD

SERVES 1 | CALORIES PER ONE SERVING OF FALAFELS 182 (3 PIECES)
CALORIES PER SERVING WITH SALAD 274 (3 FALAFELS AND SALAD)

INGREDIENTS

FALAFELS (MAKES 12)
8 T Egg whites
2 scoops Unflavored protein powder
(such as Isopure)
1 can Chickpeas (drained)
¼ C Oat flour
¼ Red onion
1 clove Fresh garlic
½ C fresh Parsley
Juice of 1 lemon
2 tsp Ground cumin
2 tsp Ground coriander
Salt and pepper to taste

SALAD
Arugula
6 Black olives – sliced
¼ Red onion – sliced
½ Cucumber – sliced
4 Yellow heirloom tomatoes – halved
1 T Creamy Avocado and Cilantro
Dressing (see Page 207)

MACROS
(3 FALAFELS / 3 FALAFELS AND SALAD)
Protein 21 g / 23 g
Carbs 18 g / 31 g
Fat 2.9 g / 9.9 g

DIRECTIONS

FALAFELS
> Preheat oven to 450° F.
> Add all ingredients to a food processor.
> Blend until the ingredients turn into a smooth mixture but not a puree.
> Line a baking sheet with parchment paper and spray it with oil.
> Form 12 patties or balls and place them on the parchment paper.
> Bake for 30 minutes or until the falafels become golden, turning the falafels over halfway through.

SALAD
> Make the Avocado Cilantro Dressing.
> Prep the vegetables.
> Caramelize the onions (cook in 1 tsp grapeseed oil for 5 minutes).
> Arrange the ingredients on a bed of arugula.
> Serve with Avocado Cilantro Dressing.

CHEF'S TIP:
You can serve falafels with a salad, or make a wrap or a sandwich. Make an open-faced sandwich for a lower carb option.

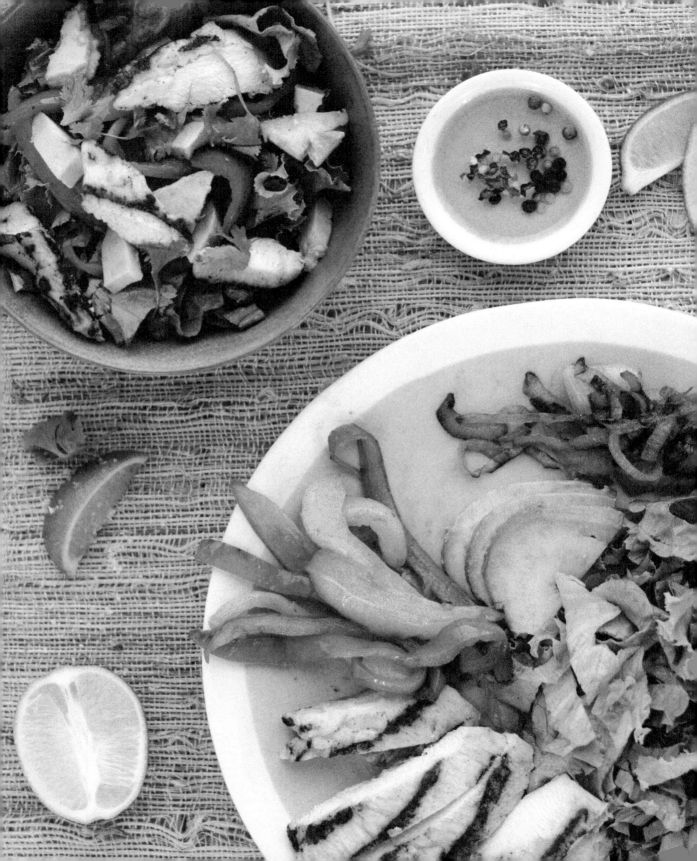

FAJITA MAMACITA SALAD

SERVES 1 | CALORIES PER SERVING 342

INGREDIENTS

¼ Yellow bell pepper
¼ Red bell pepper
¼ Orange bell pepper
⅓ Yellow onion
½ T Grapeseed oil
⅓ Avocado – sliced
Romaine lettuce – chopped
4 ozs Chicken – grilled or roasted
1 T Creamy Avocado and Cilantro
Dressing (see Page 207)

MACROS

Protein 38 g
Carbs 13 g
Fat 20 g

DIRECTIONS

> Make the Avocado Cilantro Dressing.
> Slice bell peppers lengthwise into ½"-wide strips, slice onions thickly.
> Heat a nonstick pan on medium-high heat, and cook the bell peppers and onions in the grapeseed oil for 5-7 minutes, until they get slightly browned.
> Arrange peppers, avocado, and chicken on the bed of lettuce, and add Avocado Cilantro Dressing to taste.

CHEF'S TIP:

Include bell peppers of all colors into your diet. They're very high in vitamin C, and one bell pepper may provide up to 169% of the RDA. Other vitamins and minerals found in bell peppers include vitamin K1, vitamin E, vitamin A, folate, and potassium.

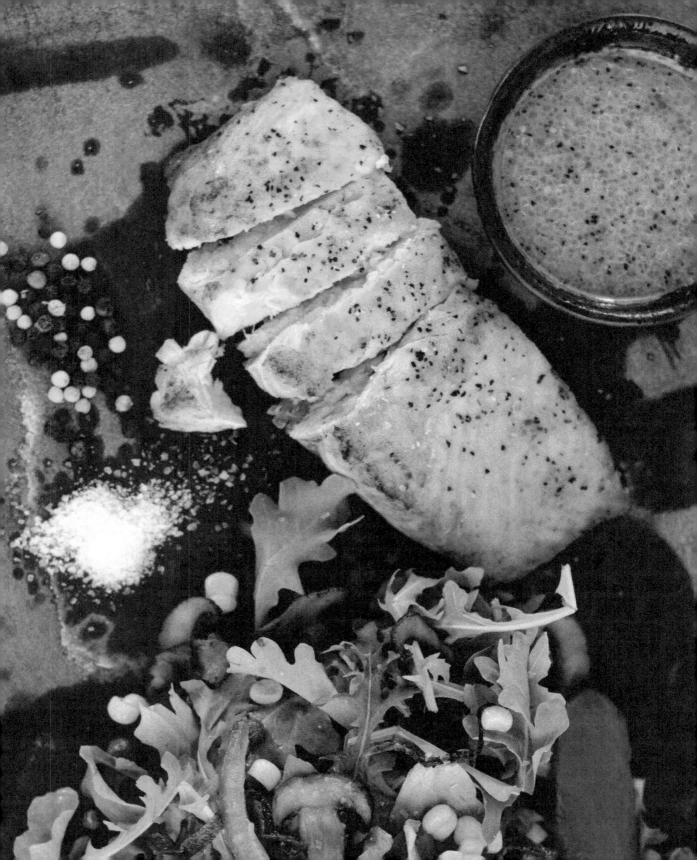

ALASKAN SALMON SALAD

SERVES 1 | CALORIES PER SERVING 443

INGREDIENTS

4 ozs Raw salmon filet
½ T Grapeseed oil
1 C Arugula
1 T Capers
2 T Corn
⅓ Bell pepper – sliced
4 Mushrooms – sliced
¼ Red onion – sliced
1 T Lemon pepper
½ tsp Salt
½ T Lemon Balsamic Dressing
(see Page 207)

MACROS

Protein 29 g
Carbs 21 g
Fat 26 g

DIRECTIONS

› Make the Lemon Balsamic Dressing.
› Preheat a nonstick skillet on medium heat and add the oil.
› Pat the salmon filet dry with a paper towel, and sprinkle with lemon pepper and salt.
› Cook the salmon on medium heat for 3-4 minutes on each side.
› Cook the peppers, mushrooms, and onion in a separate nonstick skillet on medium-high heat for 5-7 minutes (no oil needed).
› Arrange all ingredients on a bed of arugula and add Lemon Balsamic Dressing to taste.

CHEF'S TIP:

Replace the salmon with a whitefish, such as halibut or ono, to decrease the amount of fat in the dish.

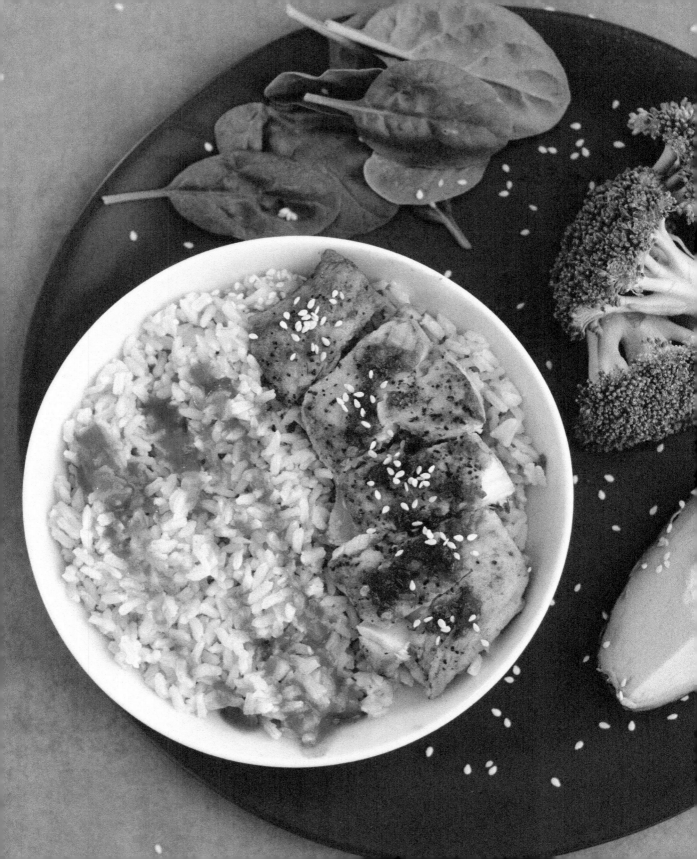

HOMETOWN TERYAKI SALMON BOWL

SERVES 1 | CALORIES PER SERVING 439

INGREDIENTS

4 ozs raw Salmon filet

½ C Brown rice – cooked

4-5 Broccoli florets

¼ Avocado – chopped

¼ C Spinach – chopped

1 T Sesame seeds

1 T Soy sauce

1 tsp Ginger – minced

1 tsp Honey

½ tsp Garlic powder

MACROS

Protein 28 g

Carbs 34.9 g

Fat 21.4 g

DIRECTIONS

> Preheat oven to 400° F.

> In a small bowl, mix the sesame seeds, soy sauce, ginger, honey, and garlic powder.

> Glaze the salmon filet with the soy sauce mixture and place the salmon on a baking sheet covered with foil. Bake for 15 minutes.

> Serve in a bowl with brown rice, broccoli, avocado, and spinach.

CHEF'S TIP:

Even though avocado, sesame seeds, and salmon are high in fat, they're also high in omega-3 fatty acids, which have a lot of health benefits and promote better heart health, as well as help keep your hair, nails, bones, joints, and skin healthy.

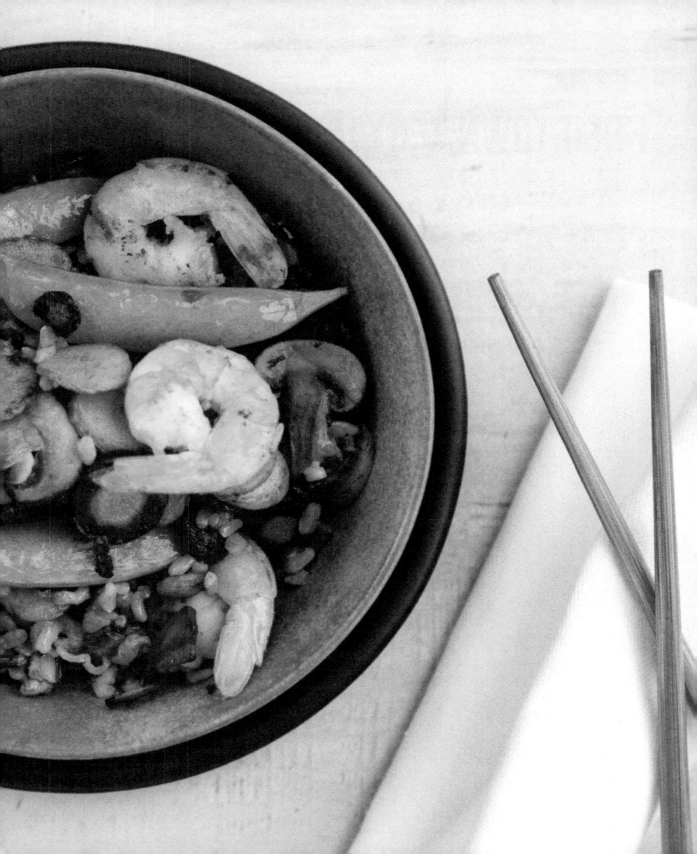

WILD SOULED SHRIMP BOWL

SERVES 1 | CALORIES PER SERVING 353

INGREDIENTS

½ C Wild rice – cooked

4 ozs Raw large shrimp (approx. 9)

½ T Grapeseed oil

5 Snow peas

3 Mushrooms – thinly sliced

¼ Yellow carrot – thinly sliced

¼ Orange carrot – thinly sliced

1 T Green onions – chopped

MACROS

Protein 28.6 g

Carbs 36.4 g

Fat 10.9 g

DIRECTIONS

› Preheat a nonstick skillet on medium heat.

› Cook snow peas, mushrooms, and carrots on medium-high heat for about 5 minutes.

› Preheat another nonstick skillet on medium heat and add the oil. Pan sear the shrimp for 2 minutes on each side.

› Serve in a bowl with wild rice and sprinkle with green onions.

CHEF'S TIP:

This dish is great for easy meal prep. It's quick to cook, and you can make enough for 4 days ahead.

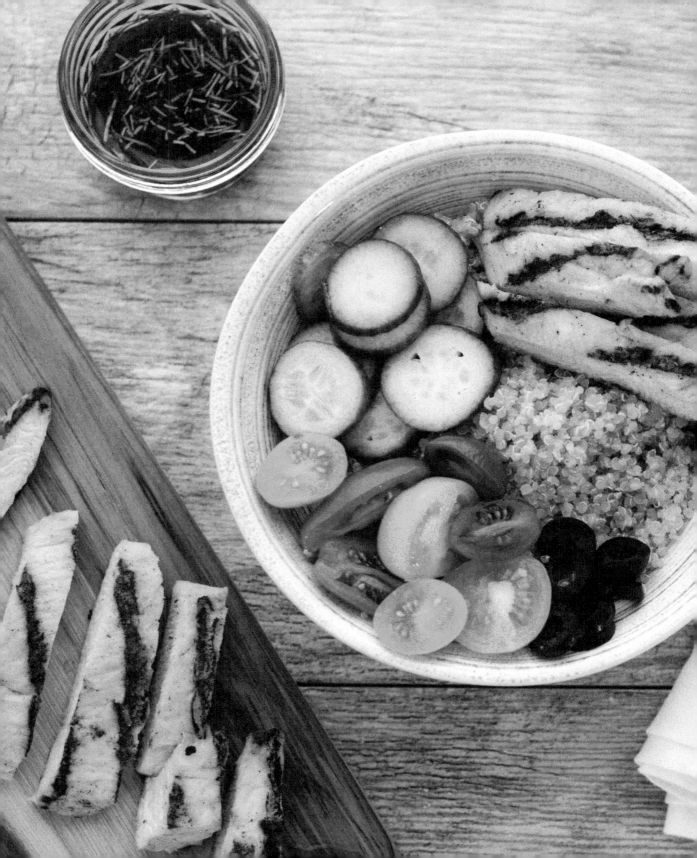

CHERRY BOMB CHICKEN BOWL

SERVES 1 | CALORIES PER SERVING 382

INGREDIENTS

4 ozs Grilled chicken – sliced
½ C Quinoa – cooked
5 Cherry tomatoes – halved
½ Cucumber – sliced
6 Black olives
Dill

MACROS

Protein 40 g
Carbs 32 g
Fat 11.9 g

DIRECTIONS

> Combine all ingredients in a bowl, add salt and pepper to taste, and sprinkle with dill.

CHEF'S TIP:

Try adding new grains into your menu. There are other grains that aren't very popular yet, but are very delicious and provide a lot of nutrients. Barley, for instance, has a rich, nutty flavor and is a very good source of molybdenum, manganese, dietary fiber, and selenium, and a good source of copper, vitamin B1, chromium, phosphorus, magnesium, and niacin. Other grains to try are buckwheat and millet.

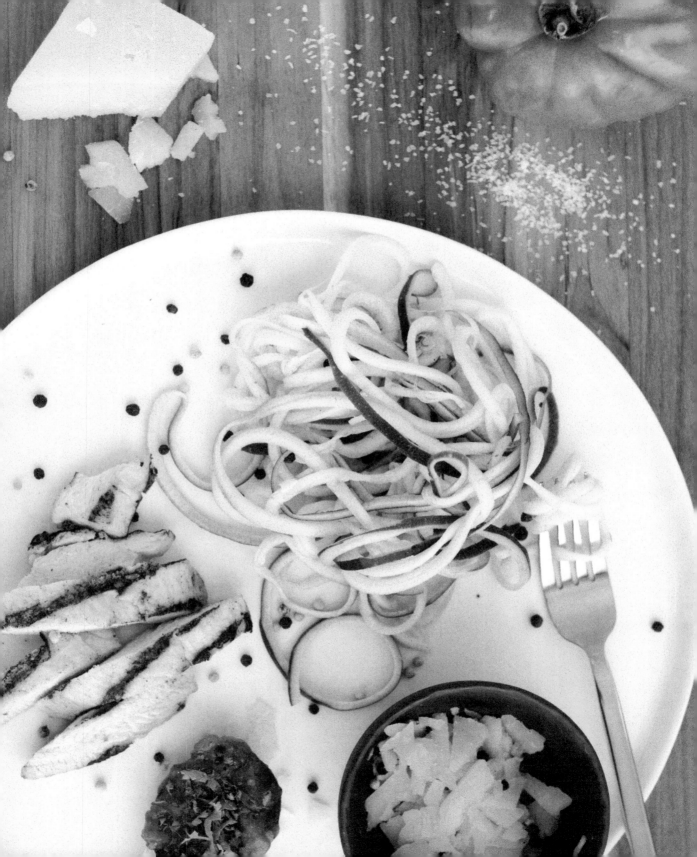

CHICKEN OODLE NOODLE

SERVES 1 | CALORIES PER SERVING 260

INGREDIENTS

1 Zucchini
4 ozs Chicken – grilled
½ oz Parmesan cheese
Tomato Mushroom Sauce
(see Page 213)

MACROS

Protein 46 g
Carbs 13 g
Fat 10 g

DIRECTIONS

> Make the Tomato Mushroom Sauce and add 1 serving to a separate pan.
> Using a vegetable spiralizer, make zucchini noodles from one zucchini.
> Add them to the pan with the Tomato Mushroom Sauce and let cook for 5 minutes, stirring twice.
> Sprinkle with grated parmesan cheese and serve with the grilled chicken.

CHEF'S TIP:

Depending on the type of your vegetable spiralizer, you can spiralize just about any vegetable, as long as it's firm and doesn't have seeds. Ideas to try instead of zucchini are sweet potato, butternut squash, hothouse cucumber, carrots, and even beets.

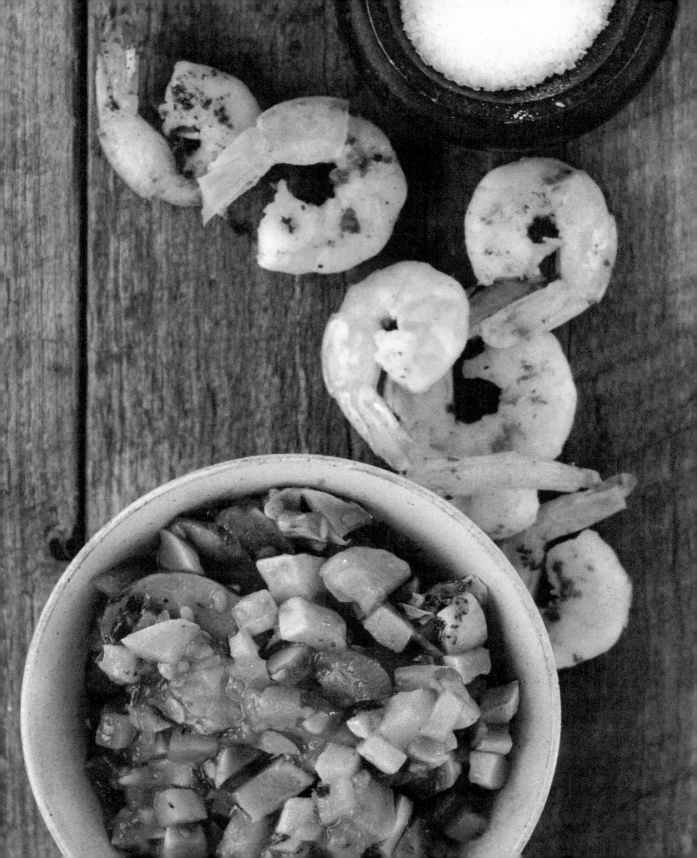

COLORFUL 'N' LEAN SHRIMP PASTA

SERVES 1 | CALORIES PER SERVING 367

INGREDIENTS

½ C Quinoa noodles – cooked
4 ozs Raw large shrimp
(approx. 9)
½ T Grapeseed oil
Tomato, Yellow Squash, and
Thyme Sauce (see Page 214)

MACROS

Protein 23 g
Carbs 41 g
Fat 12 g

DIRECTIONS

> Cook noodles according to the package.
> Make the Tomato, Yellow Squash, and Thyme Sauce.
> Preheat a nonstick skillet on medium heat and add the oil. Pan sear the shrimp for 2 minutes on each side.
> Place 1 serving of the Tomato, Yellow Squash, and Thyme Sauce into a bowl and add the cooked noodles.
> Serve with pan-seared shrimp.

CHEF'S TIP:

To lower carbs and increase protein, replace quinoa noodles with edamame or black bean noodles.

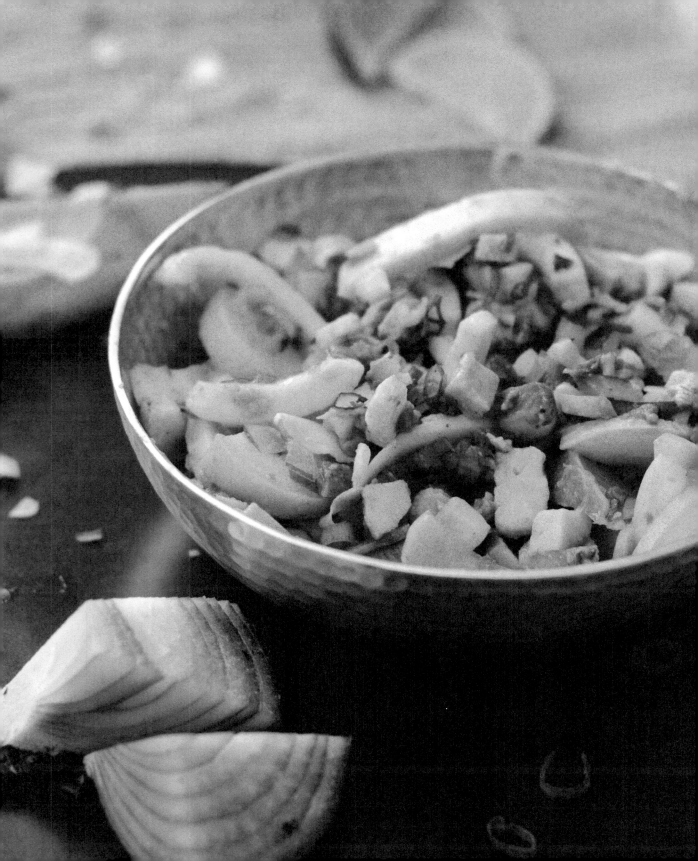

COCONUT CEVICHE
SERVES 2 | CALORIES PER SERVING 180

INGREDIENTS
1 Young (Thai) coconut
1 T Coconut – unsweetened,
(shaved)
Juice of 1 lime
2 T Fresh orange juice
1 T Green onions – sliced
1/4 Jalapeño – seeded and minced
1/2 Thin yellow squash – sliced
1/3 Avocado – chopped
1/4 C Fresh parsley – chopped
1/4 C Fresh cilantro – chopped
1 T Olive oil
Salt and pepper to taste
Pinch of cayenne pepper

MACROS
Protein 2.1 g
Carbs 19.9 g
Fat 13.4 g

DIRECTIONS
> Open the coconut, pour out the water, and scoop out the insides using a spoon.
> In a nonstick skillet, cook the shaved coconut on medium heat for 2-3 minutes or until it becomes golden.
> Slice the coconut into 1/4"-wide strips and combine with the rest of the ingredients in a bowl.
> Chill 30 to 60 minutes before serving.

CHEF'S TIP:
To make this dish a balanced meal, serve it with whitefish or shrimp (grilled or pan seared in 1/2 T oil), as they're high in protein and low in fat.

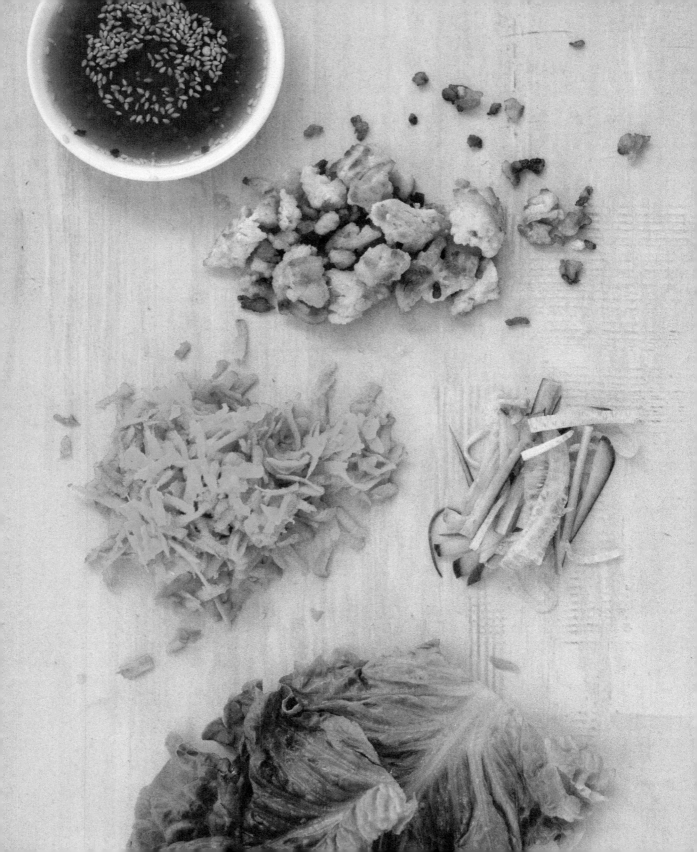

NOT YOUR AVERAGE CHANG'S LETTUCE WRAPS

SERVES 1 | CALORIES PER SERVING WITH 1 T OF DRESSING 239 (3 WRAPS)

INGREDIENTS

2 ozs Ground turkey
(I use 97% lean)
½ T Grapeseed oil
⅓ Carrot – shredded
⅓ Cucumber – shredded
Scallions – minced
3 Lettuce leaves
Asian Dressing (see Page 210)

MACROS

Protein 17 g
Carbs 7 g
Fat 16 g

DIRECTIONS

> Make the Asian Dressing.
> Heat the oil in a nonstick skillet on medium heat. Add 3 ozs of raw ground turkey, and cook for 10 minutes or until golden brown.
> Divide the ingredients between the lettuce leaves and add 1 tsp of Asian Dressing per wrap.
> Wrap, hold tight, and enjoy.

CHEF'S TIP:

You can use any type of lettuce for a wrap, but the best one is Butter lettuce because it holds the ingredients in the wrap the best.

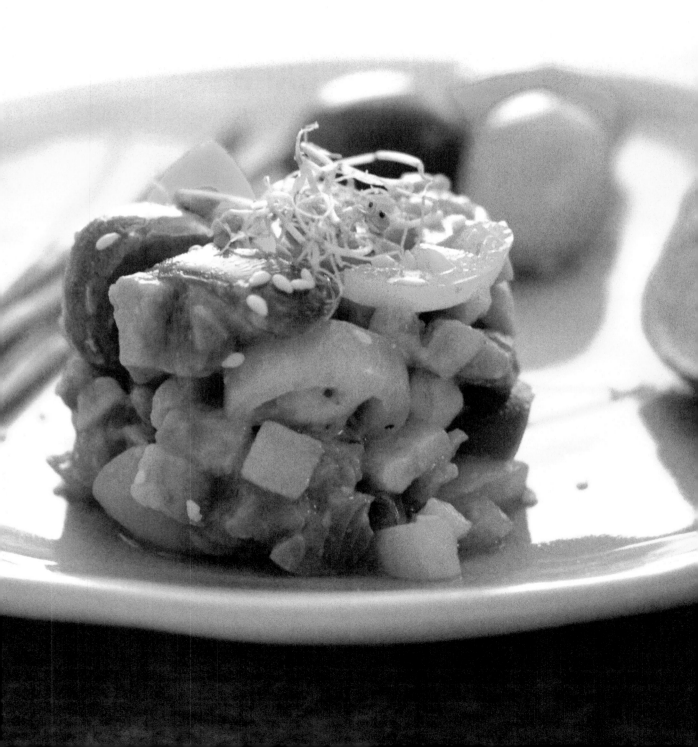

SVETLANA'S SALMON TARTARE

SERVES 1 | CALORIES PER SERVING 158

INGREDIENTS

4 ozs Raw salmon –
cut into ½"cubes
⅓ Avocado – diced
1 T Soy sauce
Juice of 2 limes
1 tsp Sesame seeds
1 tsp Sesame oil
1 tsp Chives – diced
4 Cherry tomatoes – diced
1 oz Sprouts
Salt and pepper

MACROS

Protein 13.5 g
Carbs 10.6 g
Fat 9.6 g

NOTE: You could serve
this as an appetizer
or fit into your macros
as a small snack.

DIRECTIONS

› Add the salmon to a bowl with the soy sauce, lime juice, sesame seeds, sesame oil, salt, and pepper. Mix well and refrigerate for 30 minutes.
› Dice the avocados, chives, and tomatoes.
› Add the tomatoes, avocados, and chives to the prepped salmon and mix together.
› Divide the mixture into two parts, form each into a tower, and add sprouts to the top.

CHEF'S TIP:

To make your salmon tartare look like it just came from a restaurant, you can use a plastic cup with a cut off bottom to form the towers, or even a regular glass.

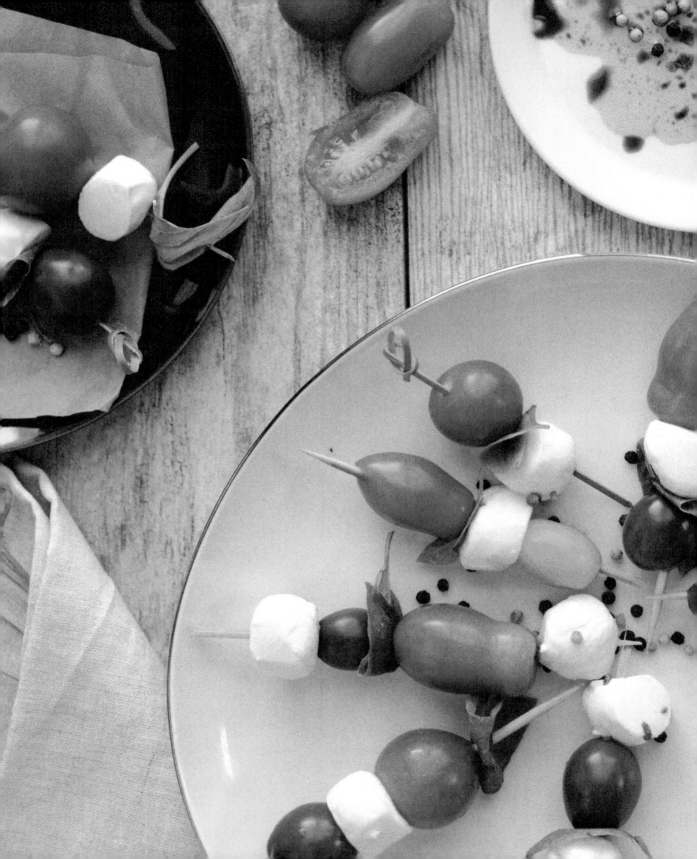

SEXY SIMPLE CAPRESE STICKS

SERVES 6 | CALORIES PER SERVING 59

INGREDIENTS

6 Fresh mozzarella balls
12 Heirloom cherry tomatoes
1 T Basil – chopped
1 T Olive oil
1 T Balsamic vinegar
6 Toothpicks
Salt and pepper to taste

MACROS

Protein 2.3 g
Carbs 3.4 g
Fat 4.1 g

NOTE: You could serve
this as an appetizer
or fit into your macros
as a small snack.

DIRECTIONS

› Put the tomatoes and cheese balls on the toothpicks, placing the cheese ball in the middle.
› Sprinkle with basil and pour the olive oil and vinegar over the sticks, and add salt and pepper to taste.

CHEF'S TIP:

You can make a whole table of appetizers on toothpicks. Some variations to try are Swiss cheese, pineapple and ham; watermelon, feta cheese, and mint; and artichokes, sundried tomatoes and cucumber.

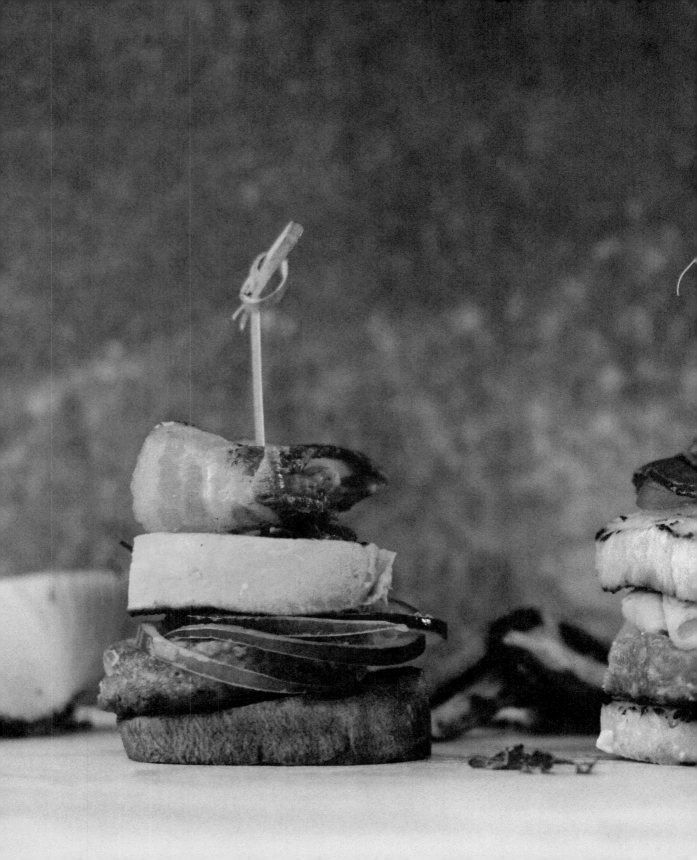

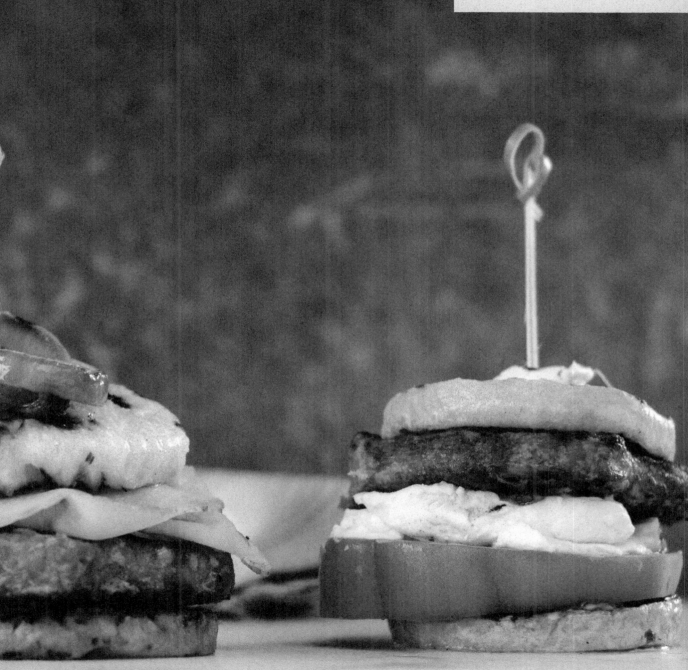

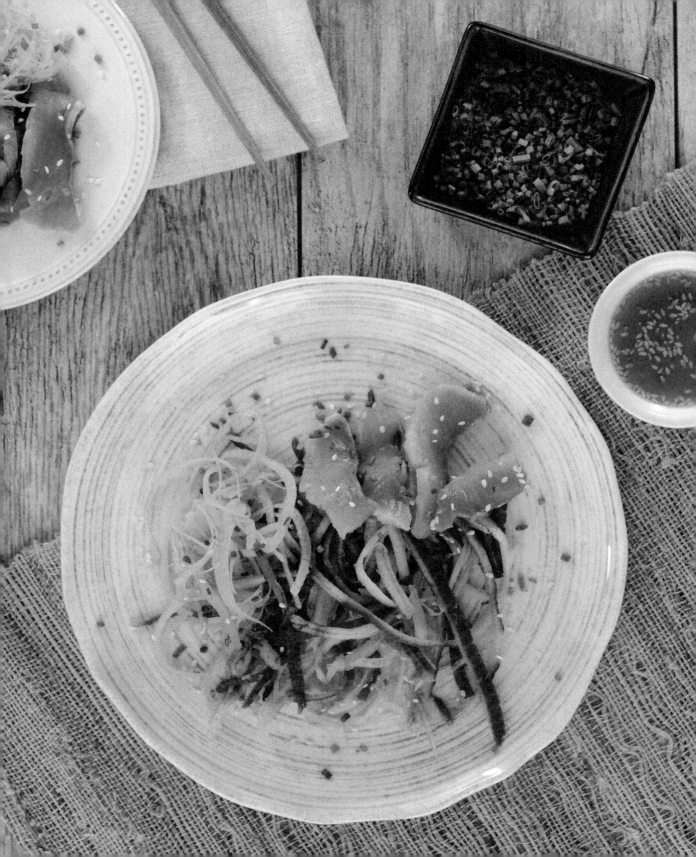

RAW AND REAL SALMON SALAD

SERVES 1 | CALORIES PER SERVING 239

INGREDIENTS

SALAD

½ Carrot – thinly sliced
½ Cucumber – thinly sliced
1 tsp Cilantro – chopped
1 tsp Scallions – chopped
4 ozs Sashimi-style salmon
1 T Asian Dressing (see Page 210)

SALMON

1 lb Salmon (skin on)
1½ T Kosher salt
1 ½ tsp Dark brown sugar
3 Lemons
1 T Rice vinegar

MACROS

Protein 26 g
Carbs 13 g
Fat 11 g

DIRECTIONS

> Make the Asian Dressing.
> To make Vera's sashimi-style salmon, add rice vinegar to the bottom of a glass container. Mix the salt with the sugar, and spread a half of it on the bottom of the container. Slice lemons, and use half to cover the salt-sugar mixture. Place the salmon (skin down) on top of the lemons. Spread the rest of the salt over the fish and cover with remaining lemons. Refrigerate overnight.
> Slice the cucumbers and carrots very thinly (you can use a spiralizer or a mandoline).
> Mix the cucumbers and carrots in a bowl, add the cilantro and scallions, and mix with the Asian Dressing.
> Serve with the salmon.

CHEF'S TIP:

If you're afraid to eat raw fish, don't worry. The salt, rice vinegar, and lemons basically "cook" the fish, so after 6-8 hours in the refrigerator the salmon isn't raw anymore.

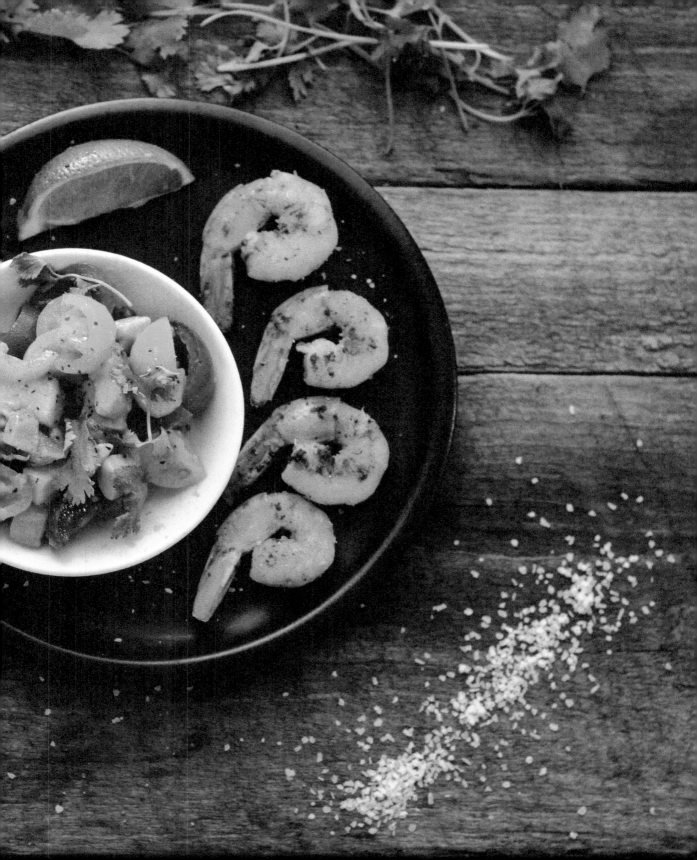

DANCING SHRIMP AVOCADO SALAD

SERVES 1 | CALORIES PER SERVING 266

INGREDIENTS

½ Avocado – sliced
½ C Yellow cherry tomatoes – halved
½ C Cilantro – chopped
4 ozs Raw large shrimp (approx. 9)
½ T Grapeseed oil
Juice of 1 lemon

MACROS

Protein 23.1 g
Carbs 15.7 g
Fat 15.4 g

DIRECTIONS

> Prep the vegetables.
> Heat the oil in a nonstick skillet on medium heat. Pan sear the shrimp for 2 minutes on each side.
> Mix the avocado, tomatoes, and cilantro with the lemon juice, and add salt and pepper to taste.
> Serve with the shrimp.

CHEF'S TIP:

If you haven't done so, include shrimp in your weekly menu. Shrimp has a VERY impressive variety of nutrients. Just 4 ounces of shrimp will provide you with more than 100% of the Daily Value for selenium, more than 75% for vitamin B12, more than 50% for phosphorous, and more than 30% for choline, copper, and iodine.

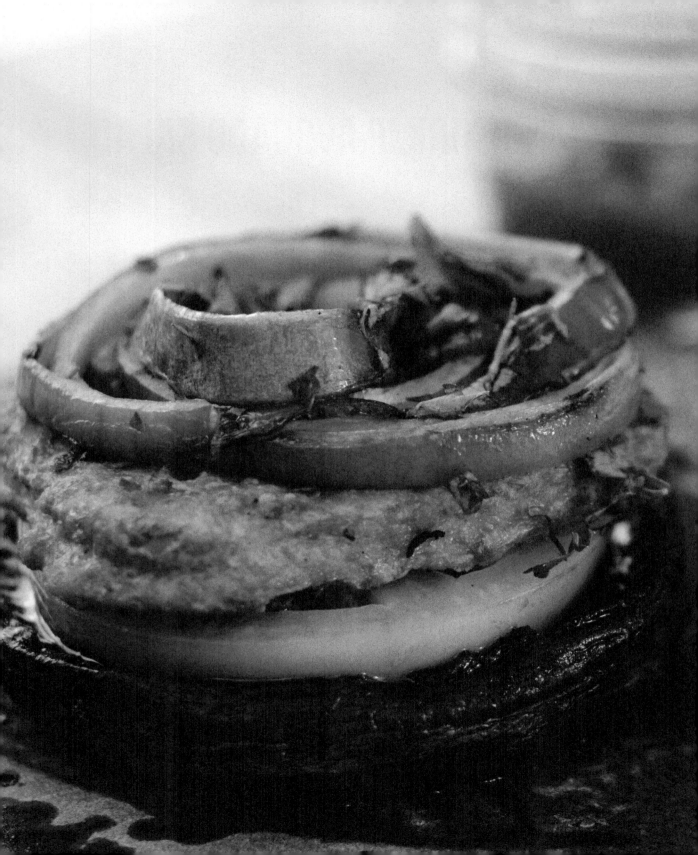

TURKEY 'SHROOMBURGER

SERVES 1 | CALORIES PER SERVING 174

INGREDIENTS

1 Portobello mushroom cap
2 slices Red onion – grilled
¼-lb Turkey burger (97% lean)
1 slice Yellow Tomato
½ tsp Parsley – diced

MACROS

Protein 29.6 g
Carbs 7 g
Fat 3.1 g

DIRECTIONS

> Grill the portobello mushroom cap and onion over medium heat for 3-4 minutes on each side.
> Cook the turkey burger (if frozen, according to the package; if made from fresh ground turkey, until a meat thermometer reaches 165° F); add the parsley to the turkey while it's cooking.
> Place the mushroom cap on a plate, place the tomato slice, then the turkey burger, and top with onions.
> Serve with a side of choice.

CHEF'S TIP:

If you don't have a grill, you can use a griddle, griddle pan, or even a regular pan. Just make sure it's nonstick and heated on medium heat.

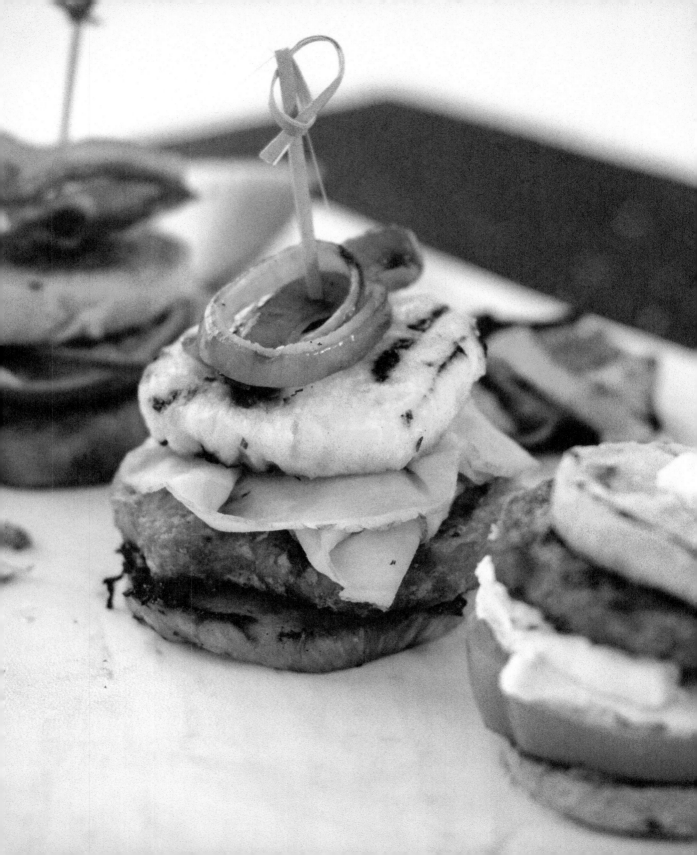

THREE BEST FRIENDS: SWEET SLIDE, ZUCCHINI MINI, PINAPPLE MAN

SERVES 1 | CALORIES PER SERVING SEE BELOW UNDER MACROS

INGREDIENTS

3 ⅛-lb Chicken burgers (97% lean)

SWEET POTATO SLIDER
2 slices ⅓"-thick Sweet potato
1 slice Bacon
1 slice Red onion

ZUCCHINI SLIDER
2 large slices Zucchini
1 slice Tomato
½ oz Goat cheese

PINEAPPLE SLIDER
2 slices Pineapple
1 oz Turkey ham
1 slice onion – grilled

MACROS (SWEET POTATO/ ZUCCHINI/PINEAPPLE)

Calories 236/172/216
Protein 30.1 g/29.5 g/30.1 g
Carbs 18.5 g/3 g/17.3 g
Fat 6.4 g/6.6 g/5.6 g

DIRECTIONS

> Grill the sweet potatoes, zucchini, pineapple, onions, and chicken burgers.
> Cook the bacon for 2-3 minutes on each side in a pan over medium heat; remove from heat and let the bacon rest on a paper towel.
> Arrange the sliders according to the picture.

CHEF'S TIP:
To prevent the vegetable slices from falling into the grill, place them in a grilling basket. They're inexpensive and a great tool to use if you grill often.

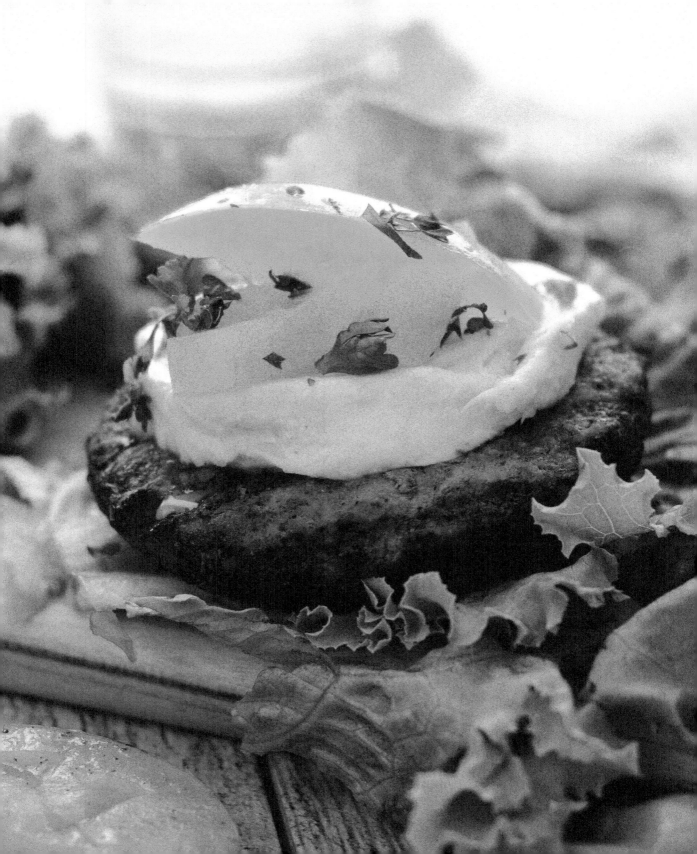

"LOOK AT ME" OPEN-FACE BURGER

SERVES 1 | CALORIES PER SERVING 258 (1 BURGER)

INGREDIENTS

1¼-lb Beef patty (97% lean)
2 Lettuce leaves
1 oz Fresh mozzarella cheese
1 slice Heirloom tomato
1 tsp Basil – chopped
2 Yellow pickled peppers

MACROS

Protein 30 g
Carbs 2.9 g
Fat 13.1 g

DIRECTIONS

> Cook the burger (if frozen, according to the package; if made from fresh ground beef, until a meat thermometer reaches 140° F for medium rare, 155° F for medium, or 165° F for well done).

> Arrange the burger on a lettuce leaf; top with cheese, tomato, basil, and peppers; and add salt and pepper to taste.

CHEF'S TIP:

Peperoncini peppers are fermented, and fermented foods are considered to be probiotics, increasing overall nutrition, promoting the growth of friendly intestinal bacteria, and aiding digestion and supporting immune function, including an increase in B vitamins (even Vitamin B12), omega-3 fatty acids, digestive enzymes, lactase and lactic acid, and other immune chemicals that fight off harmful bacteria and even cancer cells.

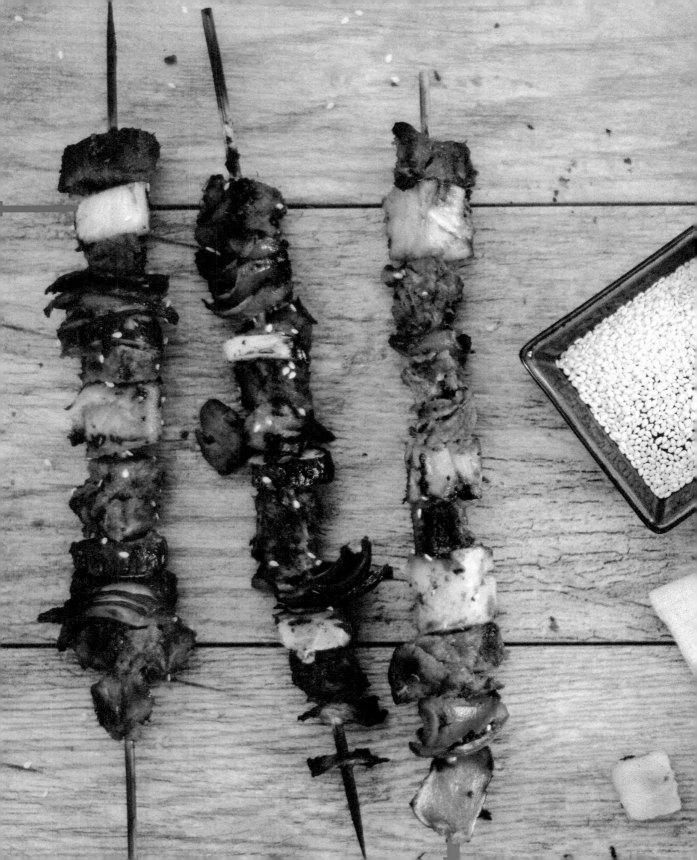

SWEET SHASHLIK KEBABS

SERVES 4 | CALORIES PER SERVING 120

INGREDIENTS

2 lbs Chicken breast –
cut into 1-1½" cubes
1 T Spiced vinegar
2 T Chili sauce
1 T Soy sauce
1 tsp Garlic powder
1 C Zucchini – sliced
1 C Onion – sliced
1 C Pineapple – cubed
Salt and pepper
Bamboo skewers

MACROS

Protein 36 g
Carbs 31 g
Fat 4 g

DIRECTIONS

> Prep the meat and the vegetables.
> Mix all of the ingredients together in a large bowl and marinate in the refrigerator for at least one hour (overnight is best).
> Soak the bamboo skewers to prevent burning.
> Put the chicken on the bamboo skewers, mix and match the vegetables between the chicken, and grill on low heat for about 12-14 minutes, turning every 3-4 minutes.

CHEF'S TIP:

You can use this recipe to make beef kebabs, as well! The recipe pictured in this photo features both beef and chicken. Also, if you want to decrease the carb count on the dish, use peppers or mushrooms as a substitute for the pineapple.

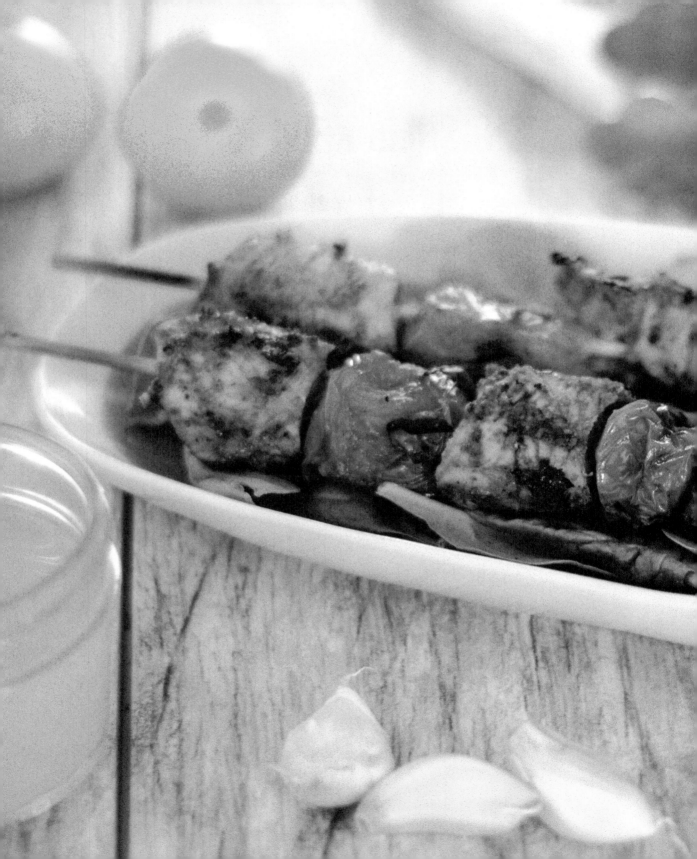

VIVA ITALIA CHICKEN PESTO KEBABS

SERVES 3 | CALORIES PER SERVING 177 (4 OZS CHICKEN)

INGREDIENTS

1 lb Chicken breast

8 ozs Yellow cherry tomatoes

4-6 Bamboo skewers – presoaked

4 T Pesto Sauce (see Page 216)

MACROS

Protein 37 g

Carbs 3 g

Fat 9 g

DIRECTIONS

› Make the Pesto Sauce.

› Cut the chicken into 1" cubes and marinate in the Pesto Sauce for 1-2 hours or overnight.

› Add chicken and tomatoes onto the skewers, alternating between the two.

› Grill on low heat for 12-15 minutes, turning 4 times.

CHEF'S TIP:

When calculating your macros for protein that has been marinated in a sauce, only count ⅓ of the marinade because most of it stays in the container, and only about ⅓ gets absorbed into the food.

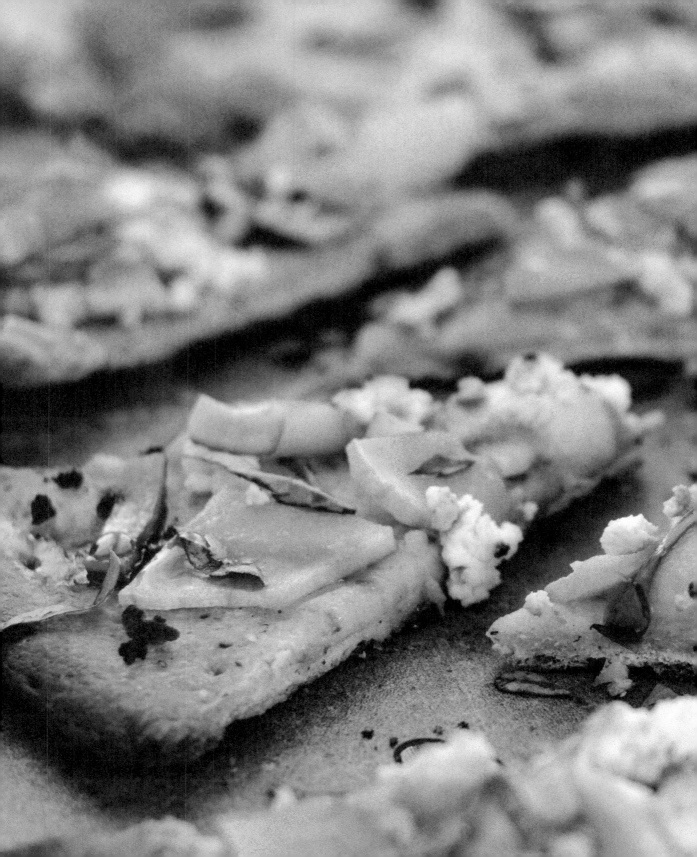

FOR THE LOVE OF PEACHES PIZZA

1 PIZZA = 6 SERVINGS | CALORIES PER SERVING 114*

INGREDIENTS

6 ozs Butternut squash
1 Nectarine
3 ozs Ricotta cheese
2 ozs Fresh Mozzarella cheese
¼ C Basil – chopped
*Pizza crust
(I use a 9" Great Low Carb Pizza
Crust, which is low in carbs and
high in protein, but you can make
your own; just don't
forget to adjust your macros.)

MACROS

Protein 9 g
Carbs 12.2 g
Fat 5.6 g

*NOTE: This value will increase
depending upon the crust
you use – add these macros
to the macros above.

DIRECTIONS

› Preheat oven to 425° F.
› Arrange the ingredients on the pizza crust.
› Bake until the crust becomes golden, and the cheese is melted.

CHEF'S TIP:

For gluten-free alternatives you can choose to use cauliflower crust, zucchini crust or sweet potato crust.

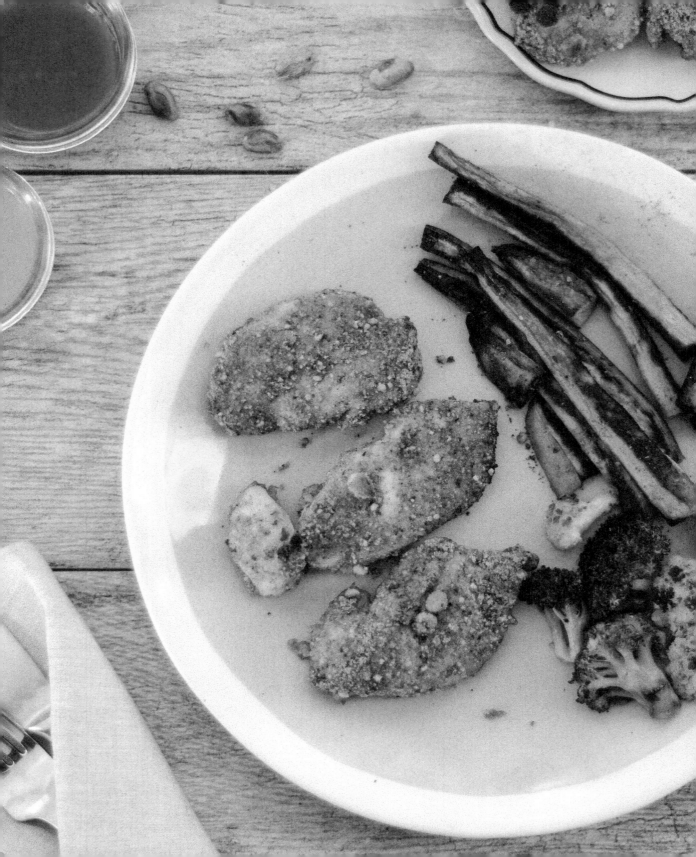

SEXYFIT STYLE CHICKEN NUGGETS + SWEETER-THAN-SWEET POTATO FRIES

SERVES 1 | CALORIES PER SERVING 390

INGREDIENTS

5 ozs Raw Chicken breast filet
½ oz Pistachios
3 ozs Sweet potatoes
4 Broccoli florets
4 Cauliflower florets
½ T Olive oil
Kosher salt
Pepper

MACROS

Protein 39.2 g
Carbs 29.5 g
Fat 14.9 g

DIRECTIONS

> Preheat oven to 400° F.
> Crumble pistachios in a food processor or with a knife.
> Evenly cover the chicken filet with crumbled pistachios.
> Add broccoli and cauliflower florets, and sliced sweet potatoes into a large bowl, add olive oil, and kosher salt and pepper to taste, and mix well.
> Place all ingredients onto a baking sheet lined with foil.
> Bake for 20 minutes or until a meat thermometer inserted into the chicken reaches 160° F.

CHEF'S TIP:

Crusting proteins in crumbled nuts not only saves you a lot of carbs macros, but it also adds some omega-3 fatty acids that all nuts have. You can use any nuts you have at home.

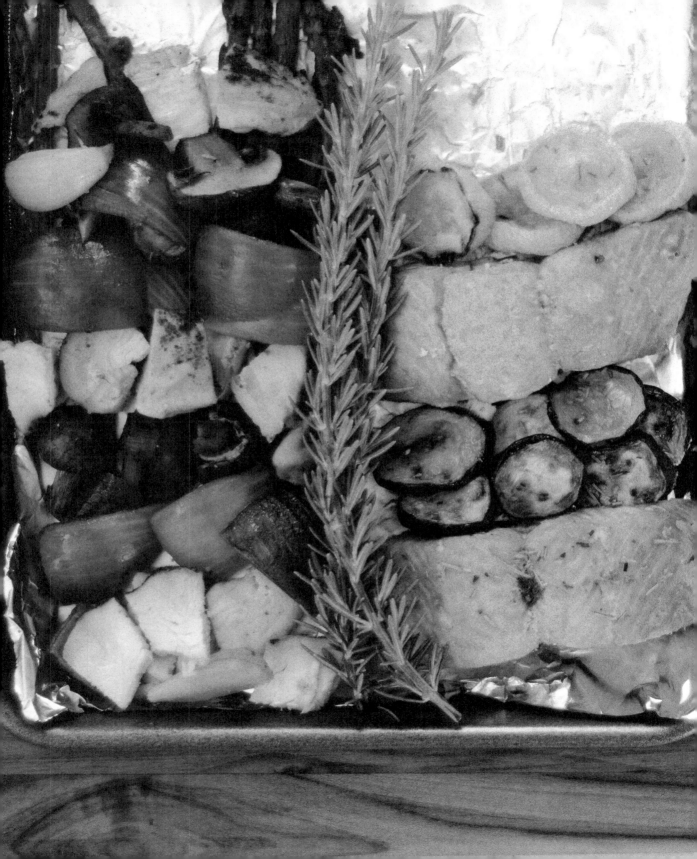

TWO BIRDS, ONE STONE: SALMON AND CHICKEN ONE PAN DISH

SERVES 2 | SALMON PAN CALORIES PER SERVING 229
| CHICKEN PAN CALORIES PER SERVING 226

INGREDIENTS

SALMON

2 5-ozs Raw salmon filets
1 Thin zucchini –
sliced in ½ oz slices
1 Thin yellow squash –
sliced in ½-oz slices
½ T Olive oil
1 T Rosemary (fresh or dried)
Juice of ½ lemon

CHICKEN

10 ozs Raw chicken breast
4 ozs Mushrooms – quartered
1 Red onion – quartered
4 ozs Asparagus
1 T Olive oil
1 tsp Paprika
1 tsp Dry garlic

MACROS
(SALMON/CHICKEN)

Protein 33.3 g/30.4 g
Carbs 7.8 g/4.4 g
Fat 8.2 g/9.8 g

DIRECTIONS

> Line two small baking pans with foil.
> Preheat oven to 450° F.
> In a large bowl, mix together the zucchini and yellow squash; add olive oil, rosemary, and mix again.
> Layer the squash mixture on a baking sheet and place the salmon filets next to the vegetables. Sprinkle the salmon with lemon juice, and add salt and pepper to the salmon and vegetables.
> In another large bowl, mix together the mushrooms, onions, asparagus, and chicken cut into 1-oz cubes; then add the olive oil and mix again.
> Transfer to the second baking pan and sprinkle with paprika and garlic, and add salt and pepper to taste.
> Bake both pans at once for 20-25 minutes.

CHEF'S TIP:

To make sure all of the ingredients on a pan cook evenly, cut them in similar size pieces and choose vegetables that are similar in texture. Salmon cooks faster than chicken, and it's always best to cook a whole filet, so choose vegetables to go with it that cook quickly, such as squash, asparagus, onions, mushrooms, or small potatoes cut in half.

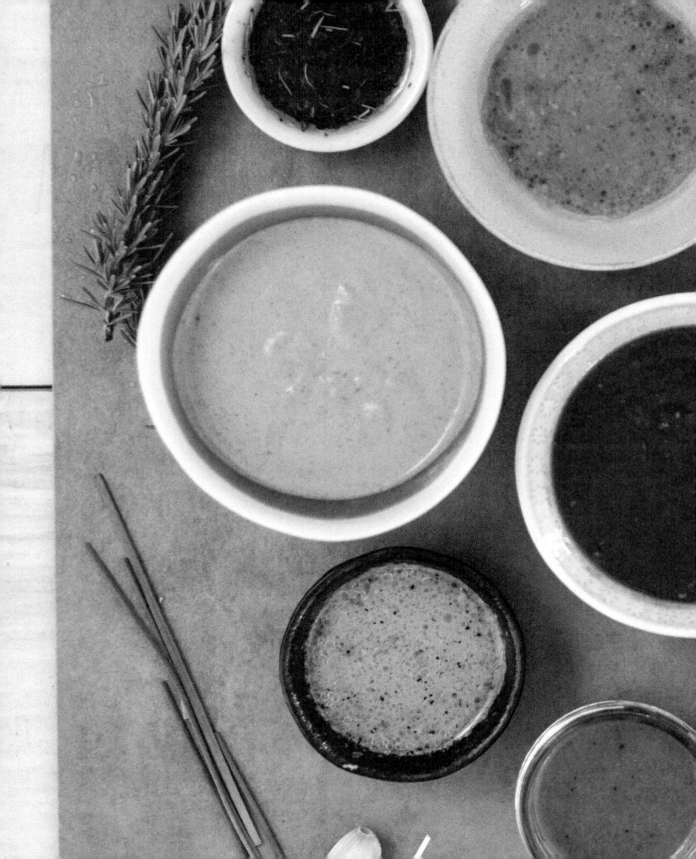

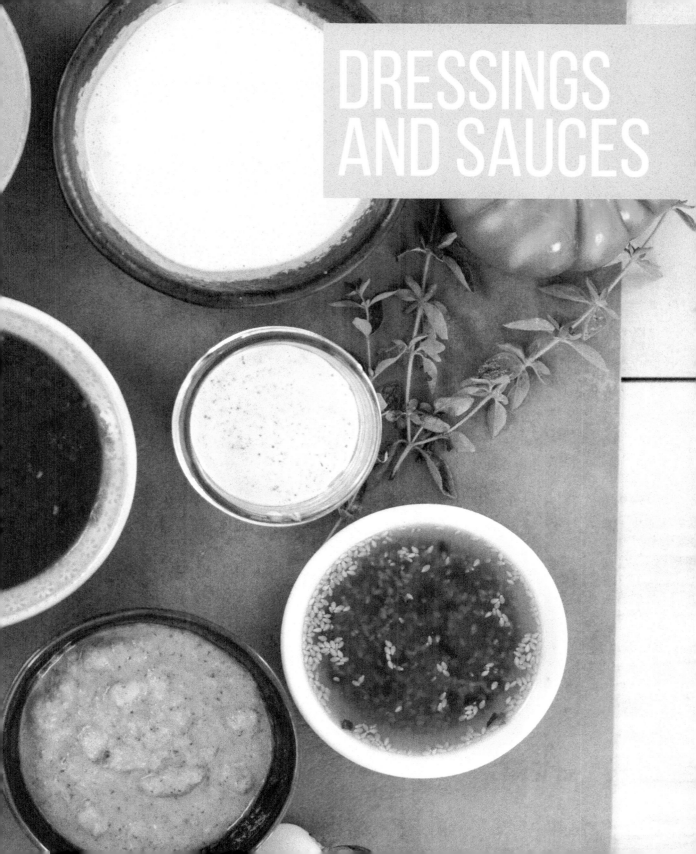

DRESSINGS AND SAUCES

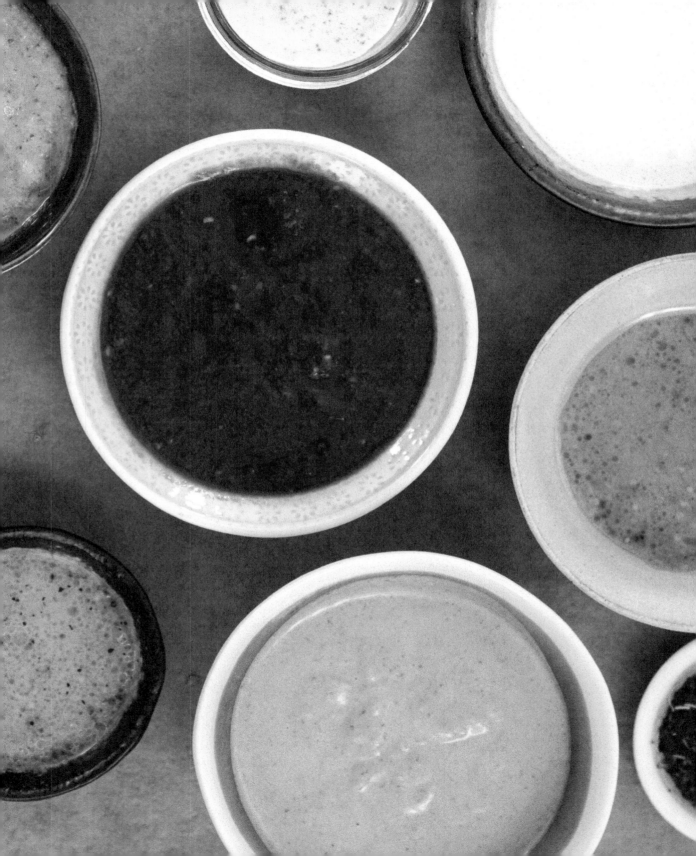

CREAMY AVOCADO AND CILANTRO DRESSING

SERVES 12 / 1 SERVING = 1 T | CALORIES PER SERVING 12

INGREDIENTS

½ Avocado
1 C Cilantro
1 Clove garlic
Juice of 1 lime
¼ C Greek yogurt
3-4 T Water
Salt and pepper

DIRECTIONS

> Add all ingredients but the water into a food processor and blend on low/ medium speed, adding water one tablespoon at a time until the dressing reaches the desired consistency.

MACROS

Protein 0.6 g
Carbs 1.1 g
Fat 1.2 g

LEMON BALSAMIC DRESSING

SERVES 10 / 1 SERVING = 1 T | CALORIES PER SERVING 53

INGREDIENTS

¼ C White wine vinegar
¼ C Olive oil
Juice of ½ lemon
Salt and pepper

DIRECTIONS

> Add all ingredients into a cup or bowl, and whisk together.

MACROS

Protein 0 g
Carbs 1.1 g
Fat 5.4 g

I'M ITALIAN DRESSING

SERVES 8 / 1 SERVING = 1 T | CALORIES PER SERVING 61

INGREDIENTS

¼ C Olive oil
¼ C Red wine vinegar
¼ tsp Dried basil
¼ tsp Dried oregano
¼ tsp Dried parsley
¼ tsp Dried thyme
Salt and pepper

DIRECTIONS

› Add all ingredients into a cup or bowl, and whisk together.

MACROS

Protein 0 g
Carbs 0 g
Fat 6.8 g

HONEY MONEY DRESSING

SERVES 11 / 1 SERVING = 1 T | CALORIES PER SERVING 53

INGREDIENTS

1 T Whole grain dijon mustard
1 T Honey
1 T Honey dijon mustard
¼ C White wine vinegar
¼ C Avocado oil

DIRECTIONS

› Add all ingredients into a cup or bowl, and whisk together.

MACROS

Protein 0 g
Carbs 1.9 g
Fat 5.2 g

SEXYFIT-STYLE HOMEMADE MAYO

SERVES 22 / 1 SERVING = 1 T | CALORIES PER SERVING 12

INGREDIENTS

2 Egg yolks
Salt and pepper
1 T Dijon mustard
1-1½ T Water
1 C Avocado oil
Juice of 1 lemon

DIRECTIONS

> Make sure all ingredients are room temperature (30-60 minutes on the counter).
> Add the egg yolks, salt, pepper, water, and mustard into a food processor and start blending on slow speed.
> SLOWLY pour the oil into the food processor as you continue blending.
> Once the mixture becomes thick, pour it out of the processor into a bowl, add the juice of one lemon, and mix with a spoon.

MACROS

Protein 0.3 g
Carbs 0.3 g
Fat 10.6 g

RANCHO SANTA FA RANCH DRESSING

SERVES 8 / 1 SERVING = 1 T | CALORIES PER SERVING 53

INGREDIENTS

¼ C Mayo (see recipe above)
⅛ C Coconut cream
1 T White wine vinegar
¼ tsp Garlic powder
¼ tsp Onion powder
¼ tsp Paprika
¼ tsp Dried parsley
¼ tsp Dried dill

DIRECTIONS

> Add all ingredients into a cup or bowl, and whisk together.

MACROS

Protein 0 g
Carbs 0 g
Fat 6 g

ASIAN DRESSING

SERVES 6 / 1 SERVING = 1 T | CALORIES PER SERVING 36

INGREDIENTS

¼ C Rice vinegar
1 T Light soy sauce
½ tsp Minced ginger
1 clove Minced Garlic
Red pepper flakes
1 tsp Sesame seeds
1 T Sesame oil
1 tsp Honey

DIRECTIONS

› Add all ingredients into a cup or bowl, and whisk together.

MACROS

Protein 0.3 g
Carbs 3.5 g
Fat 2.5 g

RASPBERRY CHIPOTLE DRESSING

SERVES 20 / 1 SERVING = 1 T | CALORIES PER SERVING 10

INGREDIENTS

½ C Raspberries
½ small can Chipotle peppers
½ C White wine vinegar
1 T Brown sugar
Salt and pepper

DIRECTIONS

› Add all ingredients into a food processor and blend together until the mixture becomes smooth.

MACROS

Protein 0.2 g
Carbs 1.6 g
Fat 0.2 g

POMEGRANATE DRESSING

SERVES 14 / 1 SERVING = 1 T | CALORIES PER SERVING 21

INGREDIENTS

½ Pomegranate
Juice of 1 lemon
Juice of 1 grapefruit
2 tsp Honey
1 T olive oil
Salt and pepper

DIRECTIONS

> Add all ingredients into a food processor and blend together until smooth.

MACROS

Protein 0.2 g
Carbs 3.1 g
Fat 1 g

PINEAPPLE HABANERO DRESSING

SERVES 12 / 1 SERVING = 1 T | CALORIES PER SERVING 50

INGREDIENTS

½ C Pineapple
1 Habanero pepper –
minced
¼ C Avocado oil
½ C Cilantro
½ Onion
2 cloves Garlic
Salt and pepper

DIRECTIONS

> Add all ingredients into a food processor, and blend on slow until smooth but not a puree.

MACROS

Protein 0.3 g
Carbs 1.9 g
Fat 4.7 g

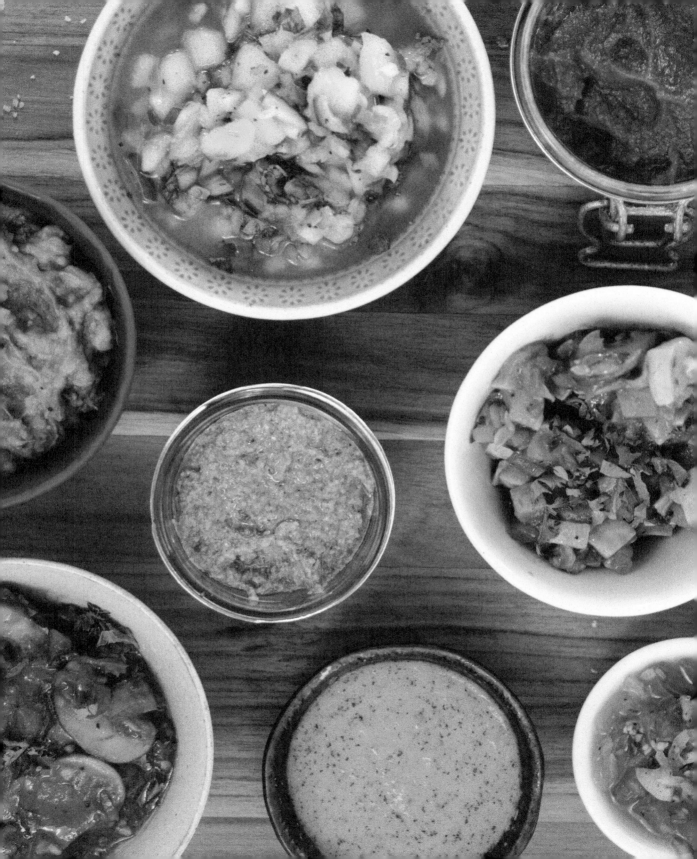

TOMATO MUSHROOM SAUCE

SERVES 6 / 1 SERVING = 1 T | CALORIES PER SERVING 66

INGREDIENTS

2 Tomatoes – chopped
½ Onion – chopped
1 clove Garlic – chopped
4 ozs Mushrooms – sliced
1 T Grapeseed oil
½ can Tomato paste
½ C Water (or vegetable broth if you have some on hand)
1 T Parsley – chopped
1 tsp Paprika
Salt and pepper

MACROS

Protein 3.2 g
Carbs 8.7 g
Fat 2.5 g

DIRECTIONS

> Heat the oil in a nonstick saucepan on medium heat.
> Prepare the vegetables and herbs.
> Saute the onions in the oil for 3-4 minutes until they become translucent.
> Add the garlic and cook for 2 more minutes.
> Add the mushrooms and tomatoes, and cook 2 more minutes, stirring a couple of times.
> Whisk together the tomato paste and water in a cup, and pour into the pan.
> Stir in the salt, pepper, parsley, and paprika; bring the heat to low and let cook for 10 minutes.

TOMATO, YELLOW SQUASH, AND THYME SAUCE

SERVES 6 / 1 SERVING = 1 T | CALORIES PER SERVING 50

INGREDIENTS

1 Tomato – finely chopped
½ Onion – finely chopped
1 Yellow squash –
finely chopped
1 clove Garlic –
finely chopped
1 T Grapeseed oil
½ can Tomato paste
½ C Water (or vegetable broth
if you have some on hand)
¼ T Thyme – finely chopped
¼ T Sage – finely chopped
Salt and pepper

MACROS

Protein 1.1 g
Carbs 5.8 g
Fat 2.7 g

DIRECTIONS

> Heat the oil in a nonstick saucepan on medium heat.
> Prepare the vegetables and herbs.
> Saute the onions in the oil for 3-4 minutes until they become translucent.
> Add the garlic and cook for 2 more minutes.
> Add the squash and tomatoes, and cook 2 more minutes, stirring a couple of times.
> Whisk together the tomato paste and water in a cup, and pour into the pan.
> Stir in the salt, pepper, thyme, and sage; bring the heat to low and let cook for 10 minutes.

SUNDRIED TOMATO GUACAMOLE

SERVES 4 / 1 SERVING = 1 T | CALORIES PER SERVING 54

INGREDIENTS

1 Avocado
2 T Sundried tomatoes
(no oil) – roughly chopped
Juice of 1 lemon
Salt and pepper

DIRECTIONS

> Peel and seed the avocado, place into a bowl, and mash with a fork or a potato masher.
> Add the chopped sundried tomatoes to the avocado.
> Add the lemon juice, salt and pepper to taste, and mix together.

MACROS

Protein 1 g
Carbs 6.3 g
Fat 6.5 g

KETCHUP

SERVES 16 / 1 SERVING = 1 T | CALORIES PER SERVING 13

INGREDIENTS

½ C Tomato paste
¼ C Apple cider
¼ C White wine vinegar
1 tsp Minced garlic
1 tsp Brown sugar
Salt

DIRECTIONS

> Heat tomato paste, cider, and vinegar in a saucepan until it starts simmering (do not boil).
> Add the remaining ingredients and whisk together. Let simmer for 5 minutes.

MACROS

Protein 0.3 g
Carbs 2.8 g
Fat 0 g

PESTO SAUCE

SERVES 14 / 1 SERVING = 1 T | CALORIES PER SERVING 97

INGREDIENTS

¼ C Walnuts
1 clove Garlic
1 C Parsley
Juice of ½ lemon
¼ C Pumpkin seeds
1 tsp Dry basil
1 tsp Dry oregano
1 tsp Dry tarragon
½ C Olive oiL

DIRECTIONS

› Add all ingredients, except the olive oil, into a food processor and start blending on slow speed.
› SLOWLY pour the oil into the food processor as you continue blending.
› Blend until the ingredients are finely chopped but not a puree.

MACROS

Protein 0.9 g
Carbs 1.2 g
Fat 10.1 g

MANGO SALSA

SERVES 4 / 1 SERVING = 1 T | CALORIES PER SERVING 27

INGREDIENTS

½ Mango – roughly chopped
½ Cucumber – roughly chopped
¼ Red onion – finely chopped
½ C Cilantro – finely chopped
1 Jalapeño – finely chopped
Juice of 3 limes
Salt and pepper

DIRECTIONS

› Prep the mango, vegetables, and herbs.
› Mix the ingredients in a bowl, add lime juice, and salt and pepper to taste. Serve cold.

MACROS

Protein 0.4 g
Carbs 7.1 g
Fat 0.2 g

CURRY SAUCE

SERVES 26 / 1 SERVING = 1 T | CALORIES PER SERVING 14

INGREDIENTS

1 T Grapeseed oil
¼ Onion – chopped
1 tsp Ginger – minced
1 clove Garlic – minced
1 tsp Yellow curry powder
½ tsp Red curry powder
½ tsp Cumin
1½ C Light coconut milk
Juice of 1 lime
Salt and pepper

DIRECTIONS

> Heat the oil in a medium saucepan on medium heat.
> Prep the vegetables.
> Add the onions to the pan and cook for 4-5 minutes until they become translucent. Add the garlic and cook 2 more minutes, stirring a few times.
> Add the remaining ingredients, stir, and bring to a simmer.
> Transfer the mixture to a blender and blend until smooth.

MACROS

Protein 0 g
Carbs 1 g
Fat 1.2 g

PICO DE GALLO

SERVES 4 / 1 SERVING = 1 T | CALORIES PER SERVING 28

INGREDIENTS

2 Roma tomatoes – roughly chopped
½ Red onion – finely chopped
1 clove Garlic – finely chopped
½ C Cilantro – roughly chopped
1 Jalapeño – finely chopped
Juice of 3 limes
1 tsp Chili powder
Salt and pepper

DIRECTIONS

> Prep the vegetables and herbs.
> Mix the ingredients in a bowl, add lime juice, chili powder, and salt and pepper to taste. Serve cold.

MACROS

Protein 0.7 g
Carbs 6.6 g
Fat 0.3 g

SPICY BARBECUE SAUCE

SERVES 10 / 1 SERVING = 1 T | CALORIES PER SERVING 29

INGREDIENTS

1 T grapeseed oil
½ Small onion – finely chopped
2 cloves Garlic – finely chopped
½ Tomato – finely chopped
½ can Tomato paste
½ tsp Paprika
½ tsp Chili powder
¼ tsp Cayenne pepper
¼ C Apple cider
1 oz can Chipotle peppers

MACROS

Protein 0.4 g
Carbs 3.5 g
Fat 1.5 g

DIRECTIONS

> Heat the oil in a medium saucepan on medium heat.
> Prep the vegetables.
> Add the onions to the pan and cook for 4-5 minutes until they become translucent.
> Add the garlic and cook 2 more minutes, stirring a few times.
> Add the tomatoes and cook 3 more minutes.
> Add the remaining ingredients, except the chipotle peppers, and bring to a simmer.
> Transfer the mixture to a blender, add the chipotle peppers, and blend until smooth.

ROASTED BELL PEPPER SAUCE

SERVES 18 / 1 SERVING = 1 T | CALORIES PER SERVING 18

INGREDIENTS

1 C Roasted bell peppers
(rinse if in oil)
2 T Olive oil
¼ Onion
1 clove Garlic
1 T Parsley
1 T Dill
Juice of ½ lime
Salt and pepper

MACROS

Protein 0.1 g
Carbs 0.9 g
Fat 1.5 g

DIRECTIONS

> Add all ingredients into a food processor and blend until desired consistency.

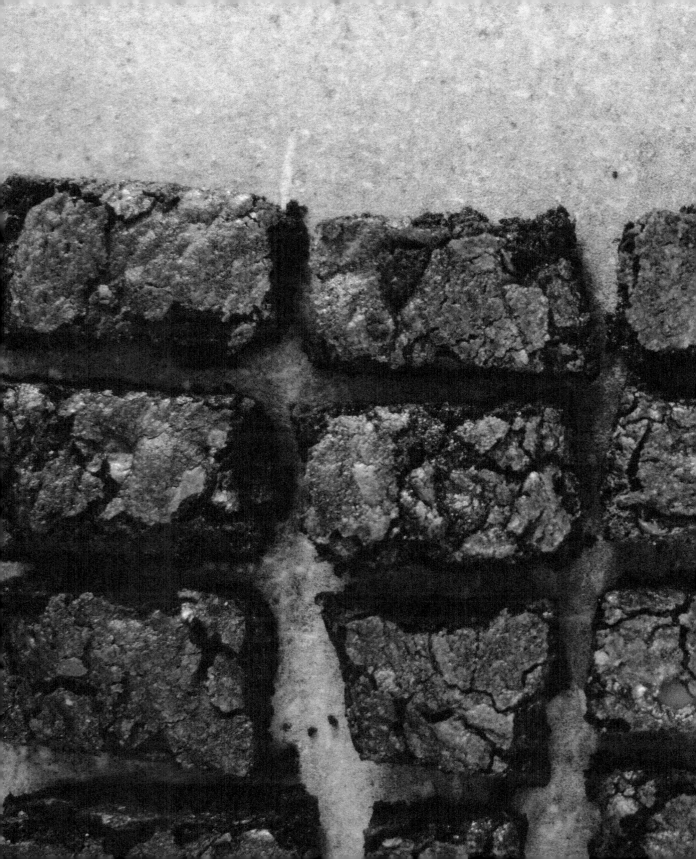

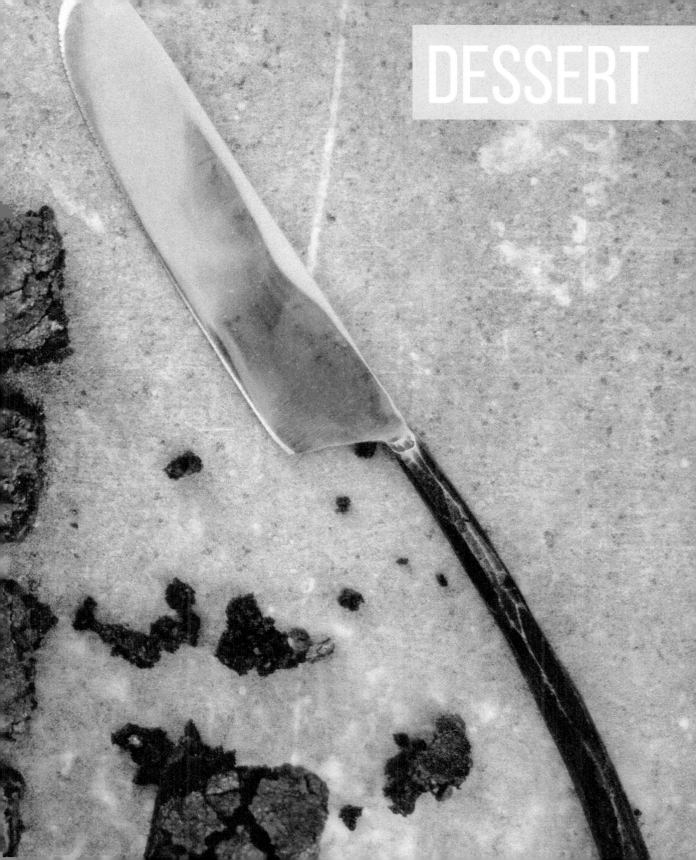

DESSERT

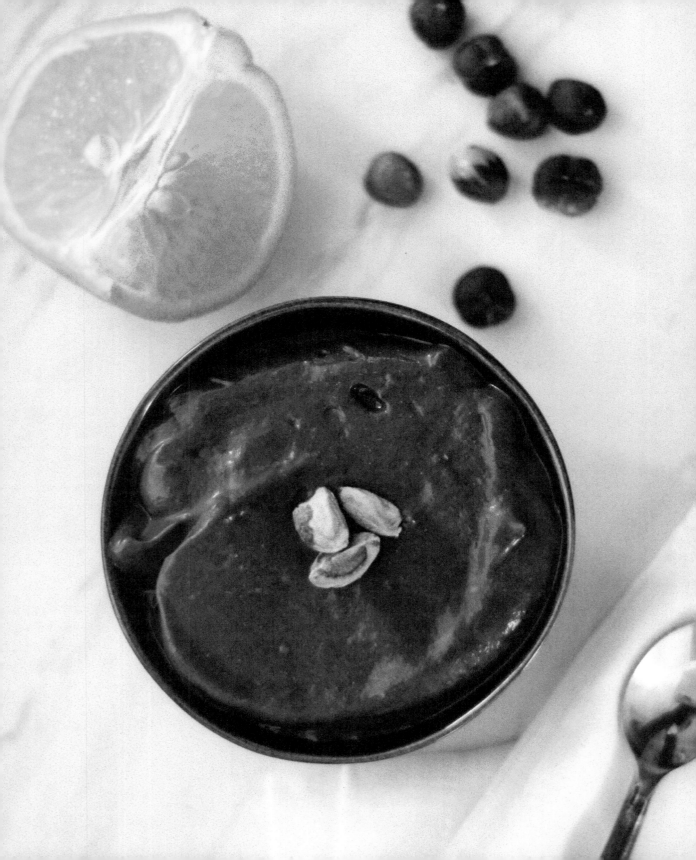

CHOCO LOCO AVOCADO PUDDING

SERVES 2 | CALORIES PER SERVING 194

INGREDIENTS

1 Avocado
⅓ C Almond milk
1 scoop Chocolate protein
powder (I use Jay Robb)
1 tsp Coconut – shaved
5 Pistachios for topping

MACROS

Protein 14.5 g
Carbs 7.4 g
Fat 12 g

DIRECTIONS

> Slice the avocado in half, remove the seed, and the peel.
> Blend the avocado, almond milk, and protein powder in a blender on medium speed.
> Transfer to a bowl, and top with shaved coconut and pistachios.

CHEF'S TIP:

If you don't have protein powder at home but still want to have a good amount of protein in your desert, you can replace almond milk with egg whites and the protein powder with 1 T of cocoa powder.

This recipes also tastes fantastic if you blend ½ banana with all the other ingredients.

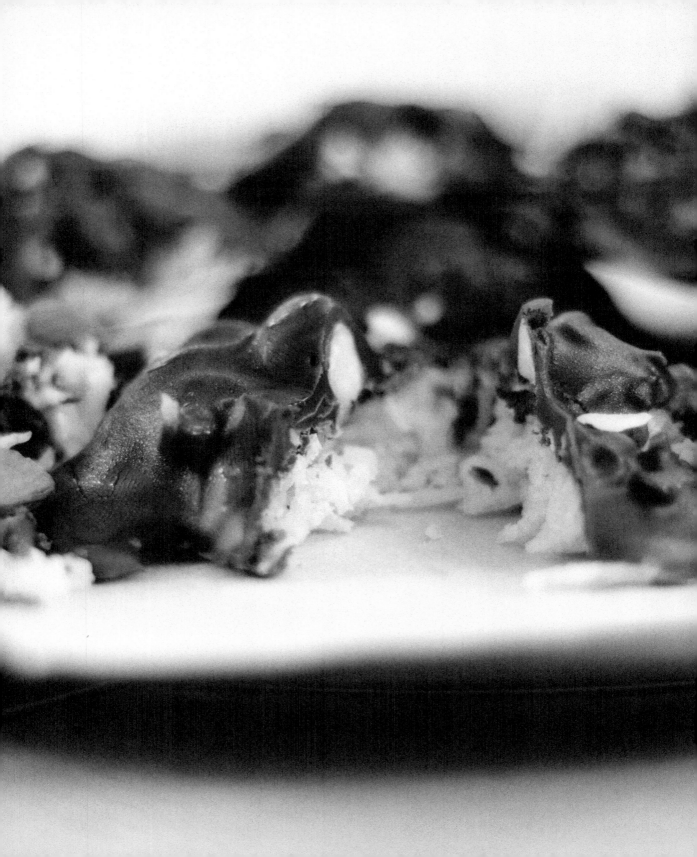

SWEET TOOTH COCONUT BITES

SERVES 10 | CALORIES PER SERVING 173 (1 CLUSTER)

INGREDIENTS

10 T Unsweetened
Coconut – shredded
2 T Honey
3 T Coconut oil
¾ C (5 ozs) Chocolate chips
10 Hazelnuts

MACROS

Protein 1.7 g
Carbs 13.7 g
Fat 14.3 g

DIRECTIONS

› Bring about an inch of water to a simmer in a saucepan. Set a heatproof bowl in the mouth of the pot, making sure the water doesn't touch the bottom of the bowl. Add chocolate chips and 1 T of the coconut oil to the pot, and stir until all of the chocolate chips are melted.

› In a large bowl, mix the coconut, honey, and remaining coconut oil. Form 10 clusters.

› Line a baking sheet with parchment paper and place the clusters on the parchment paper.

› Add one hazelnut to the middle of each cluster and press it in with a spoon.

› Pour the chocolate over the clusters with a spoon, divided evenly.

› Place in the freezer for 30 minutes.

CHEF'S TIP:

If you have a steamer pot (or double boiler), it's the best tool to melt chocolate. Just bring it to a boil and keep on simmer while the chocolate is melting.

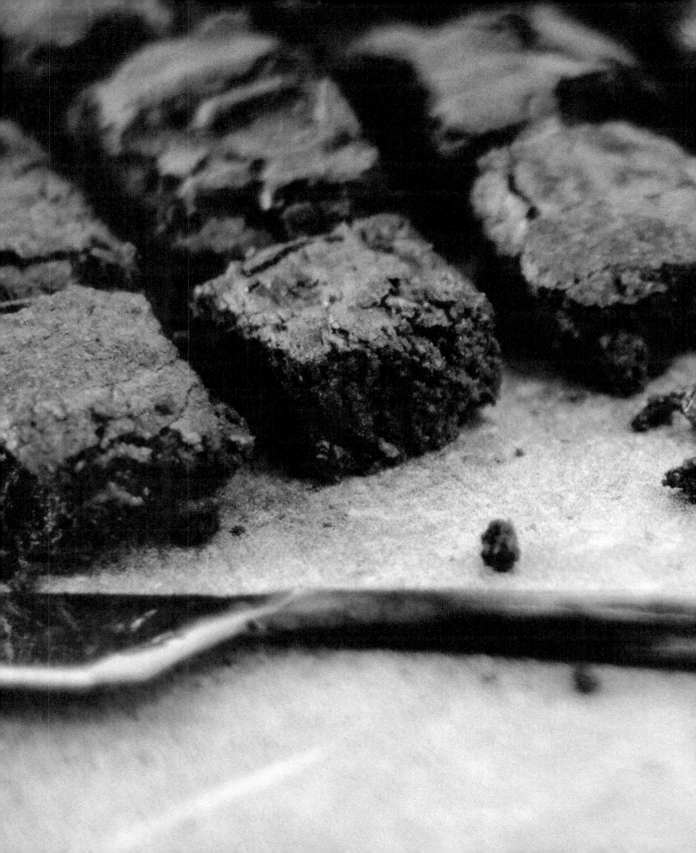

BLISSFUL BROWNIE BITES

SERVES 16 | CALORIES PER SERVING 127 (1 BROWNIE)

INGREDIENTS

3 T Coconut oil

½ C Coconut sugar

8 ozs Chocolate chips (I use Guittard – best ingredients)

2 Eggs – room temperature

1 tsp Vanilla extract

¼ tsp Salt

1 T Unsweetened cocoa powder

3 T Cornstarch

MACROS

Protein 1.8 g

Carbs 15.2 g

Fat 8 g

DIRECTIONS

› Preheat oven to 375° F. Line a 9" x 9" pan with foil and lightly spray; set aside.

› In a small saucepan over low heat, melt the oil, then add the sugar. Once the sugar is dissolved, add the chocolate chips, stirring until smooth. Remove from heat and whisk for 2 minutes. Add the eggs and the vanilla extract.

› Add the salt, cocoa powder, and cornstarch into the saucepan. Stir together, then beat the batter vigorously for 1-2 minutes (a hand mixer works best).

› Pour the batter into the pan, and bake for 25-30 minutes or until the brownies are set in the center.

› Allow the brownies to cool before cutting.

CHEF'S TIP:

If you would like to have more protein in your brownies, add 2 scoops of protein powder when adding the cocoa powder. You can use a chocolate-flavored powder or even a flavorless one.

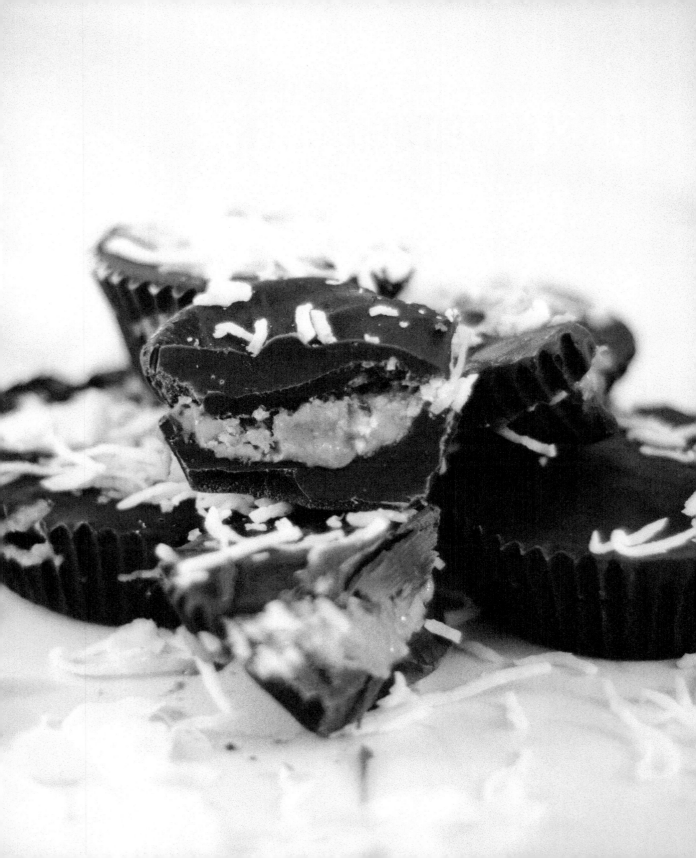

CHEER UP ALMOND BUTTER CUP

SERVES 12 | CALORIES PER SERVING 101 (1 CUP)

INGREDIENTS

¾ C Chocolate chips
1 T Coconut oil
4 T Almond butter
1 T Coconut – shredded

MACROS

Protein 1.8 g
Carbs 7.7 g
Fat 8.1 g

DIRECTIONS

> Melt the chocolate chips with the coconut oil using the method from the Sweet Tooth Coconut Bites recipe on Page 225.
> Line a mini muffin tin with cupcake liners.
> Add 1 tsp of the melted chocolate into each liner.
> Add 1 tsp of almond butter into each liner.
> Sprinkle with shredded coconut.
> Top each with 1 tsp of melted chocolate.

CHEF'S TIP:

You can use any type of nut butter you like – peanut, sunflower, cashew, hazelnut, or mixed. You can also use a high-protein peanut butter spread such as P28 or Nuts N' More.

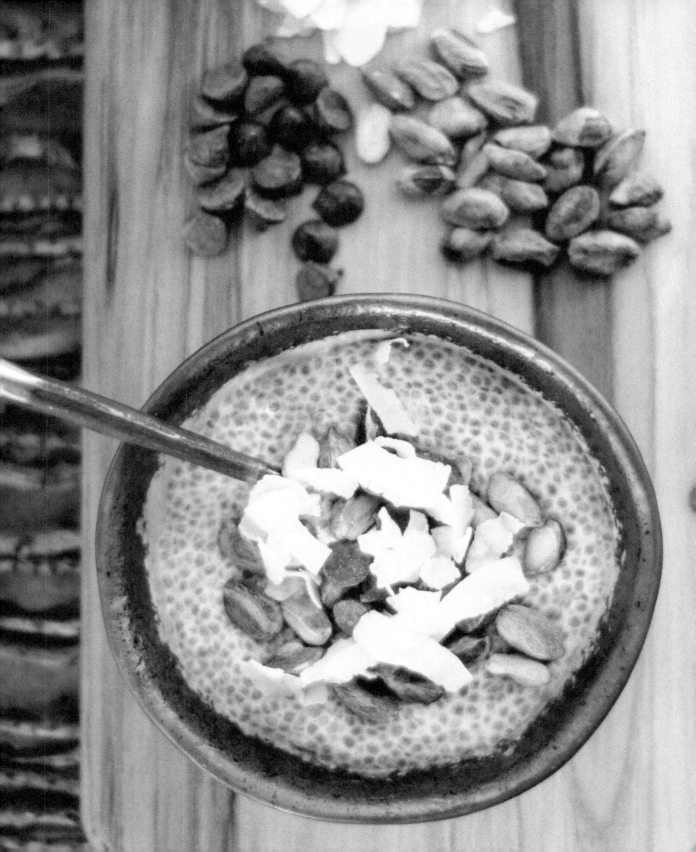

BUFF BABE CHIA PUDDING

SERVES 3 | CALORIES PER SERVING 183

INGREDIENTS

2 T Chia seeds
¾ C Light coconut milk
1 oz Chocolate chips
1 scoop Vanilla protein powder
1 T Coconut – shaved
12 Pistachios

MACROS

Protein 33.9 g
Carbs 41 g
Fat 28 g

DIRECTIONS

> Mix the coconut milk with the chia seeds, and place in the refrigerator for at least 2 hours or overnight is best..
> Move to a bowl, and add the chocolate chips and protein powder.
> Top with shaved coconut and pistachios.

CHEF'S TIP:

If you would like to reduce the fat content, replace the coconut milk with almond milk and use half of the chocolate chips.

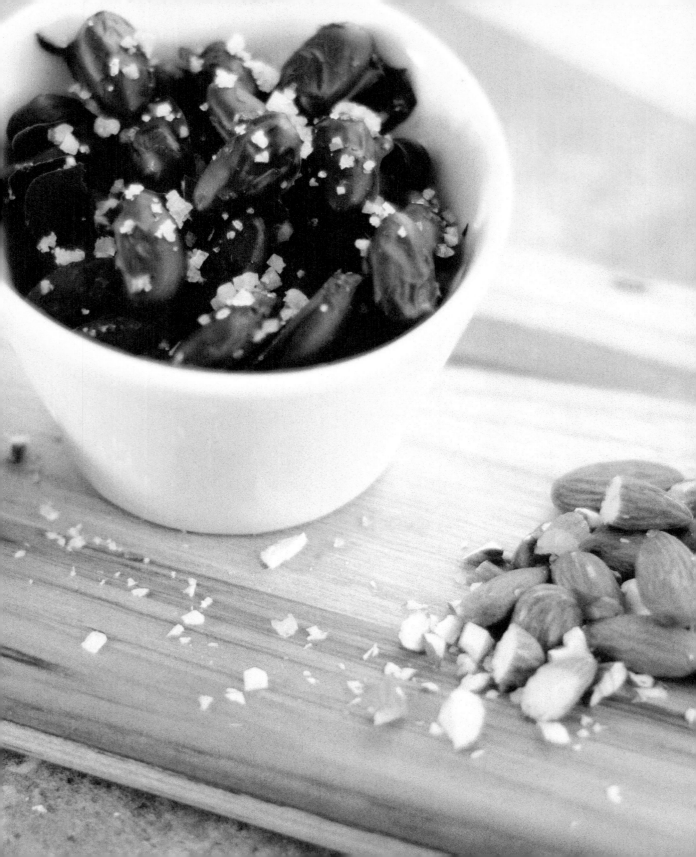

SEA SALTED ALMONDS

SERVES 4 / 1 SERVING = ¼ C | CALORIES PER SERVING 278

INGREDIENTS

4 ozs 85% dark chocolate

1 cups unsalted raw almonds

Sea salt

MACROS

Protein 40 g

Carbs 65 g

Fat 77 g

DIRECTIONS

> Melt the chocolate in a double boiler over medium heat, stirring until fully melted.

> Stir the almonds into the chocolate, and toss until well coated.

> Place the chocolate covered almonds onto a parchment covered baking sheet.

> Sprinkle almonds with sea salt, and set aside until the chocolate is set.

> Store in the refrigerator until ready to eat.

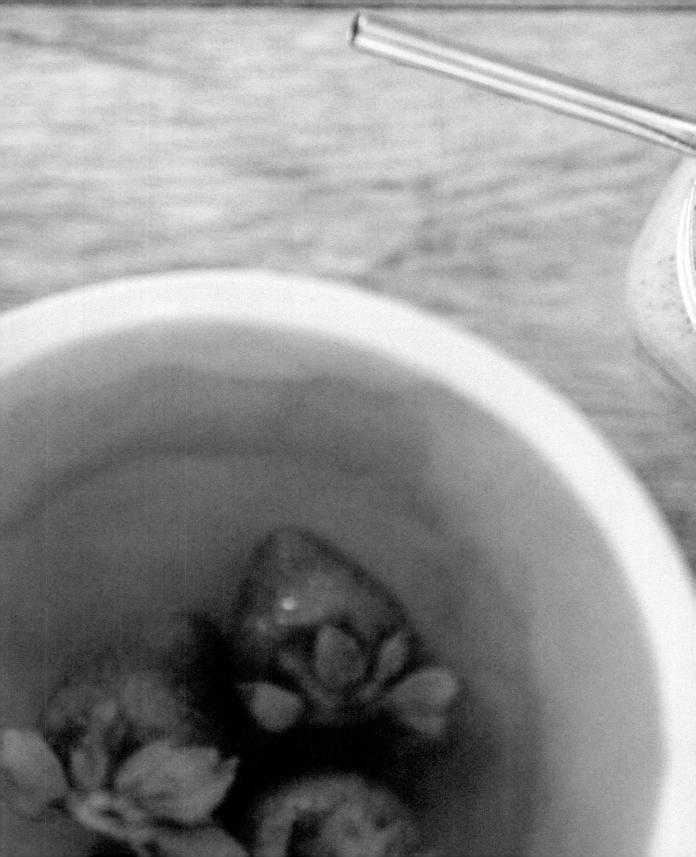

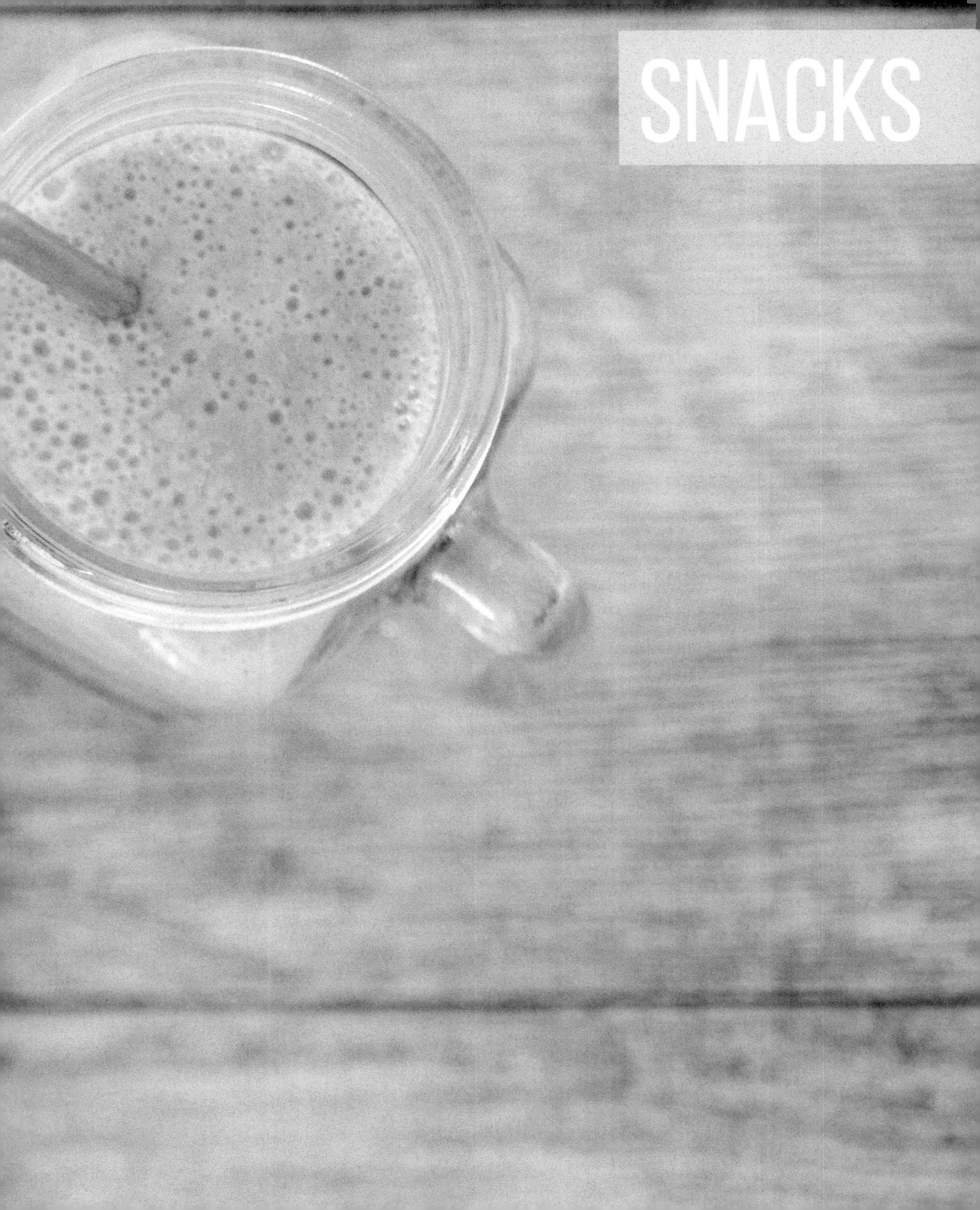

PROTEIN SHAKES

SERVES 1 | CALORIES PER SERVING SEE BELOW

> Mix or blend ingredients together with ice and place in a cup.

INGREDIENTS

1 C Spinach
1 scoop Chocolate
protein powder
1 T Almond butter
1 tsp Cocoa powder
½ T Chia seeds
1 T Flaxseed (optional)

MACROS

Calories 283
Protein 33 g
Carbs 11 g
Fat 14 g

INGREDIENTS

1 C Spinach
1 scoop Vanilla
protein powder
⅓ Avocado
½ C Mango

MACROS

Calories 232
Protein 28 g
Carbs 17 g
Fat 6 g

INGREDIENTS

½ Avocado
1 scoop Vanilla
protein powder
½ C Blueberries
½ C Raspberries
2-3 Basil leaves

MACROS

Calories 300
Protein 28 g
Carbs 25 g
Fat 11 g

INGREDIENTS

1 C Spinach
1 scoop Chocolate
protein powder
½ C Frozen cherries
1 tsp Cocoa powder
2 squares Dark chocolate
(27 g) — shredded on top

MACROS

Calories 307
Protein 29 g
Carbs 27 g
Fat 13 g

INGREDIENTS

½ C Kiwi
1 Cucumber
½ Green apple
1 scoop Vanilla
protein powder
1 T Honey
8 ozs Coconut water
2-3 Mint leaves

MACROS

Calories 300
Protein 25 g
Carbs 51 g
Fat 0 g

YOGURT AND COTTAGE CHEESE

SERVES 1 | CALORIES PER SERVING SEE BELOW

> Mix or blend ingredients together and place in a bowl.

INGREDIENTS	MACROS	INGREDIENTS	MACROS
¾ C Yogurt	Calories 369	¾ C Cottage cheese	Calories 433
½ C Blueberries	Protein 22 g	¼ C Raisins	Protein 25 g
1 oz Almonds	Carbs 24 g	1 oz Almonds	Carbs 35 g
	Fat 22 g		Fat 25 g
1 C Yogurt	Calories 293	½ C Cottage cheese	Calories 317
½ C Pineapple	Protein 22 g	¼ Avocado	Protein 17 g
½ C Peaches	Carbs 24 g	1/2 Banana	Carbs 25 g
	Fat 11 g	1 tsp Cocoa powder	Fat 19 g
		½ oz Pistachios or hazelnuts	
1 C Yogurt	Calories 377		
1T Chia seeds	Protein 24 g		
½ C Raspberries	Carbs 39 g		
1 tsp Cocoa powder	Fat 14 g		
1 tsp Honey			

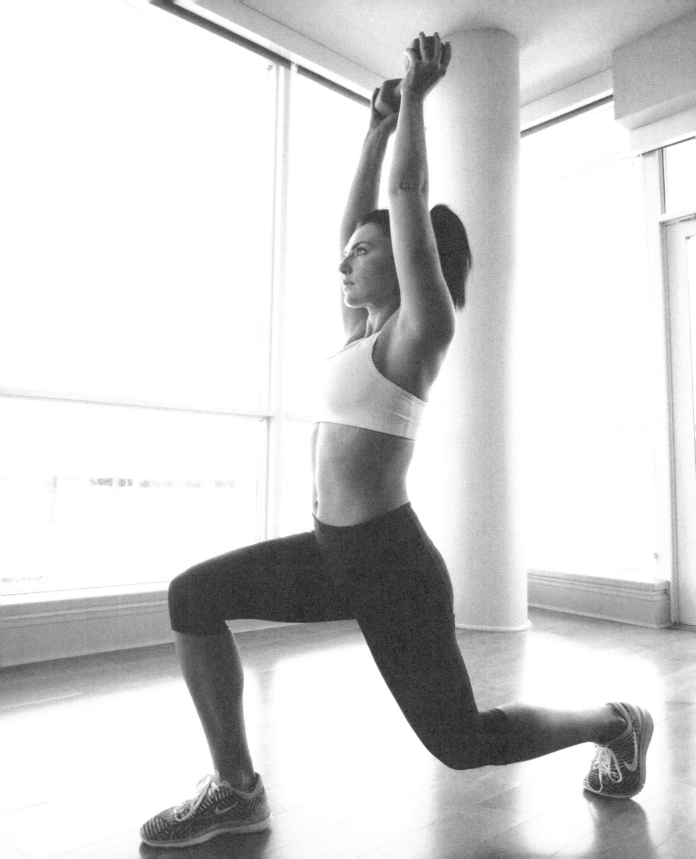

STEP III
SIMPLE FITNESS

Make fitness a lifestyle with an
effective workout method
designed for women
by a woman.

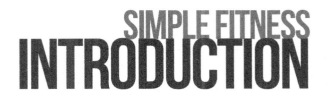

SIMPLE FITNESS INTRODUCTION

"I really regret that workout."

— Said no one ever

In the previous section, you had the opportunity to learn everything you'll need to know about nutrition and how to create complete food freedom YOUR way. In this section, I'm going to walk you through the exact method to help you get in the best shape of your life and keep those results for life.

Fitness is by FAR my most favorite topic, and putting together this section of the book was the most difficult part because there's SO much to share with you. My goal with the Sexyfit workout method is to give you the exact step-by-step strategy for an attainable and sustainable physique, both functionally and aesthetically — without compromising either. I want you to look great AND experience the external functional benefits of making fitness a lifestyle.

IN THIS SECTION OF THE BOOK:

- We'll discover what fitness is for us and create a long-lasting mental shift so we can make fitness a lifestyle.
- We'll create simple daily habits and routines to add movement and stretching into our day.
- We'll walk through the concept of lifting to get lean and discover the most efficient methods of training for our body.
- We'll understand how sleep, soreness, monthly cycle, and other lifestyle factors influence our fitness progress.
- We'll learn the best nutritional practices to maximize our results.
- We'll create a loving, kind, caring relationship with our body and learn how to get in tune with our inner guidance in regard to working out.

FITNESS IS A TOOL
CHAPTER 24

"Active living is waking up and throwing away all your excuses."

– Lorna Jane

We're going to start this section in a very similar way that we started the Nutrition section. What's your fitness story? Meaning, what is fitness to you?

For many of us, fitness has been a way to crash train into a bikini body for Hawaii next month. For others, it's a way of pushing ourselves for eating something we're not supposed to. For me, as you know, it was a way to control my environment and release stress.

Fitness is a tool.

First and foremost, the purpose of fitness is to move your body in a way that gives you energy for your daily schedule, gives your strength to go through life, and keeps you active and healthy. Having a set fitness routine allows you to thrive in your life from overflowing energy. And second, the purpose of fitness is to create the look that you desire. But that's just secondary and usually comes as a side-effect. I have to say this, we've spent quite some time in the Mindset and Nutrition chapters talking about cultivating self-love and loving your body the way it is right now. Fitness is not an outlet for punishment, self-shaming, or hating on the body you have now. You can love the body you have now and choose to exercise with purpose.

I've spent years in an environment where fitness was only praised as a look for vanity. It's a trap; don't buy into that. In fact, I ask you to detach from the visual outcome as fast as possible, and really allow yourself to see and feel the massive benefits that fitness can bring into your life. The faster you let it go, the more consistent you'll become because there's no expectation of a "perfect body." I've been there and done that sister, I look better now than I did competing because I don't care about the outcome, BUT I know exactly how my body will respond to certain types of training. The moment I realized that looks are just a side-effect of fitness and stopped objectifying my results, I got extremely grateful and present for every moment I got to spend moving my body. Every day I show up at the gym or on the road or on the mat for yoga, I'm beyond grateful for what I GET to do with my body.

One good thing about my many years of being on the competitive stage is that since I had spent so much time learning how to alter body composition in such a way that's both pleasing and symmetrical to the eye, we get the best of both worlds: function and aesthetics. I'm also beyond grateful (seriously, I'm so grateful that I feel the need to repeat how grateful I am: I'm so grateful!) for the experience I've had and get to share, so that your workouts get the best bang for your time spent.

In no way, shape, or form do I intend to tell you that some parts of your body are inadequate or not good enough. I'm simply going to talk you along the journey of how to be the most efficient with the time you'll dedicate to working out.

As a result of what I'm about to share with you in this section, you'll be sexy and fit, and your body will feel the best it has ever felt and will look it, too. I want you to feel fit, but I also want you to function better overall as a woman. It's my way of thinking about "functional training." Functional, here, is the ability for you to be a better mother, wife, boss, artist — whatever you identify as — that carries with it the responsibilities of an independent 21st-century woman.

Opening a jar without asking your partner? You got it. Being able to pick up your 3-year-old and actually holding him/her? Maybe being able to hold a curtain rod over your head while putting it up in your new apartment without getting tired? Or perhaps getting the skis out for the kids and carrying them over your head for what feels like an infinite about of time before getting to the slopes?

YOU'LL BE AN OVERALL BETTER-FUNCTIONING WOMAN WHO'S PREPARED FOR ANYTHING … even a zombie apocalypse.

Fitness is a way for you to take care of yourself and show your body that you care, you're listening, and you're paying attention. If you're just starting out, take it one day at a time, put your blinders on, and do your thing. If you've been working out periodically, getting back in the groove will feel really good, so root into that feeling and emotion to make this a long-term shift. If you've been working out for quite some time, this will be a great way to have a structured program.

💡 CHAPTER PRACTICE

Now we know that we use food as fuel. However, I want to make sure you're aware of what and how you're using exercise in your life right now. Take out your journal and answer the following questions. Once you complete this section, you will gain more clarify about your habits around fitness so you can create a lasting lifestyle shift.

I feel _____ when I'm working out.

Exercise is _____.

I exercise when _____.

IF YOU WEREN'T SUCCESSFUL:

My last exercise routine didn't stick because _____.

But really because_____.

But really, really because _____.

IF YOU DON'T EXERCISE:

I don't exercise because _____.

I use exercise to_____.

🎙 PODCAST ALERT

Reference the www.sexyfit.com/resources page to listen to the "How to Find Motivation" and "Grow into Your Sexier Self with Sexyfit Transformation Susanne Rose" podcasts.

MOVE, MOVE, MOVE
CHAPTER 25

"Every body is meant to move."
— Movemeant Foundation

Simple things first.

Fitness starts with movement. I prefer to keep things easy for you. Fitness doesn't have to be a complex task of following along with DVDs, buying a bunch of equipment, or going to the gym every single day. It can all start with a daily walk.

I know that doesn't sound fancy or sexy.

We often discount what consistent daily walks can do for us.

The best way to describe it, is to show you.

Check out Irina's transformation; she's also a thyroid cancer survivor. When we started working together, she was quite frank with me: "I hate working out, I just won't do it. I'll do the nutrition part, but fitness NOPE. I'm just not going to do it." She lost more than 30 pounds just by practicing macros and walking every morning for 30 minutes.

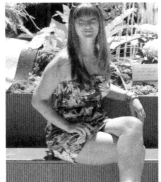

If you aren't inspired by this, I don't know what else will get you moving.

WALKING IS BEST!

It's simple, and it works. Consistency is key!

We as humans weren't designed to sit all day. Modern society is engineered for sitting — we spend more time off of our feet that ever before. We wake up and drive to work, seated; we sit at a desk all day; and when we come home from work we sit down in front of the TV, or we go to dinner with friends and sit, too.

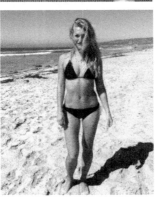

Have you ever heard of the saying, "Sitting is the new smoking"?

I think it's a bit of an overreach by Harvard researchers, but you get the point. Sitting does destroy your posture. By that, I mean it makes your stomach appear larger than it really is and weakens your core because those muscles aren't being used the way they're supposed to be. Keeping those muscles trained, fit, and functional will translate into less pain in your back, hips, and neck, since these joints will be properly supported and aligned. Studies have also connected extended periods of sitting with an increased risk of obesity, diabetes, high blood pressure, and even cancer.

If you're not up for a walk or can't even fathom a workout after a 12-hour day, think about this: Your body is like a finely tuned car. If the car is sitting in the parking lot all day with the lights on, when you come out your car will most likely be dead. If it's a newer model, sure you'll be able to keep it going for two days or so, but your car battery wouldn't last long. So what do you need to do? Jump it with some cables; meaning, put energy toward the battery. Your body works the exact same way. You can't expect to sit around all day long staring at the computer and not jumpstart your battery. You're going to move from office to couch at home and be just as tired. You need to jumpstart your battery in between.

Trust me, you do have the energy in you, and you'll only feel better afterward.

Whether you're already working out or you're just getting into it, I ask you to find a way to move any time you get a chance:

- Take a 10-minute walking break for every 50 minutes of seated working (which burns twice as many calories as sitting) or walk around.
- Stand or exercise while watching TV or working on the computer.
- Park as far away as you can in parking lots.
- "Walk and talk" rather than "sit and speak" while talking on cellphones or land lines.
- Introduce walking meetings to the work calendar (you'll be more productive and less distracted).
- If you sit at your job all day long, set an alarm on your cellphone (on low) to remind yourself to stand up for more than a minute at a time at least every two hours. Stretch, bend, or take a short walk. Better yet, recruit a walking partner to go with you.

A 30-minute daily therapeutic walk will change your life in the best way possible. At the very LEAST, you'll need to do it every day to hit a minimum of 7k-10k steps per day. You don't need to buy a $200 watch tracker for this. Just grab your iPhone and look at the health app; it'll tell you all of your stats. If you're walking at or more than 10k steps, great, congrats to you. You nailed the first part already. If you're under that, figure out how you're going to move more.

We feel like we're too busy to take a walk, but the truth is that we all have 15 minutes rather than scrolling on Facebook or Instagram. You have 20 minutes to walk; just get in the groove of doing it. This is the best way to improve body mechanics, boost your mood, and keep active.

⊙ CHAPTER PRACTICE

Sister, what I want you to do is take a look at your current daily schedule. I ask you to find a gap in your schedule where you feel low on energy or when tend to go on social media to "relax", or perhaps, reach for afternoon cup of coffee. Use this time to walk to jumpstart your internal battery. As a result, you will be more productive, more focused and your body will thank you.

Note this time in your calendar and set an alarm on you phone labeled "Time to move sister" with a cute emoji.

⊙ PODCAST ALERT

Reference the www.sexyfit.com/resources page to listen to the "Dance Away the Pounds and Radiate Rock Solid Confidence with Superstar Keaira LaShae" podcasts.

MUSCLE — THE MOTHER OF ALL TRANSFORMATIONS
CHAPTER 26

Ever wonder why fitness trainers are so obsessed with muscle? I, too, am admittedly obsessed with the art of building muscle. But sexy, toned, and the way that makes me feel and look my best.

If I could, I'd write a song dedicated to the greatness of Queen Muscle!

Muscle is FASCINATING — you can grow it, shape it, mold it into whatever you'd like. Simplest example: Have you ever seen a runner's body or a bodybuilder's body? The difference is the amount of muscle mass on that person's body.

The more muscle you have, the more definition you have.

Muscle = definition = tone

If we're going to talk about the fastest, most efficient, and most time-efficient way to create muscular composition for the sake of visible muscle, resistance training is the way to go. Resistance training — weight training, strength training, or whatever you want to call it — is also the fastest way to torch fat and increase your metabolism. You can do so by using your body weight and adding weight equipment like dumbbells, bars, bands, gym machines, TRX, etc.

How does muscle happen, you ask?

When you strength train, your muscle fibers are broken down and then rebuilt over the next 24-48 hours. While your body is rebuilding those muscles, it's recruiting more calories and energy to make the process happen (generally referred to as the "afterburn" effect or EPOC). What this means is that your metabolism operates at a faster rate, even while you're sitting on the couch after a workout.[20]

It also has a very fancy clinical term called "muscular hypertrophy" — enlargement of the skeletal muscle fibers in response to being recruited to develop increased levels of tension, such as resistance training. Progressive resistance training programs using moderate repetition protocols with high loads will result in increased hypertrophy in adults. Research has shown that resistance training protocols using moderate repetition are the most effective way to improve muscular endurance.

Anything that will add resistance to your body will add muscle. The heavier the thing, the more muscle it's going to add.

But Zlata, "I want to tone up, but I don't want to gain muscle."

Sister, TONING = INCREASING MUSCLE MASS + DECREASING BODY FAT PERCENTAGE.

Therefore, you can really have one without the other.

MUSCLE is QUEEEENNNN ... Here's why:

- The main reason is because it allows you to have a stronger metabolism. Your metabolism is essentially how efficiently your body burns energy. If your metabolism is slow, you'll burn less; if your metabolism is high, you'll burn more. The more muscle mass you have, the more calories you burn. We need a faster metabolism to use energy efficiently so we actually have energy.

- You build a strong and fast metabolism. After you lift weights, you're maximizing excess post-exercise oxygen consumption (EPOC), so will experience after-burn. This means that you'll be burning calories and consuming more energy (burning calories means that you're burning energy because calories are energy) even if you're sitting on the couch watching TV or writing a graduate school paper. Burning calories while sitting on the couch? Yes, please, I'll take it!

- Having muscle on your body increases your metabolic capacity; that is, you burn more calories. You're not increasing your metabolism when you're only focused on decreasing the number on the scale. Your body doesn't feel "firm" or tight. It's the same body, just in a smaller size. Increased muscle mass gives your body shape, firmness, and "tightness."

- Another benefit of resistance training and putting on muscle is that your body will begin to metabolize carbohydrates differently. Instead of immediately storing them as fat, it'll use them gradually for energy to fuel your workouts.

- Unfortunately, as the human body ages, we lose strength, mobility, and balance. A regular routine of strength training slows down the aging process. Women also have to worry about a reduction in bone density, called osteoporosis, that occurs naturally as we get older. Here's something crazy to think about: Lifting weights doesn't just make your muscles stronger with the addition of supporting your bones. Your bones get denser, too. Taking care of your bone health before it becomes a problem can prevent the issue from becoming worse down the line.

"Okay, cool, I'm with you on the muscle thing, but I don't want to get bulky." — you say.

The most common complaint I hear from women when I talk about building muscle is that they don't want to get bulky.

I'm with you #teamnobulk. I AM! One hundred percent. It irritates me when the industry says women don't get bulky. How do you explain the phenomenon of a woman going to the gym and gaining size in her legs that she never intended to gain?

I can look at the squat rack and gain size in my quads. Bulking is real, and I'd NEVER do that to you.

Let me explain bulking ...

BULKING: gaining more size than desired for aesthetic purposes.

WHY DOES BULKING HAPPEN?

1. You gain muscle faster than you lose fat. When you work out and your size increases rather than decreases, it simply means that you've gained muscle, but the layer of body fat is still there. Because your body likes to be prepared for emergencies, fat tends to go away slower than muscle is built, and this is exactly why you get the impression that you look bulkier. It's not the muscle, it's the excess fat. Lose the fat, and the bulk will disappear. It's actually not easy at all for a woman to achieve visible muscles. Bodybuilders — of both genders — spend their lives weight training and following a very strict nutrition regimen to get the results. It doesn't happen overnight.

2. You may be lifting too heavy for your desired outcome. When you start a workout routine, you need to know exactly what you want to achieve. Do you want to tone up? Do you want to lose fat? Do you want to become stronger? Depending on your goals, your coach (if they know what they're doing) will create an individualized fitness plan intended to reach those goals.

Yes, Zlata, I'm team no bulk, too! I want those lean, long muscles!

Hold up!

There's a whole myth going around about adding "longer muscle" or "lean muscle" or creating these mystery long, lean muscles.

You read it here first: the idea of long, lean muscle doesn't exist, and if it did, we'd be in trouble. You can't change where muscles begin and end — these are anatomically predispositioned. They begin where they begin, and they end where they end. Period. So if we could elongate muscle, that would mean that certain muscles would be longer and certain joints would begin to deteriorate. Okay, but you're thinking that you elongate your muscles by stretching in yoga or pilates, right? Wrong. Your muscles don't get longer when you stretch; it's all a matter of your brain communicating to your muscle that it's okay to stretch further. It has nothing to do with making the actual muscle longer. I didn't say that yoga and pilates are not the best way to train; you can get one heck of a workout through either. I simply used it as an example because these are the fitness industries where "long, lean muscle" seems to be a trend.

No bulk. No long muscles. Just muscle.

"So how do you build this muscle the Sexyfit way?"

I suggest that you use free weights from the very beginning to create the best outcome and habits for the time invested.

HERE'S WHAT I CONSIDER FREE WEIGHTS:

- Dumbbells
- Barbells
- High/low or adjustable pulley system
- Lat pull-down and low-row device
- Medicine balls (all types, including kettle bells)

- Ankle weights
- The human body — the ultimate free weight of all!

At Sexyfit, I rarely suggest to use any machines. After coaching hundreds of women, I've only used machines for a handful of clients who required additional support, stabilization, or were overcoming an injury.

Since I went over free weights, let me define machines:

MACHINES: awkward types of bulky metal-looking things in the middle of the gym to create confusion around getting in shape and scare women.

Don't quote me on that, but I think this should be the new official definition.

I recommend using free weights for the reason of engaging your core with every movement, and conditioning your body to work great and look great. When you're using free weights, your body is required to use more muscle and, therefore, more energy to stabilize your body.

When you're training with free weights, you also have the opportunity to equally distribute your strength, and, therefore, you won't be fighting any muscle imbalances in the future. Many machines require either legs or arms to push and pull, and you never know which body part or which side is more dominant. Machines can also cause additional joint stress, as you can only move a certain way. Each machine isn't tailored to you — your weight and your height, etc. Can a 220-pound man attain the same benefits as a 150-pound woman when working out on the same machine? It just simply makes no sense. Pick up the dumbbells and let's go.

CHAPTER PRACTICE

To make sure that everything you are learning sticks, take our your journal and answer the following questions:

1. What does muscle help you do?

2. Why is muscle important?

3. Name three ways of resistance training.

PODCAST ALERT

Reference the www.sexyfit.com/resources page to listen to the "Can Women Get Bulky? Spot Conditioning for Women" podcast.

SEXYFIT WORKOUTS TO TRANSFORM YOUR BODY
CHAPTER 27

I've coached a multitude of athletes over time. I love working with runners, powerlifters, ultra marathoners, bodybuilders. However, my most favorite athletes are women like me who go to work, enjoy time with their family, love drinking wine with their girlfriends, and want a program that works to give them results and fits their lifestyle. My theory is, if you have a body you're an athlete. As a result of coaching hundreds of women, I listened to their needs, time constraints, deciphered between excuses and real life circumstances, tweaked hundreds of individual programs, and ran group coaching with hundreds of female athletes from all walks of life. With Sexyfit, I created a method that allows you to work out at home, at the gym, use minimum equipment, is only 21 minutes long, AND gives you amazing results functionally and aesthetically. This is what women wanted, this is what I created. It took me years of research, practice, and trial and error, and I was really, really, really certain that I didn't want to compromise function or aesthetics, but wanted to give you a workout that inspires you to do more and that you'll fall in love with.

For years, women came to me asking how they could make specific areas of their body look firmer, tighter, and leaner. We've heard over and over that reducing fat in certain (spot) areas is absolutely impossible, but is it really?

I drove me a little up a wall at first because I believe we must love, respect, cherish, and be grateful for the body we have right now first and foremost. Asking to alter one body part is like criticizing a sunset for being too orange or too yellow or not bright enough. Nobody criticizes certain parts of the sunset, we love and appreciate all of it, right? Your body is your own gorgeous sunset. #rantalert I know why I was asked these questions over and over, because as a former fitness "person" and a trainer, this is what I teach, right? That's what the fast-food version of fitness is like on the covers of mags — tightER glutes, leanER arms; therefore, this is what we focus on.

I always said that you can't spot-reduce one area. Because it's just that you can't spot-reduce fat.

But ...

After a little thinking I realized that in a way this is what we do with resistance training and conditioning workouts.

Most certainly, you CAN shape your muscle in a way so that a certain area of your body looks better AND also in a way that helps your body function better. And since we as women are a bit vain and a bit stubborn so will always find a way, I felt like I was doing many of those women a disservice when I said, "NO! Not possible! BS! Workout for function." Because then, they'd go out and find some silly workout that promises "Tight Glutes in 3 Minutes a Day." In that case, nobody wins. You don't win because you're expecting tight glutes in three minutes a day, and that isn't happening; and I don't win because I failed to give you what you want.

I realized I'm here to deliver a result, and that's what most of my clients wanted, so I had better figure out how to serve and deliver a way that can do that ... and still feel good about it as a fitness professional.

So that's how the Spot Conditioning technique was born.

HOW DOES SPOT CONDITIONING WORK?
SPOT CONDITIONING (SC) — mid-volume, mid-range resistance training balanced with the incorporation of compound movements, isolated movements, and cardiovascular training to optimize fat loss, muscular balance, and overall symmetry for a female athlete's body from both a functional and aesthetic point of view, with the added bonus of an overall increase in metabolic capacity.

SPOT — muscle mass in a certain body part.

CONDITIONING — optimizing the performance of the athlete, and minimizing the risk of injury and illness.

There are a lot of new words here.

LET ME EXPLAIN:
MID-VOLUME — the number of repetitions that you'll perform of a specific exercise. In Spot Conditioning, we use a 12-15 rep range to optimize muscle endurance.

MID-RANGE — the number of sets or the number of cycles of reps you perform. In Spot Conditioning, we use 3-4 as a set range to optimize muscle hypertrophy.

COMPOUND MOVEMENTS — any exercise that engages two or more different joints to fully stimulate entire muscle groups and multiple muscles. Compound movements put a lot of emphasis on pushing, pulling, squatting, pressing, and lifting, which closely resemble the muscles we use in day-to-day life. These types of movements produce greater capability and have maximum practicality, which helps us complete daily tasks with maximum efficiency. These types of movements work multiple muscle groups simultaneously and require greater energy output — which means they burn more calories by making our body work harder to complete them.

CARDIOVASCULAR TRAINING — Any movement that gets your heart rate up and increases blood circulation throughout the body. In a regular training plan, you'll use low-intensity steady state (LISS) cardio training. In an advanced plan, you'll use high-intensity interval training (HIIT).

At Sexyfit, your time investment in your SC workouts will be three times a week for 21 minutes each, depending on your fitness level. Each workout is broken down into three blocks. Every block is seven minutes long. Workout days are divided into upper body, lower body, and whole body. This way you have enough recovery time between your workouts, and you'll be able to give it your ALL every time.

Each block has three exercises. You'll perform one exercise after the other within the block. When you're done, you'll keep repeating them until your timer shows seven minutes. After you're finished with the first block, you'll move on to the next until you finish all three blocks.

The more advanced you get, the faster you'll work through the blocks and get the ultimate fat burn as a result! Just for fun, every workout has a name, so you're able to connect with Sexyfit Community sisters and discuss your workouts.

Unless you're doing a custom program with one of the Sexyfit coaches — which, by the way is available for you to do — this is the kind of technique that you'll experience with us.

It's short, it's sweet, and it gives you results!

WHAT ABOUT CARDIO?

Oh, the almighty cardio question!

Treadmill is bad.

Walk for 30 minutes a day.

Running is good.

Running is bad for your knees.

HIIT is bad for your hormones.

HIIT is the fastest way to get in shape.

GOOD LAWDY! There's an ocean of opinions out there!

Any type of cardio that you do that's at the same pace is called LISS — low intensity steady state cardio. When you are performing LISS, your body is working at around 60% of maximum heart rate.

Here's my rule of thumb for you: If you use the treadmill/LISS to ... decompress after work (me), move your body when you're exhausted and don't feel like doing anything else (me), watch a movie (me, ha!), talk on the phone with your mom (my all-time gym crime), listen to the podcast (me), or simply because you feel like walking and it's cold outside — use the treadmill. It's not evil; it's not terrible. I hear so many trainers talk smack about others using a treadmill when they SHOULD be running or SHOULD be lifting or SHOULD be powerlifting.

We live in a world where we sit on our bum all day, I'm happy to see you on a treadmill! You showed up! You're moving your body! And that's awesome!

A treadmill is a tool; just not the best tool for efficient fat loss. If you're lapping miles in hopes of losing weight, and huffing and puffing for 40 minutes trying to lose weight, it'll work short-term ... until you stop doing it, OR until your smart, smart, smart body figures out what you're doing and adapts to that expenditure. Your body is a smart cookie when it comes to cardio. That's why to lose weight by running, you need to do more and more miles, and spend more time doing it. That's why when you're using a treadmill for weight loss it'll also suck up an enormous amount of your time. Neither running nor cardio will change your shape, but it'll be good for you to move around. If that's your goal and the outcome you desire, go for it.

CARDIO FOR FAT LOSS

The most efficient cardio for fat loss is interval cardio, formerly known as High Intensity Interval Training (HIIT). A HIIT workout alternates between short work intervals (70 to 90 percent max heart rate) and rest periods (60 to 65 percent max heart rate). I suggest incorporating HIIT 2-3 times per week for 20 minutes each if you want to achieve results at a faster rate and enjoy intense training. I would add it on the non-workout days. This will insure that you get enough recovery time.

Here's the science behind interval training, sister. Your heart is a muscle. If you keep it beating at a constant rate, never expanding it outside of its comfort zone, it'll never grow. If you do 100 bench presses with 10 pounds and don't feel it, your chest will never develop. Same thing with your heart; if it's not feeling the exertion, it doesn't have to work harder, and nothing has changed. However, when you throw some intervals in there, your heart will have to expand, pump more blood, and work hard to return to normal levels. Have a high-stress job? Wouldn't you benefit from having a heart that's used to rapid changes in blood pressure and needs? That's the kind of heart I want!

A study conducted by The University of Western Ontario gives us insight into how much more effective interval training really is. Researchers had 10 men and 10 women train three times a week, with one group doing four to six 30-second treadmill sprints (with four to six minutes of rest in between each), and the other group doing 30-60 minutes of steady state cardio (running on the treadmill at the "magical fat loss zone" of 65 percent VO2 max, [VO2 max is a numerical measurement of your body's ability to consume oxygen]).[21]

The results: After six weeks of training, the subjects doing the intervals had lost more fat.

Yes, four to six 30-second sprints burn more fat than 60 minutes of incline treadmill walking.

Although the exact mechanisms of how high-intensity cardio trumps steady state cardio aren't fully understood yet, scientists have isolated quite a few of the factors:

- Increased resting metabolic rate for upwards of 24 hours after exercise
- Improved insulin sensitivity in the muscles
- Higher levels of fat oxidation in the muscles
- Significant spikes in growth hormone levels (which aid in fat loss) and catecholamine levels (chemicals your body produces to directly induce fat mobilization)
- Appetite suppression post-exercise
- And more …

The bottom line is that high-intensity interval training burns more fat in less time than steady state cardio. But steady state cardio is also relevant and applicable for optimal health. Here's also the catch; I know a lot of us are going to hop off the couch and go straight to running intervals because it's the most efficient aka the fastest way. If you have not worked out in quite some time or fitness has never been your thing, don't make it hard on yourself at first. If your body is not used to movement, your joints, muscles, heart, and mind aren't used to the intensity — allow yourself at least 30 days of easing into the fitness plan with resistance training. Your body will take time to get used to movement, so more is not always better. Steady Freddy wins the race.

💡 CHAPTER PRACTICE

Much of your fat loss progress is related to the intensity of your workout and will depend on how quickly you are moving AND how heavy you are lifting. When it comes to fat loss, intensity NOT duration is the name of the game. Therefore, short workouts can bring enormous fat loss results. How do you determine if you are working out hard enough and maximizing the outcome? Easy, we can do so by measuring and referencing our heart rate zone. Exercising in our target heart rate zone assures that we're getting our fitness bang for our buck: burning enough calories, but not going overboard and risking injury. In other words, follow your heart.

1. We start with calculating our maximum heart rate which is very simple:
   220 – Age = Maximum Heart Rate
   Example 220 – 30 = 190 (beats per minute) as max heart rate zone.

2. Figure out what heart rate zone you want to reach and reference the chart below.

   50-60% (GREY ZONE) This is your warm-up zone for before and after the resistance-training workout. It helps to improve blood flow and circulation to your working muscles. You'll find yourself in this zone when you're doing LISS training, such as walking or leisurely biking.

   60-70% (BLUE ZONE) This is the basic endurance-training zone: comfortable, easy-breathing, light sweating. This is where the heart rate zone you would be in if you're doing some easy running or light weight training. It improves basic endurance, and you'll burn fat. You burn more calories per minute than in the healthy heart zone because the exercise is a little more intense — you're going faster and, therefore, covering more distance. In this zone, your body fuels itself with 85% fat, 5% protein, and 10% carbohydrates. You get the same health benefits and fat-burning benefits as the healthy heart zone.

   70-80% (ORANGE ZONE) This is where your workout gets hard. You'll only be able to speak in short phrases. This is also known as your endurance zone. It spurs your body to improve your circulatory system by building new blood vessels and increases your heart and lung capacity. Aiming for 20-60 minutes in this zone is believed to give the best fitness training benefits. You burn 50% of your calories from fat, 50% from carbohydrates, and less than 1% from protein. With the increase in intensity, you burn more calories in the same amount of time, as you're covering more distance in that same time. THIS IS THE BEST ZONE FOR RESISTANCE-TRAINING SPOT CONDITIONING WORKOUTS.

   90-98% (RED ZONE) Most people can't stay in this zone for more than a few minutes. The maximum amount of time recommended in this heart rate zone is one minute. You burn lots of calories per minute in this zone; 90% of them are carbohydrates, 10% fats, and less than 1% protein. This is typically the highest heart rate you are aiming for during HIIT workouts. .

🎙 PODCAST ALERT

Reference the www.sexyfit.com/resources page to listen to the "What Type of Training is Best for Female Fat Loss?" podcast.

LIFESTYLE FACTORS
CHAPTER 28

SLEEP

In the last century, we've glorified that sleeping is for the weak, and that's absolutely not true. Especially if you're a fitness enthusiast. Sister, sleep is when you recover from those workouts and shape the sexy muscles you're working on getting.

You'll notice that you're probably more sleepy when you start your fitness routine, and that's because your body is craving recovery. Start getting to bed just 15 minutes earlier every night, and it'll make a world of a difference in your overall progress. SLEEP = SEXY MUSCLES.

Another thing I want to mention is soreness.

You'll be sore; that's just the truth. When you work hard, you get sore.

I want to explain why this is happening ...

Your muscles need time to adapt to the new workout plan, new schedule, and moving forward to the new load of training. Why do you get sore? You get the DOMS, sister. Scary acronym, I know, so let me explain. It stands for delayed onset muscle soreness.

Many would believe that it has everything to do with lactic acid buildup, which is actually not true. During exercise, your body needs energy, and it breaks down molecules to get it. As a result of this metabolic process, your cells naturally become more acidic, which makes your muscles feel like they're burning. But this isn't caused by lactate. Lactate is actually a by-product of the metabolic process, serving as a buffer, and slows down the rate at which the cells become acidic. A study in Clinics in Sports Medicine found that DOMS is the result of micro-trauma in the muscles and surrounding connective tissues, which causes inflammation.[22] It's the same type of micro-trauma that'll help you grow your muscles.

I don't recommend repeatedly working out the same body part when you're sore. Not because it's bad for your body or for your metabolism, but because it isn't the most enjoyable process and you might be out of form. This can cause an imbalance and/or potential injury.

It doesn't matter how fit you are, you're still going to experience DOMS. After 10 years of training, I still get sore. According to studies, we can be no-responders, low-responders, or high-responders to soreness. If you're a high-responder, you'll experience DOMS more acutely than someone who's a no- or low-responder when given the same training load. While you can't change your genes, it's important to know where you fall on the spectrum so that you can understand how your body may respond to changes in your workouts.

STRETCHING

In order to prevent injuries, you should incorporate dynamic stretching into your workout routine, pre-workout. If you're sore 24-48 hours after a workout, the best way to get rid of the soreness is with a foam roller, stretching, massage, or a yoga class.

WATER

A hydrated body moves better. When you're hydrated, you're able to move much better and you're able to give more effort. If you're showing up to your workouts dehydrated, a side-effect is less intensity than you're capable of and making things more difficult for yourself than they need to be.

Drink at least 20 ounces of water before ANY activity, especially in the morning!

AUNT FLO

I often get asked, "Do I work out on my period?" I don't know, it's your body, it'll tell you. I always secretly wanted to roll my eyes at the women who say, "Oh, I work out because it helps me with my cramps." Yep, not me. If you're this lucky, good for you. Most of us aren't.

I suggest that you track your period so that you know exactly what your body will do at what time of the month. Plan your food and your fitness around you period. Create awareness of your habits and know what's coming because it literally comes every month! You can't fight your body, and you don't need to. If you know you'll probably be craving certain foods like chocolate or ice cream, stock up on the healthier version of those foods. And don't plan workouts for the first three days of your period if you'll feel self conscious about it the whole time.

Don't make things more difficult for yourself than you have to. If you don't feel like working out because you're experiencing a heavy flow and feel low on energy, don't force it. Stay in and take care of yourself. Go on a walk instead, take a shower, stretch. The gym isn't going anywhere.

CAPACITY AND SEASONS

There are going to be seasons in life when you can dedicate more time to fitness. For some of us, it's summertime; for others, it's winter. You'll find yourself having time, desire, and energy to work out more during those seasons. Other times, you'll find yourself looking for that motivation you once had, and kicking yourself in the ass wondering where to find the ZING and the ING again.

LOOK OUTSIDE — check out Mother Nature. Mother Nature has seasons: Sometimes it's dark and cozy, and in the spring everything literally springs back to life. Summertime energy is high, the sun is shining. Your body is the exact same way; it goes through seasons and cycles.

This is also reflected in athletes: Football has seasons, too — pre-season, playoff season, time off.

You can't expect your body to always be in season and get down on yourself because it's doing what comes natural to it.

This is our typical cycle, unless we grew up playing some competitive sport and our body is used to that schedule.

WINTER — We focus on strength-training workouts; steady cardio, if any at all; yoga, restorative movements; cycling indoors; skiing — frequency is at two to three times a week.

SPRING — We crave the outdoors and want to get outside, start to think of summer; more cardio starts to appear naturally — kick up the frequency to three times a week with something more aerobic, perhaps superset training, multi-sets, etc.

SUMMER — We relish this time with a full-on movement extravaganza; we're outside running, training intensely with intervals, kicking ass with high-intensity weight training; and just all-around kicking ass and taking names.

FALL — We slow down on high-intensity workouts; still enjoy running at times, but our workout intensity decreases, and we start to crave slower activities.

Listen, for you it might look insane to think about it this way because to this day all you have been trying to do is get a bikini body over and over for the last 5-10 years, and that's all you think fitness is good for. When you start making fitness a lifestyle, you want to know how to keep the habits that made you so sane and happy, but you can't require yourself to kill it 24/7/365. I rarely have met anyone who's killing it all year-round.

Once I understood my cycle and was able to explain cycles to my clients, it changed everything for them, from feeling less like a failure and being frustrated to something that's natural to us.

SUPPLEMENTS

I remember my mom used to tell me that I'd grow a penis if I took protein supplements; and my aunt used to tell my brother that drinking protein shakes would make his penis fall off.

Both of those statements are hilarious because neither would happen.

I waited for the Fitness section to tell you this: You need supplements. I'm not going to be one of those Instagram models pushing you detox tea that'll just help you poop your pants. I'm going to tell you these are MUST-haves for women. The best way to really know is to connect with your doc and get a micronutrient panel done, and see where you're deficient.

Here are the supplements that we most commonly suggest; if you want a better overview, go see your doctor:

VITAMIN C — helps you recover muscle and supports your immune system.

VITAMIN D — helps with fatigue if you're living somewhere dark and cold.

IRON — if you're bruising easily and have bad cravings, even if you eat enough protein, you might have an iron deficiency.

I recommend taking this on a three-weeks on/three-weeks off basis.

MAGNESIUM — 995 of us are walking around deficient in magnesium. If you're craving chocolate during your period and can't get off sweets, you're most likely deficient. Spray, tablets, etc. are available; you can also take a powdered magnesium, called "CALM," before bed.

DHEA — for anyone who's stressed out and needs an extra boost for their thyroid function. DHEA helps the production of t4 and t3 to help support metabolism.

GREENS — everyone needs powdered greens because I know that very few of us have the patience to clean a juicer; so get powder greens and use them every morning.

PROTEIN — good lord we have options! There are hundreds of brands out there offering hundreds of products. I prefer collagen protein or plant-based. The majority of protein powders on the market are complete crap. If it promises to taste like cinnamon rolls or birthday cake, toss it. If it's gross and you don't want to drink it, don't drink it. Find something you like and enjoy. I enjoy tasteless collagen for my second shake of the day and plant-based for the first shake.

What about pre-workout powders, fat burners, orange chews to provide magic "energy" in the morning? What about cleanses, wraps, waist trainers, fancy colorful chewy vitamins? ... Honestly, don't waste your money. Toss anything that's fluorescent green, orange, or purple in color and gives you anxiety-like symptoms. Your body doesn't need it. You should have enough natural energy from food.

◉ PODCAST ALERT

Reference www.sexyfit.com/resources page to listen to the "Supplements that are Actually Good for You," "How to Deal with Muscle Soreness" and "Fitness Tips for PMS Symptoms" podcasts.

HOW TO EAT AROUND WORKOUTS
CHAPTER 29

Eating before and after a workout seems to be counter-productive to many women. We think that we're working out to burn calories, so why would we eat before or after the gym? In the Nutrition section, we discussed in depth the theory of having enough nutrients from macros in order to optimize our body for fat loss and daily function. The primary focus of your nutrition strategy, as well as your workout strategy, is to give you energy for life, improve your mood, and gateway you into the body you love.

To help you figure this whole topic out, let's pretend we're talking; you're the Q and I'm the A. Here goes ...

DOES IT MATTER WHAT I EAT, OR IF I EAT BEFORE OR AFTER A WORKOUT? SHOULD I TRAIN ON AN EMPTY STOMACH? WHAT'S BETTER?

As far as the research and the science go, there seems to be a torn decision on this. Some say absolutely, yes. We must replenish our glycogen stores, which we draw energy from in order to have more energy and stimulate protein synthesis, by adding a protein supplement to improve muscle recovery. And, we must do this in the "anabolic" window of time, 15-45 minutes post-workout. Others will discredit this theory entirely and say that as long as you take in your daily macros, protein/carbohydrate timing doesn't matter.

Here's my take on pre- and post-workout nutrition, based on what I see with women on a daily basis:

Your pre-workout meal is what'll give you energy for the workout. If you're eating throughout the day and you show up at the gym fed, happy, and ready to go, don't stress too much. If you, however, are going to show up starving, hAngry, and your tummy is growling the entire workout, plus your fatigue is going to slow you down from getting the best workout ever, absolutely eat.

SO WHAT DO I EAT?

I suggest that you eat protein combined with a carb if you'd like. Or, you can just go with a carb and vegetables combo, and eat it an hour before your workout.

There's also a big conversation about the benefits of fasted training and whether working out on an empty stomach is better. There's currently conflicting information regarding to whether this style of training is best. On one hand, researchers are saying that our body catabolizes muscle (e.g., starts to use muscle for energy vs. for fat); others are going to say that in turn our body will use fat for fuel. In this regard, I also leave it up to your body and how you feel.

If you feel better training fasted in the morning and choose to have breakfast afterward, this is what works for you and your body. If you show up like a zombie to your session and have no desire, and you'd rather die than work out on an empty stomach, yet don't want to eat much, have a banana or a full-on meal, and enjoy your session. It's truly up to you.

Some of my clients choose to do fasted cardio or fasted training; some of my clients don't, and I fall into the second category.

Ninety-nine percent of the time I need fuel to get a killer workout. One percent of the time, and especially if I had a huge dinner the night before, I'm going to train fasted because I'm simply not hungry. I'd rather have you listen to your body than have a study dictate whether you should eat or not.

WHAT ABOUT POST-WORKOUT NUTRITION?
Your post-workout meal is a combination of protein and carbs. It's believed that protein will help your muscle recover faster and better if you're consuming it in a 20-60 minute window post-workout, and carbs can help with restoring your glycogen level. In my experience, taking a protein supplement, like a shake, is just a simple and easy way to meet your daily protein goals.

Strategically, it works out much better to take your shake post-workout to get your protein in and move on with your day. If you're eating dinner right after your workout, though, perhaps a protein shake isn't necessary and you can eat your calories right after the workout.

Here's what I see that works the best ...

IF YOU WORK OUT IN THE MORNING:
If you're hungry, eat a banana and rock your workout (account for this carb in your daily intake). Take a shake after you're finished.

If you aren't hungry, then work out and save your meal for afterward. No sense in stuffing yourself if you aren't hungry. Take a shake afterward if you're not a morning eater, or if you're hungry eat a full-on meal. At times, when I work out in the a.m., I'll eat a banana; work out; take a shake; take a shower; do my morning routine, like reading and meditation; and an hour later have my breakfast. It works for me but took time to learn it. Figure out what works for you.

IF YOU WORK OUT IN THE AFTERNOON ...
You can eat your lunch an hour before, work out, take a shake, and go back to business. OR, you can take a shake, work out, and then eat a meal.

IF YOU WORK OUT AT NIGHT ...
That's that interesting 4 p.m.-7 p.m. window, when we seem to make all of the crazy decisions. When I work out at night, I like to eat around 5 p.m., even if it's a quick snack, like an apple or toast with almond butter; then hit the gym, take a shake; and then prepare dinner. This is what works for me because I take my sweet time making dinner or I have dinner plans. I don't want to show up to dinner hungry because I didn't time my meals right.

PLAN ACCORDING TO YOUR SCHEDULE

A common mistake that I see with pre- and post-workout nutrition, or fitness nutrition in general, is that we don't account enough for our calories expenditure. Yoga is going to burn less calories than a high-intensity cycling class or running five times. Your nutrition is going to be different if you're following the 21-minute Sexyfit workouts or one of our builder programs.

ACCOUNT FOR YOUR EXPENDITURE.

You work out less, you eat less.
You work out more, you eat more.

It's that simple. If you're going to be running around and doing life 24/7/365, and only have time for two workouts, it's okay. Just adjust your macros to that.

If you're on a kicker and you're killing it seven days a week and you have a crazy deficit of macros, then you're on the right track to feeling weak, sad, and hungry.

If you're crashing, have no energy, or are otherwise not feeling good from your workouts, your food intake is most likely off.

This isn't something that'll come to you right away. It takes years to calculate and calibrate, but you'll just know when it's right.

🎙 PODCAST ALERT

Reference the www.sexyfit.com/resources page to listen to the ""Pre-Workout Snacks to Rock Your Workout" and "Metabolism Boosting Post-Workout Snacks" podcasts.

HOW TO "LISTEN TO YOUR BODY"
CHAPTER 30

You may have noticed that the style of my communication changed as we've been getting down to the last chapters of the workout section. I started out very assertive and to the point. Here's the thing: You must learn the basics, otherwise you're constantly going to be running in the same circle. Remember the first time you drove a car? Were you a rockstar driver or were you terrified of moving? Or perhaps you took the wheel and right off the bat knew that someday you'd be a race car driver? That's exactly what working out is like; it might be scary, awkward, weird, or, to some of us, it might feel natural. But years later, we're decent enough at it to get to work or at least hold a driver license. You get the idea.

As you're getting into fitness, I want you to create a good, solid foundation to where you feel great and look great. Muscle is key to doing this, and second is LISTENING to your body. And sister, trust me, for most of my life being active meant being actively hit in the head with a soccer ball in gym class, avoiding any form of physical fitness activities, and skipping P.E. because I was led to believe I'm not "good at sports." If I can do it, you can do it. My step-sister is still amazed that I'm a fitness professional since she was the active kid in the family with a black belt in judo. Being fit was not my story, my identity, or anything I thought I could be good at.

There's validity in the thinking that our mind won't go where our body doesn't push us. Sure, our mind is powerful, and we can visualize anything, but there's also such a thing as body limits, outside stress, fatigue, and a straight-up shitty day.

Remember, your body is your home. It'll navigate you and tell you everything you need to know. Sure, your mind will take you where you need to go, but listening to your body is critical.

Learn to tell if how you feel is a mind limit or a body limit. Here are some questions to ask yourself:

- Is this good pain or bad pain?
- What do I need right now to feel better?
- Am I in pain? Is it bad pain or does the burn feel good?
- Do I need to leave class right now, or is my mind telling me I can't?
- Or any number of other questions ... Do I need food? Do I need a hug? Do I need to push? Do I need to slow down? Can I push?

It's okay to stop and ask your body what it wants and recalibrate what you're doing. Once again we're doing the gentle dance between masculine and feminine. Having a plan is great, having a goal is wonderful, taking our body to a new level and being proud of ourselves is motivating. And it's also great to know what feels good to us and what our body needs today.

Sometimes when we think our PLAN is to work out, but our body really wants to FEEL differently, it's our job to know what it wants and what it needs. And no matter how long you have been in the game, at times we still need a reminder that our body is a smart compass to help us navigate what we need to know and do.

I'll tell you a post-adrenal fatigue story ... I was getting ready for this photoshoot for my other book cover, and I was really working hard. I was listening to my body but to be very honest, vanity got the best of me because it was a cover shoot for a fitness book. I was lifting three times a week, doing a highly popular class that integrates high-intensity training and eating what I thought was sufficient. I was also doing some occasional running with friends and hiking.

Everything was great in time for the shoot; I looked terrific, it was fabulous. When I got home, I thought I could sustain the same schedule. Three weeks later into keeping up with that schedule, I started to notice how I would get tired throughout the day, overall I was down about life, and all I wanted to do was work from my bed all day. That NEVER happens! Another week into that schedule, I walked out of class in my fancy, new studio. I stopped on the treadmill and thought I was going to pass out. My mind was doing the workouts, my body was NOT following. I was pushing, and I was ready to go for all of my mentally planned workout, except my body was saying NOOOOOO. I sat in my car and had a little powwow with myself because I was really upset with myself at first.

So I Zlata'ed myself and asked, "What does this body need today?" and closed my eyes in peace to get more present with self.

My body screamed: I NEED REST! and ice cream and cookies and I don't waannnaaaa.

It was like my cute inner 5-year-old child was crying to go to sleep and wanted comfort.

E.I.: I know that I only crave ice cream when I need to be comforted, otherwise I don't even like it.

So I wanted to stay lean at 11% body fat, but my body didn't. Over time I've learned that I'm quite comfortable at 15-16% body fat for life, and this is what I can easily maintain, have a life, fit into a dress, run a half-marathon in a matter of three weeks if I want to, lift anything, drink wine, and truly FEEL energized to run a business and life. That's my sweet spot. Anything over that, and I get frustrated with not being able to fit into my wardrobe (and it's quite expensive not to be able to), and I don't feel good because I'm not eating all that well anyhow; and anything lower, I look better, YES, but I'm a groggy, hAngry mama.

You, too, will find this sweet spot for yourself.

So listen to your inner 5-year-old child to guide you.

You have to mom yourself in a way and really listen to what your inner-child tells you. You know what's best for her—ice cream and cookies probably just means that she's tired or hungry, so feed her and let her sleep. If she's sore and needs a massage, let her stretch or go to a restorative class if it helps.

That said, you can't let yourself off the hook with "My body told me not to do anything" for six months. It's your responsibility to find what feels good to you, and what feels natural and normal to you. For some of us, lifting five times a week is natural and normal; for some, lifting two times works the best — but I do recommend two workouts per week at minimum.

Knowing what works for you and consistent effort with workouts will take time. It'll take training, practice, and patience, and at some point it'll all "click for you." You just can't quit before figuring out what it is, because you owe this level of care to yourself.

🎙 PODCAST ALERT

Reference the www.sexyfit.com/resources page to listen to the "Adrenal Fatigue — How to Recover Naturally" podcast.

21-DAY TRANSFORMATION FITNESS PLAN

Are you ready sister? I am excited for you to get rocking with your Sexyfit 21- Day Fitness Transformation Plan. As I mentioned before, your time investment in your Spot Conditioning workouts is three times a week for 21 minutes, depending on your fitness level. 21 minutes is all you need! Here's how it goes:

1. Each workout is broken down into three blocks. Every block is seven minutes long. Workout days are divided into upper body, leg day, and whole body. This way you have enough recovery time between your workouts, and you're able to give it your ALL every time.

2. Each block has two, three, or four exercises depending on the complexity of the movement. You'll perform one exercise after the other within the block. When you're done, you'll keep repeating them until your timer shows seven minutes. After you're finished with the first block, you'll move on to the next until you finish all three blocks.

3. The more advanced you get, the faster you'll work through the blocks and get the ultimate fat burn as a result!

Just for fun, every workout has a name, so you're able to connect with Sexyfit community sisters and discuss your workouts.

NOTE: To see a video example of any exercise, go to YouTube and search for "Zlata at Sexyfit." Click on the videos tab and search for the exercise by name.

BEGINNER CALENDAR: WEEKS 1-3

MONDAY	TUESDAY	WEDNESDAY	THURSDAY	FRIDAY	SATURDAY	SUNDAY
• Steps: 5,000-7,500 • Daily Abs	• Upper Body • Daily Abs	• Steps: 5,000-7,500 • Daily Abs	• Lower Body • Daily Abs	• Steps: 5,000-7,500 • Daily Abs	• Whole Body • Daily Abs	• Whole Body • Daily Abs

ADVANCED CALENDAR: WEEKS 1-3

MONDAY	TUESDAY	WEDNESDAY	THURSDAY	FRIDAY	SATURDAY	SUNDAY
• 7,500 steps • Daily Abs	• 7,500 steps • Daily Abs	• 7,500 steps • Upper Body • Daily Abs • HIIT Cardio (see Daily Abs for workout)	• 7,500 steps • Daily Abs	• 7,500 steps • Lower Body • Daily Abs • HIIT Cardio (see Daily Abs for workout)	• 7,500 steps • Daily Abs	• 7,500 steps • Whole Body • Daily Abs • HIIT Cardio (see Daily Abs for workout)

SEXYBACK

BLOCK 1

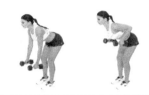

Standing Double Arm Row

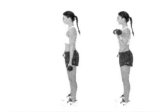

Bicep Curl

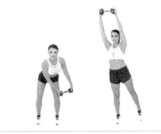

Woodchop

BLOCK 2

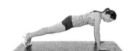
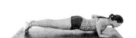

Push-Up
MODIFICATION TIP: Knee Push-Up

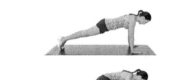

Knee to Elbow

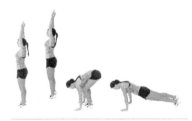

Burpee
MODIFICATION TIP: Mountain Climber

BLOCK 3

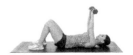
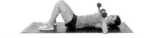

Chest Press

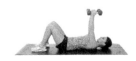
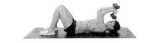

Skull Crusher

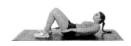
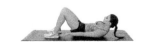

Heel Touch
MODIFICATION TIP: Crunch

BLOCK **1**

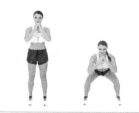

Side Lunge

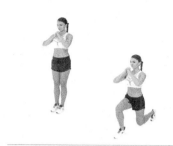

Forward Lunge

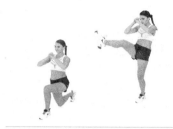

Reverse Lunge with Kick

BLOCK **2**

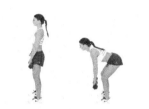

Romanian Deadlift

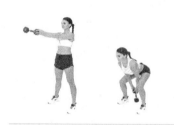

Dumbbell Swing
(or Kettlebell Swing)

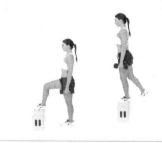

Box Step-Up with Weight
MODIFICATION TIP: Remove weight

BLOCK **3**

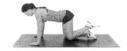
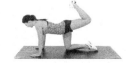

Donkey Kick

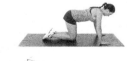
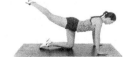

Leg Raise

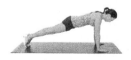
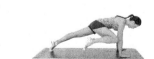

Knee to Elbow

BLOCK 1

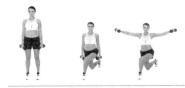

Curtsy Squat with Lateral Raise

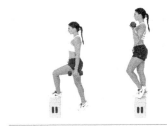

Box Step-Up with Bicep Curl

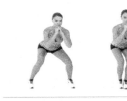

Side Shuffle

BLOCK 2

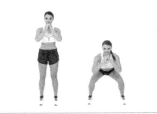

Side Lunge

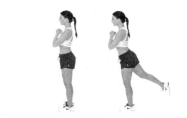

Standing Kickback

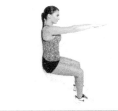

Wall Sit (hold until failure)

BLOCK 3

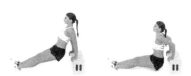

Dip

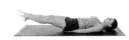
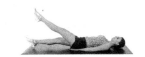

Flutter Kick

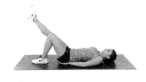
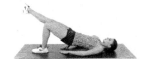

Single Leg Bridge
(hold 5 seconds each leg)

DAILY ABS

- 1 round of five exercises
- 15 reps of each exercise
- 5 seconds of rest between each exercise

Instructions

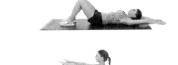

Sit-Up

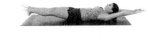
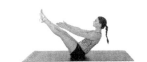

V-Up
MODIFICATION TIP: Crunch

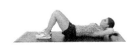
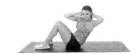

Left-side Oblique Raise

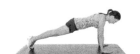
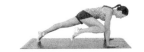

Knee to Elbow

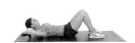
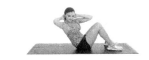

Right-side Oblique Raise

ADVANCED CARDIO HITT (10 MINUTES)

TUESDAY
- 1 minute Sprint (heart rate = orange zone)
- 1 minute Slow-pace Jog (heart rate = green zone)

THURSDAY
- 2 minutes Walk (heart rate = green zone)
- 1 minute Run (heart rate = green zone)
- 1 minute All-out Run(heart rate = orange zone)

SATURDAY
- 1 minute Run (heart rate = green to orange zone)
- 15 Burpees
- 1 minute All-out Run (heart rate = red zone)
- 15 Knee Tucks
- 2 minutes Run (heart rate = orange zone)
- 1 minute Mountain Climbers

BLOCK 1

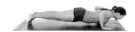

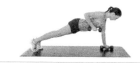
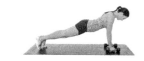
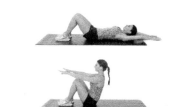

Push-Up
MODIFICATION TIP: Knee Push-Up

Plank Row
MODIFICATION TIP: Plank

Sit-Up

BLOCK 2

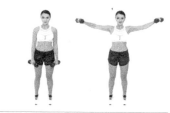
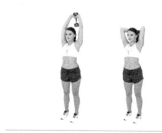
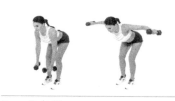

Lateral Raise
MODIFICATION TIP: One arm at a time

Overhead Tricep Extension

Rear Delt Fly

BLOCK 3

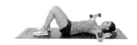
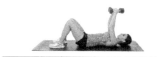
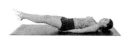
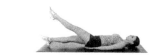
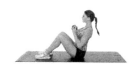
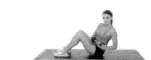

Chest Fly

Flutter Kick

Russian Twist

BLOCK 1

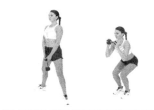

Sumo Squat with Weight
MODIFICATION TIP: Sumo Squat

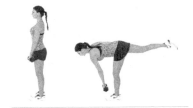

Single Leg Deadlift

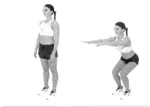

Air Squat

BLOCK 2

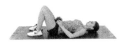
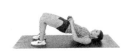

Weighted Bridge
MODIFICATION TIP: Bridge

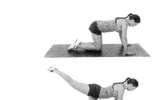

Leg Raise

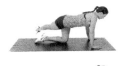
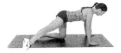

Leg Raise Side to Side

BLOCK 3

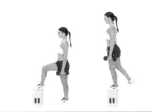

Box Step-Up with Weights
MODIFICATION TIP: Box Step-Up

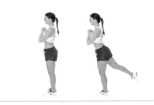

Standing Kick Back

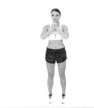

Curtsy Squat

BLOCK **1**

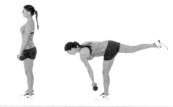

Single Leg Deadlift

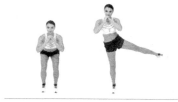

Squat with Side Kick

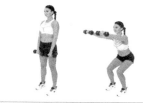

Squat with Front Raise
MODIFICATION TIP: Squat (no weights)

BLOCK **2**

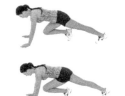

Mountain Climber

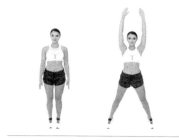

Jumping Jacks

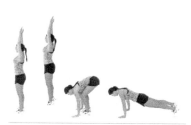

Burpee

BLOCK **3**

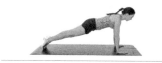

High Plank

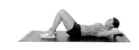
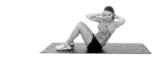

Oblique Raise (each side)

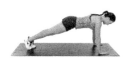
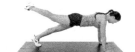

Plank with Leg Raise

DAILY ABS

- 1 round of five exercises
- 15 reps of each exercise
- 5 seconds of rest between each exercise

Instructions

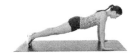
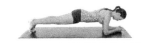

Low Plank

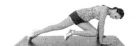
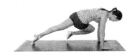

Knee to Opposite Elbow

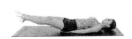
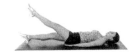

Flutter Kick

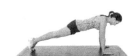
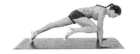

Knee to Elbow

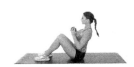
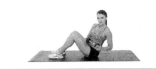

Russian Twist

ADVANCED CARDIO HITT (10 MINUTES)

TUESDAY
- 1 minute Sprint (heart rate = orange zone)
- 1 minute Slow-pace Jog (heart rate = green zone)

THURSDAY
- 2 minutes Walk (heart rate = green zone)
- 1 minute Run (heart rate = green zone)
- 1 minute All-out Run (heart rate = orange zone)

SATURDAY
- 1 minute Run (heart rate = green to orange zone)
- 15 Burpees
- 1 minute All-out Run (heart rate = red zone)
- 15 Knee Tucks
- 2 minutes Run (heart rate = orange zone)
- 1 minute Mountain Climbers

SLEEK ARMS

BLOCK **1**

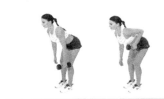

Single Arm Row

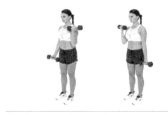

Alternating Bicep Curl

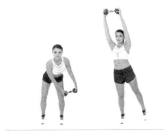

Woodchop

BLOCK **2**

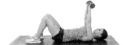
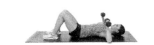

Chest Press

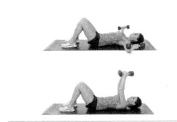

Chest Fly

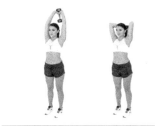

Double Arm Tricep Extension

BLOCK **3**

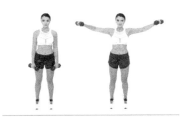

Lateral Raise

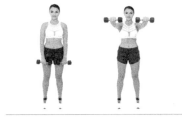

Front Raise

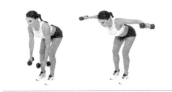

Rear Delt Fly

BLOCK 1

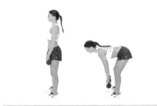

Stiff Leg Deadlift

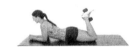

Hamstring Curl

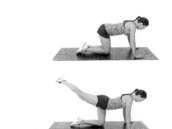

Leg Raise

BLOCK 2

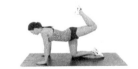

Donkey Kick

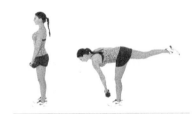

Single Leg Deadlift

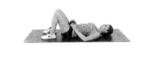
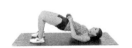

Weighted Bridge

BLOCK 3

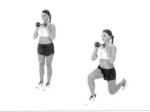

Lunge with Weight to Chest

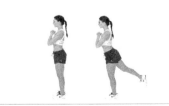

Standing Kick Back

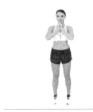

Curtsy Squat

HOT STUFF

BLOCK 1

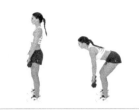

Romanian Deadlift

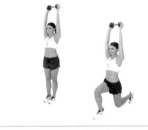

Lunge with Overhead Press

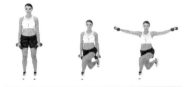

Curtsy Squat with Lateral Raise

BLOCK 2

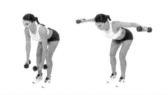

Rear Delt Fly

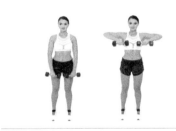

Upright Row

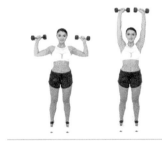

Shoulder Press

BLOCK 3

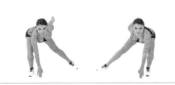

Ski Jump

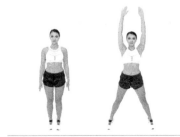

Jumping Jacks

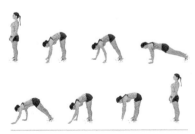

Walkouts

DAILY ABS

- 1 round of five exercises
- 15 reps of each exercise
- 5 seconds of rest between each exercise

Instructions

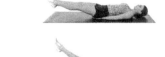

Flutter Kick

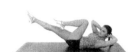
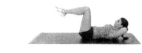

Bicycle

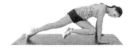
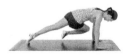

Knee to Opposite Elbow

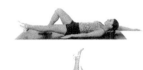
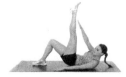

Alternating Leg Raises

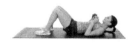
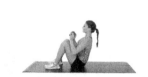

Sit-Up with Weight

ADVANCED CARDIO HITT (10 MINUTES)

TUESDAY
- 1 minute Sprint (heart rate = orange zone)
- 1 minute Slow-pace Jog (heart rate = green zone)

THURSDAY
- 2 minutes Walk (heart rate = green zone)
- 1 minute Run (heart rate = green zone)
- 1 minute All-out Run(heart rate = orange zone)

SATURDAY
- 1 minute Run (heart rate = green to orange zone)
- 15 Burpees
- 1 minute All-out Run (heart rate = red zone)
- 15 Knee Tucks
- 2 minutes Run (heart rate = orange zone)
- 1 minute Mountain Climbers

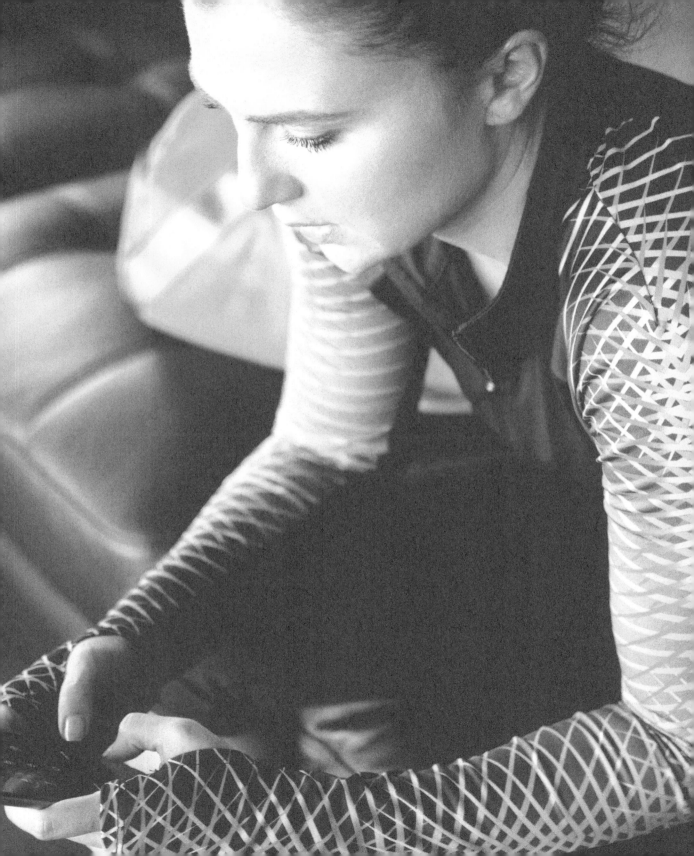

STEP IV
ACCOUNTABILITY

Unleash your potential
and stay motivated with
simple accountability
tips and tricks for
lasting fat loss.

HOW TO STAY ACCOUNTABLE WITH YOUR PROGRESS
CHAPTER 31

"Accountability is the glue that ties goals to results."

– Bob Proctor

ACCOUNTABILITY AND MEASURING SUCCESS ALONG THE WAY

You're ready to take on the new journey. You're a pro at macros, you're practically a fitness guru, and you're motivated to make "it" happen and reach your goals. To make sure that you get the results you want and keep your results for life, I'm going to show you the exact tools you need to measure progress, stay on track, and, as a result create lasting habits.

The point of accountability is really two things. One, our awareness of current patterns and willingness to analyze them and second, our ability to strategize for the upcoming week.

ANALYZE AND STRATEGIZE

ANALYZE

I can't tell you how many times I've heard women say, "Well, last week was a wash, I fell off the wagon, let's start over this week again!" But once we dive into what actually worked or didn't work, it turns out that there are quite a few wins to be proud of, and we only need to make minor adjustments and tweaks to weekly patterns, like adding a second meal prep or simply driving around with the gym bag in the car. We're so highly critical of ourselves and expect perfection that all the "losses" end up trumping the wins. Don't fall into the trap of constantly wanting to start over with high expectations of yourself to be absolutely perfect. At times **90% OF SUCCESS IS JUST SHOWING UP**, and the little wins over time add up to big changes. Analyze your past week and you'll clearly be able to see what and where you can do better and what you can celebrate. Focus on the good. Improve the rest over time.

STRATEGIZE

The second part of accountability is strategizing for the upcoming week. Guess what sister, if you don't know what's not working for YOU from the previous week, you can't strategize. Your strategy for your week builds upon YOUR schedule and YOUR lifestyle. There's nothing worse than trying to fit a fitness plan in an already jam-packed calendar to only add stress to your life. We run full schedules, I get it. Make it easy on yourself to take care of YOU and others. If you know Johnny has hockey practice, little Amy has dance recital on Friday, and there are 15 deadlines coming up at work, plan your schedule accordingly. This way you can set yourself up for success, and use fitness as a tool to relieve stress and create more energy, and you can use food to give you fuel and a boost to stay focused.

Nutrition and fitness are the foundation, the support, and the energy for your life. When things get busy, this is when you need it the most. Your accountability practices allow you to take a sober look and create a realistic strategy so you can do more in life with less effort.

Without accountability tools and celebrating our successes, we can fall into the trap of what I call the Shiny Objects Syndrome. We're surrounded on a daily basis with flashy marketing messages about magic pills helping us to lose 20 pounds in seven days, or perhaps a new magic wrap that promises tight abs and tight buns in less than 24 hours. It's easy to get trapped in unrealistic standards and ridiculous marketing schemes, and attempt to jump from product to product, diet to diet. The grass always seems to be greener on the other side of the brand-new-fad that we can rub all over ourselves. It simply doesn't work this way. The transformation that you desire, the results you want, and the change you want to see will take massive action on your part and staying constantly accountable to yourself for your actions ... all while you have blinders on from the latest workout crazes.

STAY IN YOUR LANE AND STOP SWERVIN'

You can't be chasing two rabbits at the same time because you won't catch either. Commit to one method and stay the course. I promise you it works, and it'll work for you but only if you focus.

What I'm here to do is show you a way that will actually stick. It might appear slower, but in my opinion, steady Freddy wins the race. Everyone's results will differ depending on where they start. If you think your results are too slow, I'll tell you that quitting certainly won't speed things up.

First and foremost, I urge you to break up with the scale as the validation of your success. The only thing a scale really is is the measure of gravitational pull of your body toward the planet. It's not evil, it doesn't hold the keys to your beauty, it doesn't validate your progress; it's just a number.

Merely measuring your progress by what the scale says isn't going to work. Since you're starting a new fitness plan, you're building muscle, and muscle is more dense but occupies less space than the same amount of fat, for example.

I see this happen a lot with the Sexyfit Method and when the scale doesn't more as fast as we "hoped" (expected ... expectations again). What happens? PTSS happens.

POST TRAUMATIC SCALE SYNDROME. Trust me, this is a real thing. It usually happens when we let the number on the scale define our self worth and tell us how much we've progressed. If that scale doesn't budge, then all progress goes out the window. Pretty quickly, we're back to binge eating nights, bottles of wine, and platters of cheese. "SCREW THIS fitness routine thing, I'm out!"

But not this time.

Please understand that the scale is a deeply flawed device. I don't care how much you paid for it or how well advertised it was, that scale does not account for premenstrual weight fluctuations, water retention, salt retention, or any other factors that can change your weight on a daily basis. It can be something as simple as eating a tablespoon of peanut butter late at night and you wake up three pounds heavier because it has salt in it. That can really throw you for a loop, huh? Also, the scale doesn't account for the fact that muscle is denser than fat and, therefore, occupies less space (so, yes, you get smaller, but the scale doesn't show that!).

When you move away from the scale being the only foundation of your success and move toward creating new habits for a lifestyle change, you're going to feel better and your results will come faster. Your weight loss is going to come as a side effect of having routine, discipline, and solid good habits.

Most of your success lies in consistency. I know, it's a really unsexy word and easier said than done, but it's true.

CONSISTENT ACTIONS CREATE CONSISTENT RESULTS. CONSISTENT ACCOUNTABILITY, CONSISTENT RESULTS.

Here's how we're going to measure progress and stay accountable in the **SEXYFIT METHOD**.

1. ACCOUNTABILITY SUNDAY

Every week, you'll put the concept of "Analyze and Strategize" to use during your accountability Sunday sessions. I suggest that you sit down with yourself on a weekly basis, block out 15 minutes, and really see what worked last week, what could be done better. You get a chance to pat yourself on the back for the wins and see what you can improve.

You can also see what didn't work. If you missed meal prep, for example, you ended up eating out a lot and couldn't track your macros. This gives you an opportunity to really check in with yourself and see how you're doing.

In order to strategize for the upcoming week, this is your time to plan your menu, schedule your workouts because you're able to realistically see your schedule, and feel like you're in control of your lifestyle. I'm a big fan of notebooks, journals, calendars, or any kind of tools that help you clearly see what's going on. I urge you to spend time with your MFP, calendar, and journal to really objectively see what you can do better at and what you're proud of.

In our main signature program called Sexyback, we have weekly Accountability Sundays, where you can keep yourself accountable for what happened in the previous week and strategize for the upcoming week. Our goal here is to create a set habit to analyze what worked during your week and what were some things that blindsided you.

By the way, this isn't just something you do when you're trying to get results it's an essential habit if you want to keep your results for life. Just because you achieve certain results with your new habits doesn't mean you stop doing what you need to do that got you those results in the first place! Will it always happen on Sunday? NO, sometimes it will happen on Monday and sometimes even Tuesday. But, DO NOT MISS it.

I've been exercising for over a decade. To this day, my calendar has special kinds of notes to myself set as a recurring message for Sunday.

I prefer to ask myself questions because they make me think ...

"Do you have food in the fridge?"
"What's for meal prep?"
"It's goal assessment time. It's on!"

Every week I religiously make a trip to the grocery store and set my workout schedule for the week for REALISTIC times when I'll be able to make it to my workout. No matter how busy, dead or alive, sick or blind, I'm going to make it to the gym three times. Sometimes it'll be five, sometimes three ... but never less than three. Your schedule is non-negotiable, and bosses don't cancel.

With Accountability Sunday you won't feel like you're constantly failing and starting over, you get to build upon existing good habits and keep improving consistently over time.

2. PUBLIC ACCOUNTABILITY — GO PUBLIC
It's undoubtedly difficult to start something alone and continue by yourself, and without the right support and accountability you need to follow through with your new commitment. This is why we recommend to go public with your Sexyfit journey.

Here's the science behind it ...

A weight-loss research study conducted by Ray Wu — co-founder of Weilos, a social media platform for people to talk about their weight loss and fitness goals and share selfies of their progress — showed that people who posted progress photos documenting their weight loss lost 1.2 pounds per week, compared to 0.27 pounds when they didn't use the sharing platform. Strong social circles are seen as a very effective method in combating obesity. In a 2013 research study published in "Translational Behavioral Medicine," participants who published their weight loss progress on Twitter lost more weight than those who kept their progress to themselves.

Therefore, when we go public with our new decision, we get more results in return.

We suggest you tell your friends WHY you're doing it, to help them understand how important their support is for you. You can talk about how this is different, non-restrictive, and encourage them to follow along with you on your journey. A lot of our clients end up posting fun, easy recipes, as well as workouts to inspire and motivate their friends.

Remember, you're NOT an annoyance; you're an inspiration to those who need it most. Feel free to use #sexyfit in your posts so I can easily find your first post and your journey along the way.

If you want to create a really great habit, create a separate IG account, and ask your new friends and followers to check in with you on Sundays or Mondays.

3. BODY MEASURING GUIDE
I suggest that you take measurements before you start the program. You're going to take all measurements according to the directions in the file and write them down on that piece of paper. You can also do this in the notes on your phone if you like. It doesn't matter; just write them down somewhere safe. I ask that you do your measurements weekly for the duration of the 21-Day Transformation Plan and monthly thereafter every week on Accountability Sunday.

4. PROGRESS PICTURES

Instead of weighing yourself every day, I prefer that you start taking pictures of yourself once per month instead. To keep you honest, though, and to make sure these pictures serve their purpose, here are a few guidelines ...

- Wear the same swimsuit every time. This way you'll be able to see everything.
- Always take pictures in a very well-lit room. The best time is first thing in the morning, right after you wake up and before you have breakfast.
- Use a full-length mirror and always stand the same distance from it.
- Don't forget to smile: It's proven that smiling makes you look leaner and just generally better.
- Try to look natural. Don't suck everything in too much. That belly is going to go, and it won't do any good hiding it now.
- Take a picture from three angles: front, side, and back. It might be helpful if you have someone else take the pictures so you don't have to twist your body into all sorts of crazy shapes to get the right shot.
- Only take a picture once per month.

If you follow these guidelines, you'll get the most accurate progress photos possible, allowing you to see how every part of your body is changing. I've had clients who after seeing how much they progressed, regretted the fact that they didn't take their "before" photos. Really, they missed out on the opportunity to experience how much more proud they may have been of all their hard work and the transformation they had made.

Photos and measurements are the only way to accurately track how your body is changing and where you're losing weight. It appears to be downright traumatizing for some of us to take those photos of our body. Your body is incredible, take the photos, store them on your phone and move on. This is just a task, nothing to be overly emotional about. Your body is gorgeous and will be even healthier and happier after the program is over. Remember to take your photos in the same outfit, with the same lighting, and during the same time of the day.

Also, AGAIN, remember that the scale is not an accurate measure of success! You're only using the scale monthly, IF that, to objectively adjust your macros.

Muscle is more dense than fat and occupies more space. Therefore, if you're burning fat and building muscle (especially if you're working out), the scale is going to fail you nine out of 10 times. I recommend taking progress photos in the beginning and at the end. You're going to see dramatic changes and a huge difference in how your clothes fit.

4. BODY FAT TEST

What is a body fat test? In its simplest form, body fat is the amount of fat in your body compared to everything else. Everything else includes your organs, muscles, bones, tendons, water, and so on. Fat mass varies considerably between individuals in terms of absolute amount. Fat mass consists of 20% water and 80% adipose tissue.

Here's a chart to show you different body fat percentages. I didn't create this; it's a standard chart from the American Council of Exercise. I can only attempt to explain what these labels actually mean, so here goes ...

ESSENTIAL BODY FAT: Required by the body to function properly. It's responsible for the regulation of body temperature, optimal functioning and cushioning of the internal organs, and also as an emergency source of energy during illness. This essential body fat has a measure of 2-4% for men and 10-12% for women. Any measurement below these levels poses a serious risk to the health of the individual.

ATHLETES: You're an athlete if you're competeing, belong to a sports league, or if you're consistently working out four times per week with weights and have your nutrition dialed in. Ideally, you'll end up in this range with Sexyfit. I currently hover at 14-15% body fat, while eating out twice per week and having one glass of wine. I don't say no to popcorn at the movies or dark chocolate. So this range is very possible for anyone.

ACCEPTABLE BODY FAT PERCENTAGE

DESCRIPTION	MALE	FEMALE
Essential Fat	10-12%	2-4%
Athletes	14-20%	6-13%
Fitness	21-24%	14-17%
Acceptable	25-30%	18-25%
Nonessential (obese)	31%+	26%+

FITNESS: This is where active women usually start if they're working mostly on their feet and eat an unprocessed diet. I would call this range healthy and active.

ACCEPTABLE: Typical for women who work a desk job and live a lifestyle with a variety of food choices. Most women start here.

NONESSENTIAL BODY FAT: Can be dangerous and lead to serious health problems, and is associated with type 2 diabetes, hypertension, and hyperlipidemia.

5. SKINNY JEANS OR YOUR CLOTHES

You and I both know that hidden deep within your closet there's a pair of skinny jeans that you love and just can't bear to get rid of, even though they stopped fitting three years ago. Bust those puppies OUT and put them in a nearby pile or better yet, make them the first thing you see in the morning. Try them on weekly and see how they fit. Every week it'll be easier and easier to fit into them. I promise you that. This is a much better indication of your progress than that stupid scale.

6. BUDDY SYSTEM — YOUR RIDE OR DIE

It's always easier with two of you. I highly suggest that you enlist the help of one friend who can walk this journey with you. It's simply easier to do things together, and at those times when we "don't feel like it" or are starting to lose sight of our goals, your buddy can always be there to lift you up. It's best to communicate on a daily basis about what you're planning to do, what you're eating, and how you're feeling.

Note that it's important that you both stay as positive and as encouraging to each other every day. Beware of the kind of energy and the kind of support you want to receive, and mirror that with your partner. If you do need to "vent" or share something negative, apply the 90-second rule. You're free to vent for 90 seconds, and after that the issue or situation no longer has any validity in the relationship. Keep your communication to 10% negative and 90% positive interactions.

In other words "Kale sucks" and "Screw this workout" aren't acceptable communication because you're projecting your negativity onto someone else, which, in return, won't get you the positive outcome you're looking for.

More about this in the next section titled "Community."

7. COACH

Are you familiar with Michael Phelps, 10x Olympic medalist? Or Serena Williams, award-winning tennis player. Grammy Award-winning singers Usher? Pitbull? Taylor Swift? Do you know what makes these great names great? They all have a coach. What does Michael Phelps NOT know about swimming? Or do you think Serena Williams doesn't know how to serve or Taylor Swift doesn't know how to hit notes? They achieved incredible heights because they've enlisted the help of a trained professional to take their skillset and mindset to a whole new level. Coaches see what you don't see. Coaches elevate your vision. And they create a simple step-by-step system so you can walk the path with ease, grace, and certainty.

When I hired bodybuilding coaches, I won or placed in the top five in 26 competitions.
When I hired a business coach, we tripled our income that year.
When I hired a life coach, I actually got a balanced life.
Now I'm working with a love coach. Can you guess how this will turn out? #callingintheone

If you have the opportunity to accelerate your rate of success, why wouldn't you do it? If there's someone holding a blueprint for success for you that you know and trust, take a step toward a rapid accelerated transformation, take advantage of it.

Hiring a coach brings up an array of emotions. Usually the logical side of us says, "Nah, I got this," but as they say in the 12-step program, your best thinking got you here. If you've previously read every book under the sun and nothing has worked, get help and get it now because you don't want to have the same issue 10 years from now when you can just solve it right now.

Our emotional side can get embarrassed to come clean and trust someone. We might not feel safe to share, or we're afraid that we won't be perfect so hide behind the idea that we don't have time, or don't have money, and that we'll do it later when the kids grow up.

I invested in myself when I couldn't afford to because I couldn't afford NOT to. I hired coaches when I didn't necessarily have the resources to do so. We always find time and money for those things we truly know we need. Your fitness transformation is typically your gateway to reclaiming not only your body but living your best life. So invest in coaches, trainers, and those who believe in you and speed up your progess tenfold.

Sister, remember that at the end of the day the best accountability you can experience is based on how you feel in your body and about your body. All of the tools I shared with you are a good way to keep yourself accountable as long as you need to before the Sexyfit lifestyle becomes your autopilot behavior. Yes, photos, measurements, and body fat testing are very helpful in terms of seeing your improvements, but the most important goal of your transformation is that you grow happier, more proud, and more excited with your relationship with self and your body every day. The more you become consistent, the more you show your body love and respect; the more you cherish all parts of yourself and accept your body, the less accountability you'll need because ultimately how you feel is all that matters.

💡 CHAPTER PRACTICE

1. Please reference the measuring guide on the next page, and mark the dates and all the measurements before you begin the 21-Day Transformation Plan. You'll revisit this guide every week for 21 days and every month for the next six months.

2. Reference the picture outlines below for how to take progress photos. Please follow directions as closely as possible from page 287. Take your photos and make sure to mark the dates you took them for comparison. **DON'T SKIP THIS STEP.**

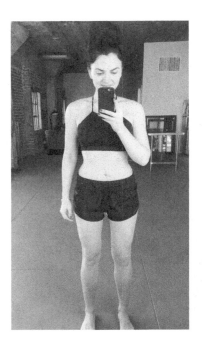 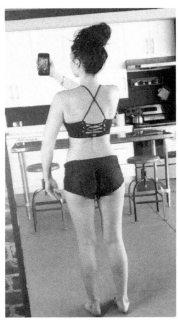 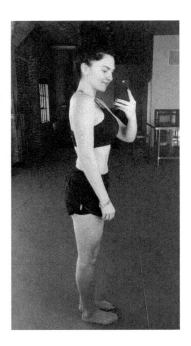

MEASUREMENTS CHART:

DAY 1

DATE _____

Chest _____

Right Arm _____

Left Arm _____

Waist _____

Hips _____

Left Thigh _____

Right Thigh _____

Weight _____

DAY 21

DATE _____

Chest _____

Right Arm _____

Left Arm _____

Waist _____

Hips _____

Left Thigh _____

Right Thigh _____

Weight _____

RECORD THE DIFFERENCE
FROM YOUR START DATE
TO END DATE.

Chest _____

Right Arm _____

Left Arm _____

Waist _____

Hips _____

Right Thigh _____

Left Thigh _____

TOTAL LOSS

Inches _____

Weight _____

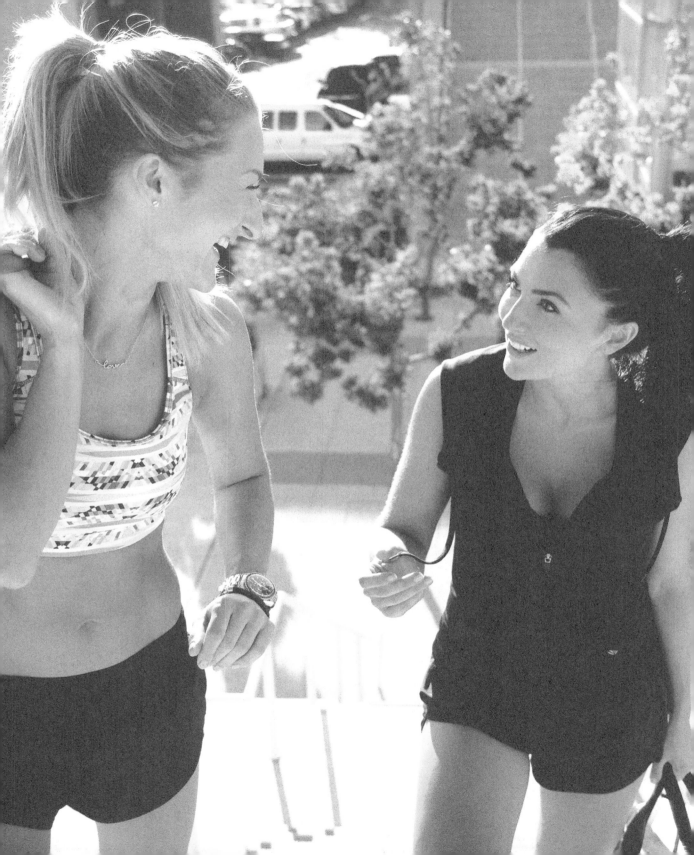

STEP V
POWER OF COMMUNITY

Create a supportive community,
find joy in the journey and,
stay sexyfit for life.

STRONG TOGETHER
CHAPTER 32

"Alone we can do little; together we can do so much."
— Helen Keller

The final, and perhaps most important, step of the entire Sexyfit Method is creating a supportive, like-minded group of women who are going to walk along this journey with you. We made it a point to cultivate a sense of community with Sexyfit from the very beginning, and this concept has proven itself time and time again to support women on their journey to success.

NOBODY GETS IN SHAPE ALONE, and those around us determine our rate of success on our journey to a lasting transformation. I experienced the power of community first hand when I started competing, and the bodybuilding community welcomed me with open arms, and shared their knowledge and support with me. Being included and connected to a group of equally committed women who desire the same level of change as we do creates a powerful force that drives the group toward achieving our goals.

What I also find incredibly interesting is that it's scientifically proven that women crave an authentic, vulnerable connection with other women. Drs. Laura Klein and Shelley Tailor, researchers, found that when we spend time with other women, our body reacts in a magical way where it releases a hormone called oxytocin. Oxytocin helps us live a longer, healthier life, but most importantly it's a natural stress reliever. In bond, oxytocin with release of estrogen counteracts stress, and helps us manage stress and anxiety in a natural way.[23]

We can find this connection face to face or virtually. While the world of high-speed internet and on-demand movies has caused a fair share of separation between us, it has given us the opportunity to connect with others with similar interests all over the world. In fact, it's easier than ever to find a community online to begin our journey with and then cultivate the kind of environment around us in person.

At the foundation of every program, every book, our podcast, events, retreats, any "thing" you'll ever see us share, our community is going to be at the core, the heart of everything we do.

We recognize the power of sisterhood early on, and we attribute our high program completion rates to having this kind of bond. This is why Sexyfit has an astonishing success rate where 93% of our clients successfully complete their coaching courses. **THAT'S 93%!**

INDUSTRY STANDARD SUCCESS RATE = 62%
COMMUNITY-BASED COACHING SUCCESS RATE = 93%

Women — we're tribal beings. We can't fight it, it's simply nature. We once lived in the culture where the women raised children together, did laundry together, cooked together, and helped each other laugh through the ups and downs of life. It's only in the last few decades that we started celebrating the fierce epitome of the strong, independent woman who "doesn't need nobody."

Strong doesn't mean alone. Strong means a part of a sisterhood and an honest, kind bond. You've heard the saying, **"BEHIND EVERY STRONG WOMAN IS A TRIBE OF STRONG WOMEN TO LIFT HER UP."**

I stand behind this statement 100%.

When you cultivate a tribe of women around you, you're able to grasp the significance of the changes you're making, and analyze and feel through the transformation you're experiencing. Not to mention that you get to share and celebrate your wins fully.

Your community becomes the gatekeepers for your vision, and you're able to share freely what you're feeling and experiencing. In a way, when we have a tribe of women we trust, we're able to break free from the fearful patterns of appearing "perfect" with our other friends, coworkers, and/or family, and this added layer of accountability makes it easy to analyze and recognize our own self-destructive patterns. When we have a friendly, kind, and loving environment where deep connection is appreciated and welcome, our community can hold our vision of transformation with us. There are quite a few moving pieces here, from releasing old patterns, facing our fears, learning how to navigate macros, and making fitness a part of our life. At times it might seem overwhelming and difficult to execute, and life happens in such a way where we think taking a break is the only way. In a way, your sisters don't let you off the hook, and are able to comfort you and re-route you on the right track. Being "checked out" is a choice that's easier to make when we don't have the support of the community because we can rationalize how taking a break for now, spending time with ourselves, and choosing not to keep our cup half full makes perfect sense. It's easy to default to fear, perfectionism, excuses, and negative self-talk, and stay in that place for quite some time before we have an abrupt awakening again to get back on the program. A strong circle of support is there to help us stay faithful to the journey we committed to.

HAVING A COMMUNITY SHORTENS THE GAP BETWEEN FAILURE AND FAST-TRACKS OUR SUCCESS. PERIOD.

Motivation, goal-setting, and commitment to self can only take us so far. When we feel connected and accountable with a group of others, we feel the need and desire to contribute to them and ourselves on a bigger scale. There's a big difference between holding onto a vision by ourself and doing so with the help of others who can sustain that vision with us, and even for us, during times of despair and self-doubt.

This is beyond motivation. This is the power of connection.

So how do we cultivate and grow a tribe?

First and foremost, we're the mirror reflection of the five people we surround ourself with. If five of our friends have no goals, eat junk food, talk smack about their body, and don't move further than grabbing another bottle of wine, we're most likely going to be the sixth friend. It's the same with money, too; if we have five broke friends, we'll most likely be the sixth. It's the simplicity of the law of proximity.

HERE'S WHERE I WANT US TO START. I highly encourage you to take inventory of everyone who's actively influencing your decision-making patterns in your life and the choices that you make that could affect your transformation. If you already have a group of friends that you typically spend time with, I want you to journal your top five friends noting how they make you feel the next time you hang out. Do you feel uplifted, supported, and encouraged when you share, or do you feel guilt, frustration, and like you want to throw your hands in the air, saying, "Why don't you get what I'm doing?" and spinning your wheels?

Think of your community as a bus ride. Think of what you want this bus ride to be like and who you want to invite to take this journey with you through the fun times and the dark times. Who are your "ride or die" friends who will be there regardless of the circumstances? Do you want to feel uplifted, supported, and encouraged or constantly frustrated?

Not everyone is going to be willing to come on our bus ride with us, and this is okay. As we evolve, grow, and transform, some of our friends, loved ones, and even family won't be able to handle our growth. I bet that you're going to piss off a fair share of your friends when you start to see changes in your physique and your attitude, and distance yourself from habits and activities that no longer serve you. Remember, this has nothing to do with you and has everything to do with them. As individuals, we're inherently selfish beings, and we don't like change. When we see someone we love changing and becoming someone different, it becomes uncomfortable for us.

To find the right tribe, right community, and right women will require one magical action: to be unapologetically yourself and let those who are on your wave rise up to you. You don't need the validation of running around and proving to everyone that you're still worthy of their love when you're 20-30-50-100 pounds lighter. The truth is that you will change and you will change for the better, and not everyone will want to ride that bus with you. Feel free to make a pit stop and let those off the bus who are killing the vibe.

We change, and this is something to celebrate!

Another thing about mirrors: Our friends are also a mirror reflection of who we are. If we want to find new friends who mirror our new mindset, we must act as if we're already those friends.

If you want to find supportive friends, **BECOME SUPPORTIVE**.
If you want your friends to call you more often, **CALL THEM FIRST**.
If you want healthy friends, **BECOME THE HEALTHY FRIEND**.

We can't complain about not having supportive, loving friends in our life if we're NOT that friend. It doesn't work that way. Your vibe attracts your tribe. You must embody those qualities in order to attract those people into your life. I'm always wary of women who say their friends are catty, unsupportive, and start drama. In a way, I know that they're internally projecting the same attitude, which attracts like-minded people. So if everyone around you is a negative Nancy, judgmental Judy, dramatic Dani, skeptical Sally, and bitchy Betty, most likely this is the energy that you project into the world which is mirroring back to you.

In other words, be the change you want to be in the world and the community around you.

I know that you might not have the most supportive friends or want to keep your Sexyfit friends separate from others, and you're probably wondering, "How in the world am I going to create this community you speak of Zlata?" Sister, remember that there are seven billion people in the world, so I'm sure you can find someone who wants to be your loving, kind, and supportive friend. The online world has made it possible for us to connect with like-minded individuals all over the globe. I caution you against trying to mold someone and get her to your level of commitment to the journey. At times we want others to want to experience what we're going through and desperately try to get them to commit to our community. Despite how open, excited, loving, and supportive you attempt to be, others can only meet you as deeply as they have met themselves. If you feel like you're trying too hard, remember that those who are ready will meet you when they're ready. Keep encouraging, loving, and spreading the message but keep this at heart.

Here are the qualities that you're looking for in your community members in order to create a powerful force fueled by authentic connection and driven toward success. The qualities might look familiar to you since these are a mirror reflection of the qualities you cultivated within yourself in the first section of this book.

ACCEPTANCE

In order to create an authentic connection, we must accept who WE are, where we are, and who our community members are and where THEY are right now. We tend to default to judgment to try to find common ground or give a compliment. Like, if you're part of a group of more fit women, "Oh, look at you, you're as thin as a stick; look at me!" or, "Oh, honey, you really have a lot of work to do." I ask you to look at everyone in your group as though you've seen them for the first time, EVERY time you meet or connect. This way you're able to move away from judgment, and move toward acceptance and support.

DESIRE AND ACTION

A strong sense of desire to take action must be present among all members of the community. This doesn't mean that everyone must share a specific common goal, but all must share a common desire and be willing to take action to achieve the transformation. Desire is what ultimately drives us to make choices, sacrifices, demonstrates perseverance, and shows the willingness to do what's required of us to grow into the women we're trying to become. It's fairly simple to measure someone's desire. You'll clearly see who's willing to take action and who's only willing to talk about it.

TRUST

Trust is a variable that's going to evolve and grow the longer your community spends time together. An essential piece that's going to create a high trust circle is the ability to share openly what we feel and what we're experiencing on our journey. Some of us might be faced with experiences from the past where we don't feel others are trustworthy enough to share our emotions with. We must open up to experience the full beauty of what having a community is like and share vulnerably from the heart. In recent years, we chose the path of silent suffering, and as a result chose to keep everything "bottled up" inside, attempting to appear strong on the outside. It's not fair to you to not open up and create a deeper bond with others. It's very selfish to keep everything inside and not let others into your world.

If you've been through betrayal, loss, or anything where your trust bond has been influenced negatively by the behavior of others (recent or childhood), you can't let those experiences shape your future—you're disallowing yourself to have the best experience based on the past. Anger, resentment, unforgiveness, and unfinished business are what typically hold us back from creating a lasting and meaningful connection with those around us. Don't let your past experiences shape your future. That's not wisdom—that's prison. You can trust again, you can be open again, you can love a friend again. Being closed for business of authentic connection is our denial of love and support from others that we emotionally crave.

NOTE: There's no room for gossip or talking about group business with others who don't belong in your community.

RESPECT
Remember, the purpose of a group is to support one another on the transformation journey. Everyone's transformation is going to take a different shape and take a different amount of time, and we must let our community members have their own experiences. You shouldn't coach anyone and avoid the temptation to parent others, but rather treat them with respect to their feeling, emotions, and choices. This isn't therapy. Really be careful with the kind of language and energy you project on others. There's no "You should do" language in your community. If you want someone to solve something and you continuously see the same situation presenting itself that's negatively influencing one of the members, ask them more questions to get to the bottom of why they feel and do things a certain way.

If you desperately want to "fix" something in someone, look within yourself for the wound that you're trying to heal within yourself first and foremost. Nobody needs fixing; this is a broken mindset projected from the deep core of whom we are, a gentle nudge to direct our attention toward that particular issue. Respect others and yourself to let them make the right decisions for themselves.

LOVE—COMPASSION, KINDNESS, POSITIVITY
Spread love, kindness, positivity, and love likes its confetti! As I mentioned in the first part of this book, we have two mental preconditions: to think from a place of love or a place of fear. Always default to love, kindness, and positivity, and look for the light in every situation toward yourself and others. There's no reason to get angry at anyone because they're not meeting yours or their own expectations. There's no reason to be frustrated with others, no reason to rush, push, and control. You're here to share the love with one another and support each other in the most loving way possible.

AND ... FUN!
I'm talking about pure, child-like JOY when you see each other, or meet for workouts or meal prep. HAVE FUN! I can write a whole book on how we all could use a little fun in our life. We all have the power to choose our outcome and the journey we take there. You can struggle your way into success, or you can sing, dance, jump, laugh, and make your journey be filled with joy. Some of this stuff isn't fun, so it surely won't be fun if you aren't having any fun. Your community is your tribe to vibe with. Make sure that you aren't just meeting to complain over snacks you can't have, or turn every gathering into a whine and complain fest. Create opportunities to have a great time so everyone is having fun.

💡 CHAPTER PRACTICE

Here are the directions for how you can form your community for the duration of the 21-Day transformation plan and beyond.

STEP 1: GET YOUR MEMBERS TOGETHER AND HOSTING

I suggest that you make this a close group. This means that you should look for members who are willing to commit to the five weeks and potentially beyond the initial challenge. I say five weeks because you need your first meeting before the challenge and last meeting afterwards. Four to eight members is the most effective number of women if you're going to meet in person. If you're forming a virtual community, you can always do a larger online group if you'd like. We've seen up to 100 members still be effective to jumpstart a transformation. However, since your 21-day duration is a just a jumpstart to your journey, choose women to get on the bus with you who are in it for the long haul. The best way to see who has the most desire is to ask if they'd be willing to commit to a six-month transformation together. This will help you weave out who's actually serious about this and who isn't.

I suggest that you have a community leader starting this group and planning the first meeting. After the first meeting, your leader can pass the token to the next member to host the meeting (virtual or in person).

After the first five weeks when you finish the 21-Day plan, you can allow members to introduce one new friend into your existing group — virtual or in person. In order to be respectful toward the members of the group, please introduce your friend ahead of time and ask if she's a good fit. When your friend enters the group, make sure she makes an introduction and also reads this book right away. Remember, it's important that everyone has the same level of desire, acceptance, trust, respect, and love for one another. If you add a bunch of random friends who are NOT all in, it dilutes the purpose of the community.

STEP 2: CHOOSE A TIME, PLACE

To help ensure success, set a time and meeting place in advance of your first meeting and keep them consistent. If you're doing weekly Accountability Sunday meetings in person, you can pick any day – Saturday … Sunday … Monday – it doesn't matter, just so long as you all check in. If you're hosting a virtual group, set your Sundays to be the main time to connect and follow up with everyone to be accountable. Facebook groups work really well when it comes to hosting virtual communities. Feel free to check in with those you haven't heard from within 48 hours. If they're "checked out," be kind and ask how you can help. Don't let your members use "I fell off the wagon" as an excuse NOT to Analyze and Strategize.

STEP 3: PLAN THE MEETING TOPICS

Reserve your initial meeting as a "Meet and Greet" to get your journals in order and set your goals. For the next three, check in with each others' journals and workout schedule, and discuss what worked and what the group members are learning. For the fifth meeting, get together one week after the challenge to see how the new habits are sticking and how the new routine is working. During this last meeting, determine the new meeting arrangements, which I recommend to be biweekly or once per month.

Remember that the purpose of your tribe is to connect and create a powerful support system for your goals while you're having fun. We've had members send us pictures from group meal preps because they preferred to spend time cooking together to connect. We received feedback that members chose to break up the first chapter of this book into five weeks to meet for meditations. There's no right or wrong way to do the community. Just make sure you're authentically connecting, keeping it positive, and have a set meeting schedule. You can manage your community in a group message or Facebook group to make it easier to stream.

EPILOGUE

"The course of true love never did run smooth."
– William Shakespeare, *A Midsummer Night's Dream*

Sister, I want to thank you from the bottom of my heart. I'm beyond grateful for your readership and your dedication to your new Sexyfit lifestyle. I can imagine that as you've moved through the pages of this book you've hit some obstacles. But obstacles are almost always a detour in the right direction. Everything in the world happens for a reason, and as they say, life is 10% what happens to you and 90% how you react to it. Your Sexyfit journey is no exception.

The best news is that you're beyond the toughest part of the journey to creating awareness of your old patterns and thoughts, and of your old ways of being. An open road to create an amazing relationship with self, feeling sexy in your skin, and creating your best life is ahead of you. However, your journey is exactly that: a journey. Not a sprint to a destination. As much as you may like to believe it doesn't stop and it's a 24/7 job, it's up to you to create the journey you can and will enjoy with every step. I've given you the blueprint to do exactly that.

I've worked with hundreds of women during my time as a coach, and it has become clear that there are two types of outcomes that manifest themselves. The majority of women choose to take on this path to self-discovery with an open heart, find joy in every step of the journey, embrace their imperfections, and commit to self-love to help them use health and fitness as a foundation for their success in life. And then there's the second type of woman with a vast knowledge and all of the tools at her fingertips, who will choose to fold under pressure, and allow fear and doubt to speak louder than faith and light. This is the kind of woman who will always be phased by distractions of the next best shiny object and simply isn't ready to commit to radical self-love quite yet. I pray that I've inspired you and given you everything you need to be the woman who reaps all of the benefits of the Sexyfit lifestyle and expands your capacity to grow in the proportion of your courage to take this journey to heart.

It has been my true pleasure and joy to guide you on your journey to transformation. It's my hope that you have enjoyed it so much that you'll pass it along.

With love.

SOURCES

1. Woodward Thomas, Katherine. Calling in "The One": 7 Weeks to Attract the Love of Your Life. Harmony, 2004.

2. LaPorte, Danielle. The Desire Map: A Guide to Creating Goals with Soul. Sounds True, 2014.

3. Feinman, R. and Fine, E. (2004, July). Nutrition Journal 2004 3:9. Retrieved from http://nutritionj.biomedcentral.com/articles/10.1186/1475-2891-3-9

4. http://nutritionj.biomedcentral.com/articles/10.1186/1475-2891-3-9

5. Frayn, K. (2014, May). Oxford Textbook of Medicine (5 ed.) Retrieved from http://oxfordmedicine.com/view/10.1093/med/9780199204854.001.1/med-9780199204854-chapter-1101

6. Osterweil, N. (2004). The Benefits of Protein. Retrieved from http://www.webmd.com/men/features/benefits-protein#1

7. European Food Safety Authority (EFSA) (2010). Scientific Opinion on Dietary Reference Values for carbohydrates and dietary fibre. EFSA Journal 8(3):1462.

8. http://home.trainingpeaks.com/blog/article/the-importance-of-carbohydrates-and-glycogen-for-a

9. Horton, T.J, Drougas, H, Brachey, A, Reed, G.W, Peters, J.C and Hill, J.O. (1995, July). The American journal of clinical nutrition 62(1): 19-29. Retrieved from https://www.ncbi.nlm.nih.gov/pubmed/7598063

10. Tessari, P, Inchiostro, S, Biolo, G, Vincenti, E and Sabadin, L. (1991, July). The Journal of clinical investigation 88(1):27-33. Retrieved from https://www.ncbi.nlm.nih.gov/pubmed/2056121

11. Holt, S.H, Miller, J.C and Petocz, P. (1997, November). The American journal of clinical nutrition 66(5):1264-76. Retrieved from https://www.ncbi.nlm.nih.gov/pubmed/9356547

12. McDevitt, R.M, Bott, S.J, Harding, M, Coward, W.A, Bluck, L.J and Prentice, A.M. (2001, December). The American journal of clinical nutrition 74(6):737-46. Retrieved from https://www.ncbi.nlm.nih.gov/pubmed/11722954

13. Bodyecology. The 6 Benefits of Monosaturated Fats (MUFAs). Retrieved from http://bodyecology.com/articles/6_benefits_monosaturated_fats.php

14. American Heart Association. http://www.heart.org/HEARTORG/

15. Kollias, H. Leptin, Ghrelin and Weight Loss. Precision Nutrition. Retrieved from http://www.precisionnutrition.com/leptin-ghrelin-weight-loss

16. Teta, J (2015, December). T Nation. A Lifter's Guide to Alcohol. Retrieved from https://www.t-nation.com/diet-fat-loss/lifters-guide-to-alcohol

17. Arnal, M.A, Mosoni, L, Boirie, Y, Houlier, M.L, Morin, L, Verdier, E, Ritz, P, Antoine, J.M, Prugnaud, J, Beaufrère, B. and Mirand, P.P. (2000, July). The Journal of nutrition 130(7):1700-4. Retrieved from https://www.ncbi.nlm.nih.gov/pubmed/10867039

18. Whigham, L, Watras, A. and Schoeller, D. (2007, May). The American journal of clinical nutrition 85(5):1203-11. Retrieved from http://ajcn.nutrition.org/content/85/5/1203.long

19. Fogelholm, G.M, Tikkanen, H.O, Näveri, H.K, Näveri, L.S. and Härkönen, M.H. (1991, March). British Journal of Sports Medicine 25(1): 41-44. Retrieved from https://www.ncbi.nlm.nih.gov/pmc/articles/PMC1478808/

20. National Strength and Conditioning Association. Is EPOC Large Enough to Cause Weight Loss? Retrieved from https://www.nsca.com/Education/Articles/Hot-Topic-Role-of-EPOC-in-Weight-Loss/

21 Macpherson, R. E., Hazell, T. J., Olver, T. D., Paterson, D. H., Lemon, P. W. (2011). Medicine & Science in Sports & Exercise, 43, 115-122. doi:10.1249/MSS.0b013e3181e5eacd. Run sprint interval training improves aerobic performance but not maximal cardiac output.

22 Ingraham, P. (2016, November). PainScience.Com. Delayed Onset Muscle Soreness (DOMS). Retrieved from https://www.painscience.com/articles/delayed-onset-muscle-soreness.php

23. Berkowitz, G. (2002). UCLA Study on Friendship Among Women. Retrieved from http://www.anapsid.org/cnd/gender/tendfend.html

CPSIA information can be obtained
at www.ICGtesting.com
Printed in the USA
LVOW06*1159120217
523989LV00008B/14/P